T0142083

Web Information Systems Engineering and Internet Technologies Book Series

More information about this series at http://www.springer.com/series/6970

Ning Zhong · Jianhua Ma · Jiming Liu
Runhe Huang · Xiaohui Tao
Editors

Wisdom Web of Things

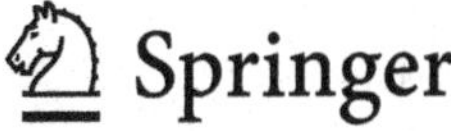

Editors
Ning Zhong
Department of Life Science and Informatics
Maebashi Institute of Technology
Maebashi
Japan

and

Beijing Advanced Innovation Center for Future Internet Technology
The International WIC Institute
Beijing University of Technology
Beijing
China

Jianhua Ma
Faculty of Computer and Information Sciences
Hosei University
Tokyo
Japan

Jiming Liu
Department of Computer Science
Hong Kong Baptist University
Kowloon Tong
Hong Kong

Runhe Huang
Faculty of Computer and Information Science
Hosei University
Tokyo
Japan

Xiaohui Tao
Department of Mathematics and Computing
University of Southern Queensland
Toowoomba, QLD
Australia

Web Information Systems Engineering and Internet Technologies Book Series
ISBN 978-3-319-83008-7 ISBN 978-3-319-44198-6 (eBook)
DOI 10.1007/978-3-319-44198-6

Softcover reprint of the hardcover 1st edition 2016

Printed on acid-free paper

This Springer imprint is published by Springer Nature
The registered company is Springer International Publishing AG
The registered company address is: Gewerbestrasse 11, 6330 Cham, Switzerland

To Artificial Intelligence and our pioneers who have been working hard to make it happen—without them we would not have as much excitements as we have today.

Preface

This book is the first monograph on Wisdom Web of Things (W2T) coherently written by multi-authors. The book contains 15 chapters structured into four parts: W2T foundation, W2T and humanity, W2T technologies, and future vision of W2T. The book has presented the recent study on the framework and methodology of W2T, as well as applications of W2T in different problem domains such as intelligent businesses, brain informatics, and healthcare. Aiming at promoting people's understanding of W2T and facilitating the related research including the holistic, intelligent methodology, the book has addressed emerging issues such as: "*What are fundamental issues and challenges in W2T?*", "*Where are the solutions lying on?*", and "*What are potential applications*?"

We would like to specifically dedicate this book to the celebration of the 60th anniversary of Artificial Intelligence (AI). Aiming at creating computers and computer software capacity of intelligent behavior, throughout the sixty years of journey many amazing achievements have been made, including the recent AlphaGo, an intelligent computer program that beat Lee Sedol, a 9-dan professional player in a five-game match of Go. Such a task was considered an impossible mission if looking back in just a decade ago. Web Intelligence (WI) has extended and made use of Artificial Intelligence for new products, services, and frameworks that are empowered by the World Wide Web. Wisdom Web of Things is then born as an extension of the Web Intelligence research in the IoT/WoT (Internet of Things/Web of Things) era. The book is recommended by the Web Intelligence Consortium (WIC, www.wi-consortium.org) as a consecutive book to the Web Intelligence monograph published by Springer in spring 2003. The WIC was formed in spring 2002 as an international, nonprofit organization endeavoring to advance worldwide scientific research and industrial development in the field of Web Intelligence. The scope of its activities covers encouraging deep collaborations among the WIC research centers around the world, supporting organizational and individual members, steering advanced research and technology showcases at the international IEEE/WIC/ACM conferences and workshops, and producing official publications. The book is a collaborative effort involving many leading researchers and practitioners in the field of WI who have contributed chapters on their areas of expertise. We wish to express our gratitude to all authors and reviewers for their contributions.

We are very grateful to people who joined or supported the W2T-related research activities, in particular, the WIC Advisory Board members, Edward Feigenbaum, Setsuo Ohsuga, Joseph Sifakis, Andrzej Skowron, Benjamin Wah, Philip Yu, and all the WIC Technical Committee members. We thank them for their strong and constant support—without such, this book is impossible.

Last, but not least, we thank Jennifer Malat of Springer US and Yanchun Zhang for their helps in coordinating the publication of this monograph and editorial assistance.

Maebashi, Japan
May 2016

Ning Zhong
Jianhua Ma
Jiming Liu
Runhe Huang
Xiaohui Tao

Contents

Contributors

Yuichiro Anzai Japan Society for the Promotion of Science, Tokyo, Japan

Enzo Brunetti Neurosystems Laboratory, Institute of Biomedical Sciences, Faculty of Medicine, University of Chile, Santiago, Chile

Jianhui Chen International WIC Institute, Beijing University of Technology, Beijing, China; Department of Computer Science and Technology, Tsinghua University, Beijing, China

Jing Chen School of Information Science and Engineering, Lanzhou University, Lanzhou, China

Francesco Chiti Università degli Studi di Firenze, Firenze, Italy

Wesley Deneke Department of Computer Science and Industrial Technology, Southeastern Louisiana University, Hammond, LA, USA

Yue Deng The Industry Innovation Center for Web Intelligence, Suzhou, China

Akihiro Eguchi Oxford Centre for Theoretical Neuroscience and Artificial Intelligence, University of Oxford, Oxford, UK

Romano Fantacci Università degli Studi di Firenze, Firenze, Italy

Yang Gao Department of Computer Science, Nanjing University, Nanjing, China

Jian Han The International WIC Institute, Beijing University of Technology, Beijing, China

Yuzhong Han China Academy of Building Research, Beijing, China

Bin Hu School of Information Science and Engineering, Lanzhou University, Lanzhou, China

Jiajin Huang International WIC Institute, Beijing University of Technology, Beijing, China

Runhe Huang Faculty of Computer and Information Science, Hosei University, Tokyo, Japan

Zhisheng Huang International WIC Institute, Beijing University of Technology, Beijing, China; Department of Computer Science, Vrije University Amsterdam, Amsterdam, The Netherlands

Andrzej Jankowski The Dziubanski Foundation of Knowledge Technology, Warsaw, Poland

Marcel Just Carnegie Mellon University, Pittsburgh, USA

Taihei Kotake The Department of Life Science and Informatics, Maebashi Institute of Technology, Maebashi, Japan

Ali Li University of Science and Technology Beijing, Beijing, China

Wenbin Li Shijiazhuang, China

Youjun Li The International WIC Institute, Beijing University of Technology, Beijing, China

Yuefeng Li Faculty of Science and Technology, Queensland University of Technology, Brisbane, QLD, Australia

Hong Liu Engineering Laboratory, Run Technologies Co., Ltd. Beijing, Beijing, China

Jiming Liu International WIC Institute, Beijing University of Technology, Beijing, China; Department of Computer Science, Hong Kong Baptist University, Kowloon Tong, Hong Kong SAR

Pablo Loyola Web Intelligence Centre, Industrial Engineering Department, University of Chile, Santiago, Chile

Jianhua Ma Faculty of Computer and Information Science, Hosei University, Tokyo, Japan

Pedro Maldonado Neurosystems Laboratory, Institute of Biomedical Sciences, Faculty of Medicine, University of Chile, Santiago, Chile

Gustavo Martinez Web Intelligence Centre, Industrial Engineering Department, University of Chile, Santiago, Chile

Philip Moore School of Information Science and Engineering, Lanzhou University, Lanzhou, China

Hung Nguyen Department of Computer Science and Computer Engineering, University of Arkansas, Fayetteville, AR, USA

Huansheng Ning University of Science and Technology Beijing, Beijing, China

Kazuhiro Oiwa National Institute of Information and Communication Technology, Koganei, Japan

Gabriella Pasi Università degli Studi di Milano Bicocca, Milan, Italy

Shinsuke Shimojo California Institute of Technology, Pasadena, USA

Andrzej Skowron Institute of Mathematics, Warsaw University, Warsaw, Poland; Systems Research Institute, Polish Academy of Sciences, Warsaw, Poland

Xiaohui Tao Faculty of Health, Engineering and Sciences, The University of Southern Queensland, Toowoomba, Australia

Craig Thompson Department of Computer Science and Computer Engineering, University of Arkansas, Fayetteville, AR, USA

Francesco Tisato Università degli Studi di Milano Bicocca, Milan, Italy

Juan D. Velásquez Web Intelligence Centre, Industrial Engineering Department, University of Chile, Santiago, Chile

Zhijiang Wan The International WIC Institute, Beijing University of Technology, Beijing, China; The Department of Life Science and Informatics, Maebashi Institute of Technology, Maebashi, Japan

Dongsheng Wang The International WIC Institute, Beijing University of Technology, Beijing, China; Institute of Intelligent Transport System, School of Computer Science and Engineering, Jiangsu University of Science of Technology, Zhenjiang, China

Guoyin Wang Chongqing University of Posts and Telecommunications, Chongqing, China

Haiyuan Wang International WIC Institute, Beijing University of Technology, Beijing, China

Hui Wang International WIC Institute, Beijing University of Technology, Beijing, China

Ningning Wang The International WIC Institute, Beijing University of Technology, Beijing, China

Bo Yang School of Computer Science and Technology, Jilin University, Changchun, China

Laurence T. Yang Huazhong University of Science and Technology, Wuhan, China; St. Francis Xavier University, Antigonish, Canada

Yiyu Yao International WIC Institute, Beijing University of Technology, Beijing, China; Department of Computer Science, University of Regina, Regina, SK, Canada

Stephen S. Yau Arizona State University, Tempe, USA

Neil Y. Yen School of Computer Science and Engineering, The University of Aizu, Fukushima, Japan

Feng Zhang China Academy of Building Research, Beijing, China

Xiaowei Zhang School of Information Science and Engineering, Lanzhou University, Lanzhou, China

Yaoxue Zhang Key Laboratory of Pervasive Computing, Ministry of Education, and Tsinghua National Laboratory for Information Science and Technology, Department of Computer Science and Technology, Tsinghua University, Beijing, China

Xin Zhao Faculty of Computer and Information Science, Hosei University, Tokyo, Japan

Han Zhong The International WIC Institute, Beijing University of Technology, Beijing, China

Ning Zhong Department of Life Science and Informatics, Maebashi Institute of Technology, Maebashi, Japan; Beijing Advanced Innovation Center for Future Internet Technology, The International WIC Institute, Beijing University of Technology, Beijing, China

Erzhong Zhou International WIC Institute, Beijing University of Technology, Beijing, China

Acronyms

AI	Artificial Intelligence
EEG	Electroencephalogram
IRGC	Interactive Rough Granular Computing
IT	Information Technology
W2T	Wisdom Web of Things
WaaS	Wisdom as a Service
WI	Web Intelligence
WWW	World Wide Web

Part I
Foundation of Wisdom Web of Things

Chapter 1
Research Challenges and Perspectives on Wisdom Web of Things (W2T)

Ning Zhong, Jianhua Ma, Runhe Huang, Jiming Liu, Yiyu Yao, Yaoxue Zhang and Jianhui Chen

Abstract The rapid development of the Internet and the Internet of Things accelerates the emergence of the hyper world. It has become a pressing research issue to realize the organic amalgamation and harmonious symbiosis among humans, computers and things in the hyper world, which consists of the social world, the physical world and the information world (cyber world). In this chapter, the notion of *Wisdom Web of Things* (W2T) is proposed in order to address this issue. As inspired by the material cycle in the physical world, the W2T focuses on the data cycle, namely "from things to data, information, knowledge, wisdom, services, humans, and then back to things." A W2T data cycle system is designed to implement such a cycle, which is, technologically speaking, a practical way to realize the harmonious symbiosis of humans, computers and things in the emergin hyper world.

N. Zhong (✉)
Department of Life Science and Informatics, Maebashi Institute of Technology, 460-1 Kamisadori-Cho, Maebashi-City 371-0816, Japan
e-mail: zhong@maebashi-it.ac.jp; zhongn@bjut.edu.cn

N. Zhong
Beijing Advanced Innovation Center for Future Internet Technology, The International WIC Institute, Beijing University of Technology, Beijing, China

J. Liu · Y. Yao · J. Chen
International WIC Institute, Beijing University of Technology, Beijing 100124, China

J. Liu
Department of Computer Science, Hong Kong Baptist University, Kowloon Tong, Hong Kong SAR
e-mail: jiming@comp.hkbu.edu.hk

Y. Yao
Department of Computer Science, University of Regina, Regina S4S 0A2, SK, Canada
e-mail: yyao@cs.uregina.ca

J. Chen
Department of Computer Science and Technology, Tsinghua University, Beijing 100084, China
e-mail: chenjianhui@bjut.edu.cn; chenjhnh@mail.tsinghua.edu.cn

N. Zhong et al. (eds.), *Wisdom Web of Things*, Web Information Systems Engineering and Internet Technologies Book Series,
DOI 10.1007/978-3-319-44198-6_1

1.1 Introduction

The Internet connects dispersive computers into a global network. On this network, the World Wide Web (Web) provides a global platform for information storage, resource sharing, service publishing, etc. An information world, called the cyber world, comes into being between the social and physical worlds.

In recent years, advanced information technologies accelerate the development of the cyber world [38, 39]. On one hand, various new Internet/Web based technologies, such as semantic Web [3, 11, 12], grid computing [13, 14], service-oriented computing [51], and cloud computing [2, 17], make the cyber world become not only a research/service platform but also a global communication and cooperation space in which various virtual communities, associations and organizations have been established. The cyber world is constantly expanding towards a social world. On the other hand, embedded technologies, automated recognition based on Radio Frequency Identification (RFID) technologies, wireless data communication technologies and ubiquitous computing technologies impel the forming of the Internet of Things (IoT) [5, 62]. A large number of sensor nets, embedded appliance nets and actuator nets (SEA-nets) have been constructed. Transparent computing technologies [55, 71–73, 85] ensure the effective deployment and publishing of resources/services on these heterogeneous nets. Furthermore, these SEA-nets are integrated and connected into the Internet through various gateways. The Web of Things (WoT) [10, 52] is emerging on the IoT to integrate the sensor data coming from various SEA-nets into the Web. The cyber world is also extending towards a physical world.

At present, various Internet/Web and IoT based applications, such as Web 2.0 [47, 48], Web 3.0 [20, 30], smart world [39, 45], smart planet [24], green/eco computing [29, 64], etc., accelerate the amalgamation among the cyber, social and physical worlds. It can be predicted that the cyber world composed of computers will be gradually syncretized with the social world composed of humans and the physical world composed of things in the near future. A *hyper world* [28, 37] will come into being on the IoT/WoT. It consists of the cyber, social and physical worlds, and uses data as a bridge to connect humans, computers and things. Such a data based hyper world will bring a profound influence in both work and life to the whole human

J. Ma · R. Huang
Faculty of Computer and Information Sciences, Hosei University,
Tokyo 184-8584, Japan
e-mail: jianhua@hosei.ac.jp

R. Huang
e-mail: rhuang@hosei.ac.jp

Y. Zhang
Key Laboratory of Pervasive Computing, Ministry of Education, and Tsinghua National Laboratory for Information Science and Technology, Department of Computer Science and Technology, Tsinghua University, Beijing 100084, China
e-mail: zhangyx@mail.tsinghua.edu.cn

society and every member in it. Multi-domain experts should closely cooperate to cope with the subsequent research challenges and opportunities.

The core research challenge brought by the hyper world is to realize the organic amalgamation and harmonious symbiosis among humans, computers and things using the Internet/Web based technologies, ubiquitous computing technologies and intelligence technologies, i.e., to make every thing in the hyper world more "intelligent" or "smart" by computers or cells with storage and computing capabilities, to provide active, transparent, safe and reliable services for individuals or communities in the hyper world. Though various theories and technologies have been developed to realize different levels of intelligent services on the Internet/Web and various SEA-nets, they do not fit well in the hyper world that is built on top of the IoT.

This chapter proposes the notion of *Wisdom Web of Things* (W2T) that represents a holistic intelligence methodology for realizing the harmonious symbiosis of humans, computers and things in the hyper world. A W2T data cycle system is also designed to implement such a cycle, namely "from things to data, information, knowledge, wisdom, services, humans, and then back to things." The W2T provides a practical technological way to realize the harmonious symbiosis of humans, computers and things in the emerging hyper world. The rest of the chapter is organized as follows. Section 1.2 discusses fundamental issues on intelligence in the hyper world. Section 1.3 proposes the W2T as a holistic intelligence methodology in the hyper world. For realizing the W2T, Sect. 1.4 describes a W2T data cycle system. Three use cases are introduced in Sect. 1.5. Finally, Sect. 1.6 gives concluding remarks.

1.2 Intelligence in the Hyper World

1.2.1 Web Intelligence (WI) and Brain Informatics (BI)

The Web significantly affects both academic research and daily life, revolutionizing the gathering, storage, processing, presentation, sharing, and utilization of data/information/knowledge. It offers great research opportunities and challenges in many areas, including business, commerce, marketing, finance, publishing, education, and research and development.

Web Intelligence (WI) [67, 74, 77, 81, 83] may be viewed as an enhancement or an extension of Artificial Intelligence (AI) and Information Technology (IT) on a totally new domain—the Web. It focuses on the research and development of new generations of Web-based information processing technologies and advanced applications to push technologies towards manipulating the meaning of data and creating distributed intelligence.

The tangible goals of WI can be refined as the development of Wisdom Web [75, 76], which is involved with the following top 10 problems [34, 35]:

- Goal-directed services (best means/ends),
- Personalization (identity),

- Social & psychological context (sensitivity),
- PSML, i.e., Problem Solver Markup Language (representation),
- Coordination (global behavior),
- Meta-knowledge (planning control),
- Semantics (relationships),
- Association (roles),
- Reproduction (population),
- Self-aggregation (feedback).

Though many efforts [16, 22, 31, 53] have been made to solve these problems, it is difficult to develop the Wisdom Web by using only the existing AI and IT technologies.

Brain Informatics (BI) [79, 80, 82] is an emerging interdisciplinary field to study human information processing mechanism systematically from both macro and micro points of view by cooperatively using experimental, theoretical, cognitive neuroscience and WI centric advanced information technology. It emphasizes on a systematic approach to an in-depth understanding of human intelligence. On the one hand, WI based portal techniques (e.g., the wisdom Web, data mining, multi-agent, and data/knowledge grids) will provide a new powerful platform [78] for BI; On the other hand, new understandings and discoveries of human intelligence in BI, as well as other domains of brain sciences (e.g., cognitive science and neuroscience) will yield new WI researches and developments. At present, some new human-inspired intelligent techniques and strategies [69, 70] have been developed to offset the disadvantages of existing intelligence technologies, especially logic-based technologies.

1.2.2 Ubiquitous Intelligence (UI) and Cyber-Individual (CI)

The development of RFID technologies and wireless data communication technologies impels the forming of IoT. The real physical things are called u-things if they are attached, embedded or blended with computers, networks, and/or some other devices such as sensors, actors, e-tags and so on [38]. The IoT makes it possible to connect u-things dispersed in various SEA-nets and ubiquitous computing applications for realizing a Ubiquitous Intelligence.

Ubiquitous Intelligence (UI) [39, 59], generally speaking, is that intelligent things are everywhere. It means pervasion of smart u-things in the real world, which would evolve towards the smart world filled with all kinds of smart u-things in a harmonious way [38–40]. The construction of smart u-things is a core issue in the UI. So-called smart u-things are the active/reactive/proactive u-things, which are with different levels of intelligence from low to high. Ideally, a smart u-thing should be able to act adaptively and automatically. Its construction is involved with the following 7 challenges [38, 40, 41]:

- Surrounding situations (context),
- Users' needs,

- Things' relations,
- Common knowledge,
- Self awareness,
- Looped decisions,
- Ubiquitous safety (UbiSafe).

Constructing such a smart u-thing is involved with various challenging topics, including the collecting and mining of logs [42], context modeling [21, 26, 27, 58], user modeling [4, 18, 19, 56], etc. However, there are many challenges due to the real world complexity. For realizing the UI, the human essence in the cyber world needs to be re-examined and analyzed. The research of Cyber-Individual (Cyber-I or CI) [63] is emphasized on re-examining and analyzing the human essence and creating cyber individuals in the cyber world. A Cyber-I is a real individual's counterpart in the cyber space. It is a unique and full description of human being in the digital world. On the one hand, ubiquitous computing technologies make it possible to collect individual's information anytime and anywhere. With the increasing power of computers, networks, ubiquitous sensors and massive storages, it is no longer a dream that everyone on this planet can have a Cyber-I going with and even beyond his/her own whole life. On the other hand, a comprehensive and exact Cyber-I can effectively guide smart u-things to provide active and transparent services for realizing the UI.

1.2.3 The Holistic Intelligence in the Hyper World

For realizing the harmonious symbiosis of humans, computers and things, u-things in the hyper world should be intelligent and able to provide active, transparent, safe and reliable services. This intelligentizing will realize not only individual intelligence but also holistic intelligence, i.e., all of related u-things can intelligently cooperate with each other for each application. Realizing such holistic intelligence will bring new challenges and opportunities for intelligence researches:

- The hyper world is involved with heterogeneous networks, service types, data forms and contents, efficiency/accuracy requirements, etc. Thus, it is impossible to realize holistic intelligence in such a complex environment by only separately using the WI, BI, UI and CI. For WI supported by BI, though the ubiquitous computing oriented data/services have been mentioned at the beginning, its related researches and developments are mainly focused on Web based data/services because of lacking the IoT and WoT, which can provide an effective approach to dynamically and largely gather the real-time sensor data coming from different SEA-nets, and realize active and transparent services anytime and everywhere. For the UI supported by the CI, though recent studies begin to focus on mining a large number of historical data for providing higher quality of services, related researches and developments were mainly oriented to specific applications and data because of lacking effective technologies and strategies to organize, manage, mining and utilize the multi-aspect real-time data and historical data, as well as

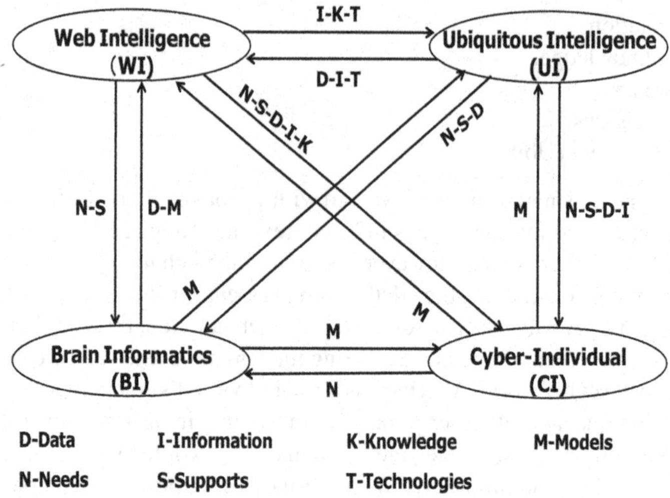

Fig. 1.1 The holistic intelligence research in the hyper world

information and knowledge derived from the data. Thus, the holistic intelligence research in the hyper world will present new research challenges to WI, BI, UI and CI.

- The infrastructure of hyper world consists of the Internet and a number of SEA-nets. It is possible to continuously and dynamically gather both real-time sensor data and historical Web data in the hyper world by the IoT and the WoT. Moreover, grid computing, cloud computing and transparent computing also make it possible to integrate the powerful storage and computing capabilities on the IoT for effectively storing, managing, mining and utilizing the gathered data, as well as the information and knowledge derived from data. Based on such an infrastructure, the hyper world will provide significant opportunities to the holistic intelligence research. It will integrate the WI, BI, UI and CI to develop a new holistic intelligence methodology for realizing the harmonious symbiosis of humans, computers and things in the hyper world.

In summary, the hyper world makes it possible and necessary to integrate separate intelligence researches into a holistic research. As shown in Fig. 1.1, in this holistic research, WI, BI, UI and CI are independent but promote each other. Finally, a holistic intelligence methodology with its associated mechanisms can be developed to realize the harmonious symbiosis of humans, computers and things in the hyper world.

1.3 Wisdom Web of Things

The Wisdom Web of Things (W2T) is an extension of the Wisdom Web in the IoT age. The "Wisdom" means that each of things in the WoT can be aware of both itself

Table 1.1 A comparison between the Web and W2T

	World Wide Web	W2T
Infrastructure	Internet	Internet of things
Function	A sharing platform and communication space	An environment to provide active, transparent, safe and reliable services for the harmonious symbiosis of humans, computers and things in the hyper world
Storing and computing medium	Different types of computers	All electronic media with the capabilities of storage and computing (including different types of computers, PDAs, mobile telephones, embedded chips, and so on.)
Data characteristic	Reliable data sources and relatively stable data streams	Various data availabilities, data stream modes, and data gathering strategies
Modeling	Data and user preference modeling	Not only data and user preference modeling but also space modeling (including environment modeling, thing modeling, context modeling, user behavior modeling, etc.)
Formal knowledge	Domain knowledge for the data and computing integration	Both domain knowledge and common sense knowledge for guiding the Web and ubiquitous computing
Awareness mode	A human centric mode (i.e., users choose the appropriate services based on individuals' judgments about the current Web environments.)	A ubiquitous awareness mode (i.e., all of humans, computers and things can be aware of themselves and others dynamically for providing active and transparent services.)
Computing mode	Computing on the Internet/Web	Computing in everywhere
Service mode	Passive services	Both active services and passive services

and others to provide the *right service* for the *right object* at a *right time* and *context*. Thus, the W2T is not a copy of the Web on the IoT. As shown in Table 1.1, it is different from the existing Web in many aspects, including infrastructure, function, data characteristic, modeling, and so on. Such a W2T is impossible to construct by using only the existing intelligence technologies that are oriented to specific humans, computers, things.

The nature is based on materials. An effective material cycle ensures the harmonious symbiosis of heterogeneous things in nature. Similarly, the hyper world is based on data. Thus, constructing the W2T for the harmonious symbiosis of humans, computers and things in the hyper world requires a highly effective W2T data cycle:

- Things to Data: Various data of things are collected into a distributed integrated data center through the WoT. These data include the real-time data of things coming from the sensors in SEA-nets and measuring equipments (such as MRI, EEG, CT), the Web accessible historic data of things stored on the Web, and the data of Web produced on the Web.
- Data to Information: After data cleaning, integration and storage, both sensor data and Web data are analyzed and re-organized to generate multi-aspect and multi-granularity data information by various data mining/ organization methods. The obtained data information is also described and stored in the data center.
- Information to Knowledge: The valuable knowledge is extracted from the data information by various modeling. Other related knowledge is also gathered and described using knowledge engineering technologies. All of knowledge is stored in the data center.
- Knowledge to Wisdom: Based on the obtained knowledge, the top 10 problems of Wisdom Web mentioned in Sect. 1.2.1 and 7 characteristics of smart u-thing mentioned in Sect. 1.2.2 are studied to develop the key intelligence technologies and strategies.
- Wisdom to Services: An active and transparent service platform is constructed on the integrated data center using the developed intelligence technologies and strategies. It can provide active, transparent, safe and reliable services by synthetically utilizing the data, information and knowledge in the data center.
- Services to Humans: The service platform provides various active and transparent services to individuals and communities by a variety of sensors and actuators.
- Humans to Things: During the process of receiving services, humans continues to influence the things around him/her and brings the changes of things. Finally, the data reflecting these changes are collected into the integrated data center.

As shown in Fig. 1.2, a variety of sensors, storage and computing terminals in the IoT provide a data storage and conversion carrier for implementing the data cycle. The emerging WoT provides a transmission channel of data cycle. Therefore, the core problem of data cycle construction is to develop a highly efficient data cycle system.

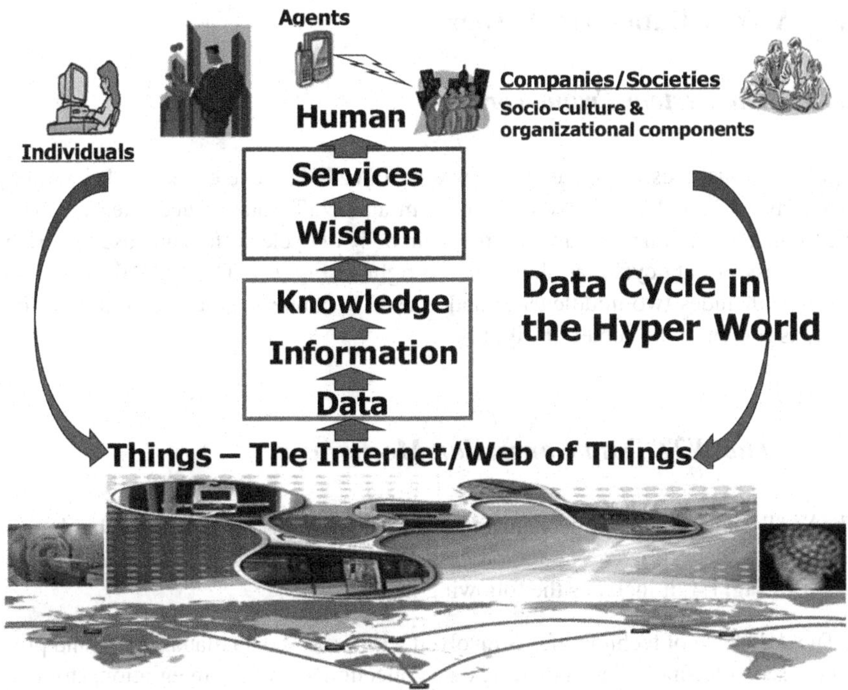

Fig. 1.2 A data cycle in the hyper world

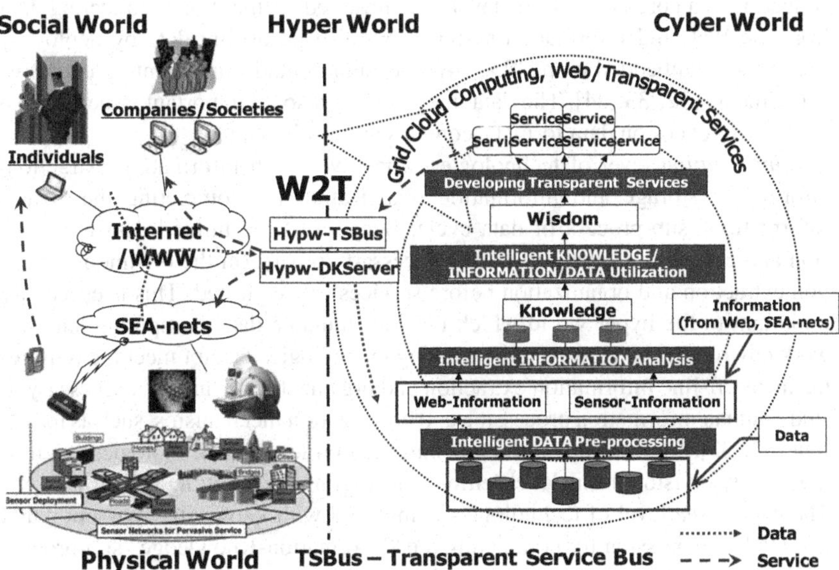

Fig. 1.3 A W2T data cycle system

1.4 A W2T Data Cycle System

1.4.1 The System Framework

Figure 1.3 illustrates the system framework of W2T data cycle system. It includes two parts, W2T data conversion mechanism and W2T data/service interface. The W2T data conversion mechanism is the main body of cycle system and used to drive the process of data cycle, as shown in the right of Fig. 1.3. The W2T data/service interface includes two middlewares and is used to connect the cycle system to the WoT, as shown in the center of Fig. 1.3.

1.4.2 The W2T Data Conversion Mechanism

The W2T data conversion mechanism includes a group of information technologies to transform data forms along the process of the W2T data cycle. As shown in the center of Fig. 1.4, it includes the following five levels:

- The *data* level of technologies is involved with various data management and preprocessing technologies, including data collection, cleaning, integration, storage, etc., for completing the "Things-Data" sub-process of the data cycle. Because the objective data include sensor data, Web accessible data and Web data, the data collection is a core issue at this level. It is involved with not only collecting data from the Web and information systems, but also producing data by deploying sensors and embedded chips [23, 54] or designing and implementing cognitive experiments [32, 33, 84]. The data integration is also an important issue because of the differences on data formats, contents and applications.
- The *information* level of technologies is involved with information extraction, information storage and information organization for completing the "Data-Information" sub-process of data cycle. Because of the limited data transmission and computing capabilities, it is necessary to perform the off-line information extraction and organization before services are requested. This is especially important to the hyper world which includes mutable data, computing and network environments. However, the existing technologies cannot meet the requirements of off-line information extraction and organization. Thus, it is necessary to study human information processing and organization mechanisms, such as induction [32, 33], for developing the new information level of technologies, such as granularity division, basic level setting, and starting point setting [69, 70].
- The *knowledge* level of technologies is involved with knowledge extraction and knowledge expression for completing the "Information-Knowledge" sub-process of data cycle. The core issues include model, common sense and knowledge retrieval. The studies of human knowledge expression and storage are also imple-

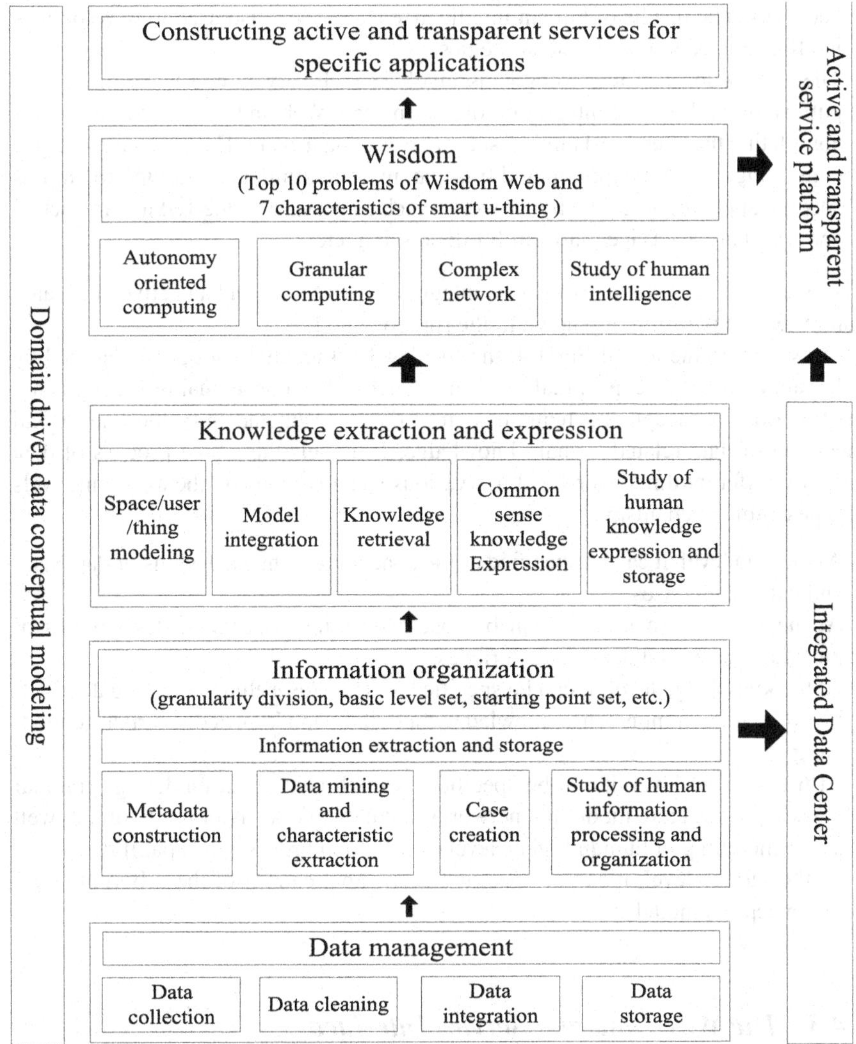

Fig. 1.4 The W2T data conversion mechanism

mented to develop the more effective technologies of knowledge expression and storage.

- The *wisdom* level of technologies mainly focuses on the top 10 problems of Wisdom Web and 7 characteristics of smart u-thing for completing the "Knowledge-Wisdom" sub-process of data cycle. The autonomy oriented computing [36], granular computing [66, 68], and complex network [57] are three core theories for realizing "Wisdom" on the WoT which includes enormous data and heterogeneous

networks. The results of human intelligence studies are also used to develop new intelligence technologies and strategies.
- The *service* level of technologies is involved with service construction, service publishing and service integration on the Internet/Web and various SEA-nets for completing the "Service-Human" sub-process of data cycle. They are based on grid computing, cloud computing and transparent computing, and oriented to various specific applications in the hyper world, such as pervasive elderly/kid care, active and transparent service platform for depression, etc.

These technologies are realized as an integrated data center and an active and transparent service platform, as shown in the right of Fig. 1.4.

As shown in the left of Fig. 1.4, the five levels of technologies are integrated by a domain driven data conceptual modeling. Such a data conceptual modeling is not the traditional conceptual schema design of databases/metadata or the ontological modeling of data related domain knowledge. It models the whole process of data cycle by different dimensions and has various specifications on the different levels of conversion mechanism:

- At the data level, it can be specified as the conceptual schema designs of databases and data warehouses.
- At the information level, it can be specified as the conceptual descriptions of metadata, cases and data characteristics.
- At the knowledge level, it can be specified as space/user/thing conceptual modeling, domain/common-sense knowledge modeling, and knowledge structure modeling.
- At the wisdom level, it can be specified as intelligent agent modeling, granular knowledge structure modeling, networks and network behavior modeling, as well as the modeling of human higher-level information processing capabilities.
- At the service level, it can be specified as the applications of the different levels of conceptual models.

1.4.3 The W2T Data and Service Interface

The W2T data and service interface includes two middlewares, hyper world data/knowledge application server (Hypw-DKServer) and hyper world transparent service bus (Hypw-TSBus). They are used to connect the data cycle system to the WoT for making it "Wisdom".

The Hypw-DKServer is a software middleware for the service publishing on the WoT. It can support centralized or distributed data/model/knowledge publishing and respond to data/model/knowledge requests coming from the Internet and various SEA-nets. Different from the existing Web based application servers, such as Weblogic, Tomcat, Jboss, etc., the Hypw-DKServer is an entirely new WoT based application server, as shown in Table 1.2.

Table 1.2 A comparison between Web application servers and the Hypw-DKServer

	Web application servers	Hypw-DKServer
Environment	The Web on the Internet	The WoT on the IoT
Operating system	Operating systems in computers (such as Windows, Unix, Linux, etc.)	New-style network operating systems on various networks
Main function	Supporting the establishment, deployment and management of static and dynamic Web applications	Supporting the establishment, deployment and management of data/model/knowledge services
Protocol	Standard Web protocols (such as HTTP, FTP, SOAP, WSDL, UDDI and so on.)	New-style standardized protocols for data/model/knowledge communications, descriptions and publishing
External interface	Database interfaces for main database systems such as Oracle, SQL Server, DB2, and so on.	Database interfaces for main database systems, and knowledge/model base interfaces for the existing/developed description languages of knowledge/models

The Hypw-TSBus is a software middleware for the service integration on the WoT. It can support dynamic service discovery, service evolution, service composition, and security validation for meeting various service requests on the Internet/Web and SEA-nets. Different from the existing Enterprise Service Bus (ESB), such as WebSphere ESB (WESB), BizTalk Server, etc., the Hypw-TSBus is an entirely new WoT based service bus, as shown in Table 1.3.

1.5 Case Studies

In this section, we present three use cases to demonstrate the usefulness of the proposed W2T methodology.

1.5.1 A W2T Based Kid Care Platform

An interesting survey [50] recently made in Japan reported that 72.5 % parents worried about their kids, 82.3 % parents felt tired in caring their kids, and 91.9 % parents had no enough time well taking care of their kids. Although the survey data may vary from country to country or from region to region, it shows that caring kids is not an

Table 1.3 A comparison between ESB platforms and the Hypw-TSBus

	ESB platforms	Hypw-TSBus
Environment	The Web on the Internet	The WoT on the IoT
Operating system	Operating systems in computers	New-style network operating systems on various networks
Main function	Providing a Web oriented infrastructure for the process-description driven service discovery and integration	Providing a WoT oriented infrastructure for the purpose-driven dynamic service discovery, evolution and integration
Other function	Supporting message routing, message conversion, message expansion, protocol intermediary, security validation, event handling, service scheduling, etc.	Supporting message routing, message expansion, security validation, event handling, etc.

easy work and it does consume a lot of time/energy to many parents. In fact, parents have been putting lot of efforts to ensure their children's safety. However, unexpected matters sometimes still happen. In other words, it is impossible for parents to keep eyes on their kids and give them prompt helps 24 h a day. Fortunately, with the rapid advancing of ICT and ubiquitous computing, not only kids can enjoy the fruits of developments brought by IT like digital games, real time animations, multimedia contents, but also their parents benefit from the advanced technologies. This section presents the W2T based kid care platform on top of which kid care systems are built. With the support of kid care systems, parents benefit from the supporting systems and can be relieved more or less from their various worries regarding to kid cares, especially to those working couples.

The issue of kid care is important to a family but it is also an ordinary and common activity. It has not been receiving much attention from research communities although there have been some research going on [23, 39, 54]. Kids as a specific group of humans, it is necessary to have a thorough study. With the rapid advancing of ubiquitous computing [5, 60, 61] and wireless communication technologies, developing kid care systems with ubiquitous sensors and wireless communications become feasible. This research field has received increasing attention. Based on related research results, we will develop a W2T based kid care platform, as shown in Fig. 1.5, which can be described as follows.

To take care of a kid, the first step is to know the kid. A system has to first record all the kid's activities and get to know the kid by analyzing his/her activities that just like a parent is doing in the process of caring children. A kid's activities are recorded via SEA-nets in the physical world. The recorded data are classified and stored in life-log, space-log, and thing-log, respectively. For example, Bob comes back from school, he watches TV in the living room from 2:30 pm to 3:30 pm, then studies in the study room from 3:30 pm to 5:30 pm. The recorded data are classified according Bob's

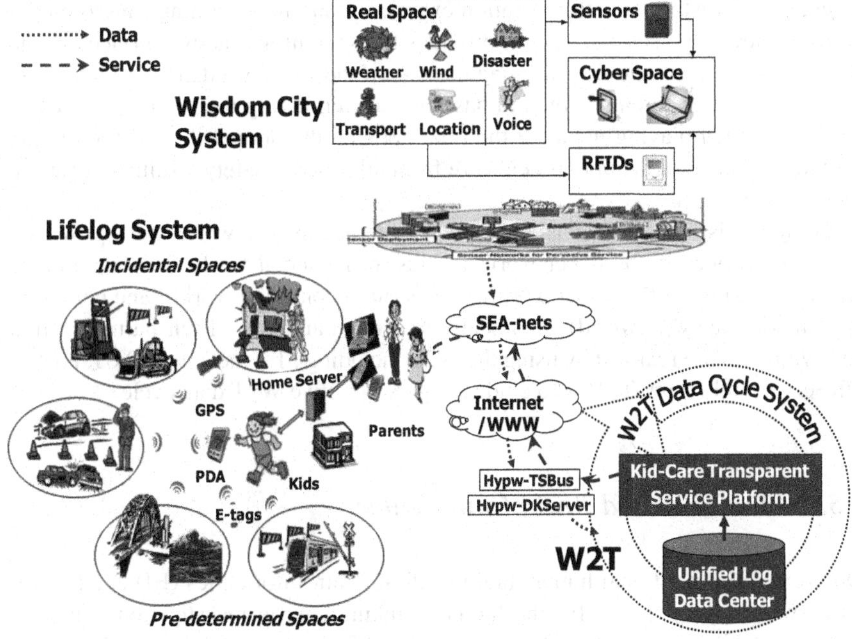

Fig. 1.5 The W2T based kid care platform

identification, physical location Bob has been, and devices he has been using into life-log (Bob-id), space-log (Bob-id,(living-room (2:30–3:30), study-room (3:30–5:30))), thing-log (Bob-id,TV (2:30–3:30), book (3:40–4:40), pen (4:40–5:10), ...). The log data are transferred via the Internet/WWW and SEA-nets to the Unified Log Data Center as shown in Fig. 1.5.

Each unified log database is a well-organized data structure and their relationships, such as the relationships regarding who, where, what, when in a 4-W hierarchical structure are implicitly preserved and accessible in an organized relational structure in the outer layer. To any situation in which a kid is, a node with its branch in the structure corresponding to the situation represents a knowledge set which is derived and composed from the log database. The knowledge set about a kid and for handling a certain situation that the kid is in, can be envisaged as a grape branch, its structure varies from a situation to a situation.

The processes from being aware of a situation or a context to derivation of a knowledge set and from the knowledge set to provision of transparent and active services to the kid are two important cores. The former requires mechanisms to extract, retrieve, and analyze data/information in the log database along the time axis or at a certain time section. The relational data/information is linked in a way that a kid's situation and context that the kid is in are represented either explicitly or implicitly. The relationships may be expressed in a n-dimension relational matrix. To be aware a situation and a context, a knowledge set can be dynamically composed together with history situation-solution experience and new learning. Based on the derived knowledge set, the system provides transparent and active services to the kid. For instance, providing a warning message if the kid is in a dangerous situation, informing his/her parents if the kid has fever, or reminding the kid to study when he/she has been playing game all the time, locking the door if the kid forgot, etc. To sum up, the system supports kid care from all aspects, safety, health, education, security, etc.

From acquisition of raw data via SEA-nets in the physical world to the provision of active services in the cyber world to kids in the social world, it is a complete data cycle. Kids (in the social world), things (in the physical world), and computer systems (in the cyber world) are actually integrated an entity. Their harmonization and symbiosis are realized by using the W2T including SEA-nets, IoT, WoT, Hypw-DKServer, and Hypw-TSBus to guide a highly effective W2T data cycle.

1.5.2 A W2T Based Brain Data Center

Different from traditional human brain studies, Brain Informatics (BI) emphasizes on a *systematic* approach for the human thinking centric investigation, which is complex and involved with multiple inter-related functions with respect to activated brain areas and their neurobiological processes of spatio-temporal features for a given task. Based on a systematic methodology of experimental design, a series of cognitive experiments are designed to obtain multiple forms of human brain data, which are involved with multiple granularities and aspects of human thinking centric cognitive functions. A systematic analysis methodology is also proposed to analyze these data comparatively and synthetically. For supporting such a systematic BI study, a brain data center needs to be developed to realize not only data storage and publishing oriented data management but also systematic analysis oriented management. This section presents the W2T based brain data center which is a global BI research platform for supporting the whole process of BI study. Guiding by this brain data center, various BI experimental studies and BI data analysis studies can be integrated to realize a systematic BI investigation.

The issue of brain database construction is a long-time focus in brain science. Although various brain databases [1, 15, 44, 46] have been constructed to effectively store and share heterogeneous brain data, especially EEG (electroencephalogram) data and fMRI (functional magnetic resonance imaging) data focused by present BI studies, these brain databases mainly focus on data storage and publishing. They cannot effectively support the systematic BI study. Based on all of the fundamental considerations, we will develop a W2T based brain data center, as shown in Fig. 1.6, which can be briefly described as follows.

BI is a data-centric scientific study whose process can be generalized as a BI data cycle, including data production, data collection, data storage, data management, data description, data mining, information organization, knowledge extraction, knowledge integration, and knowledge utilization. All of BI research activities

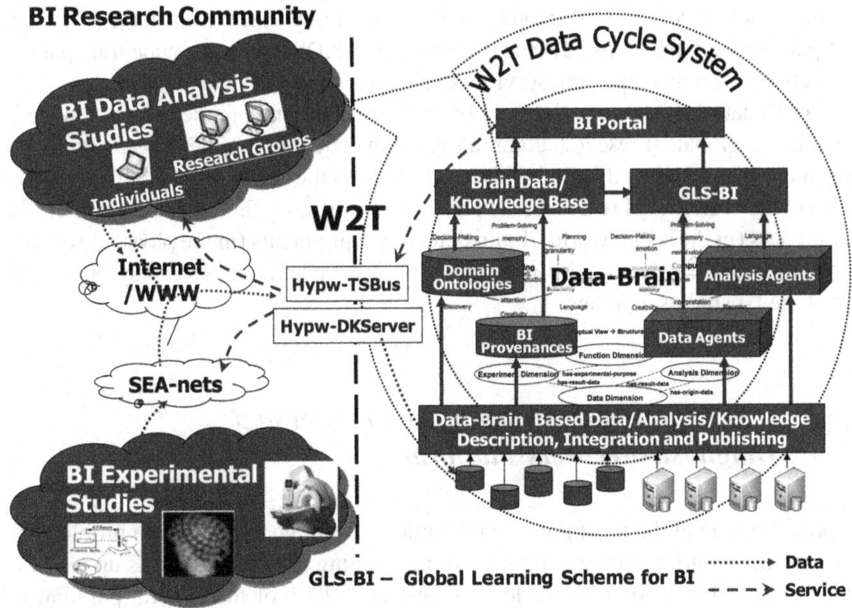

Fig. 1.6 The W2T based brain data center

apply themselves to impel this data cycle. Thus, to support the systematic BI study, the first step is to collect heterogeneous brain data, including not only experiment data obtained by BI experimental studies but also derived data, information and knowledge obtained by BI data analysis studies. These data, information and knowledge are transferred via the Internet/WWW and SEA-nets to distributed brain databases as shown in Fig. 1.6.

A new conceptual data model, named Data-Brain [6, 7], is used to integrate the data, information and knowledge stored in brain databases. The Data-Brain models the four aspects of systematic BI methodology by four dimensions. Related domain ontologies are also integrated into these dimensions. Based on the Data-Brain, the information and knowledge derived from data are integrated and organized as Data-Brain based BI provenances and sub-dimensions of Data-Brain, respectively. They provide multi-granularity and multi-aspect semantic descriptions of brain data for data understanding and utilization. The Data-Brain, BI provenances and brain data form a multi-level brain data-knowledge base, which provides data, information, and knowledge services for BI researchers and other research assistant systems, such as the Global Learning Scheme for BI (GLS-BI) [8]. The GLS-BI is a brain data analysis platform which models BI experimental and data analysis studies, as well as available BI data and computing resources. It is implemented as a multi-agent system with various data agents and analysis agents to support multi-aspect brain data analysis by various assistant functions, including dynamical mining process planning, workflows filter and performance, etc. Finally, all of the functions provided by the brain data-knowledge base and the GLS-BI are enclosed as services on the BI portal and published by the Hypw-TSBus and the Hypw-KDServer to provide transparent and active research supporting services during the whole BI research process.

As a BI data cycle system, the W2T based brain data center guides a complete data cycle in the global BI research community, from acquisition of heterogeneous data, information and knowledge in the physical world to the provision of active services in the cyber world to BI researchers in the social world. By this brain data center, BI researchers (in the social world), brain detecting equipments (in the physical world), and data/computing resources (in the cyber world) are harmonious and symbiosis to impel the BI studies together.

1.5.3 A W2T Based Depression Data Center and Diagnosis-Recovery Platform

Depression, one of the most prevalent disorders, is a huge public-health problem. It is a chronic, recurring and potentially life-threatening illness that affects up to 20 % of the population across the world. An estimated 20 % of the general population will suffer depression sometimes in their lifetimes. About 15 % of patients with a mood disorder die by their own hand, and at least 66 % of all suicides are preceded by depression. Depression is expected to be the second leading cause of disability for people of all ages by 2020 [43, 65]. The increasing of depressed patients will burden the family and society heavily. Even if treatment with medication and/or electroconvulsive therapy (ECT) and psychotherapy are performed, it is still a long-term process which needs the support of information technologies. This section presents the W2T based depression data center and diagnosis-recovery platform on the top of which depression diagnosis-recovery systems are built. These systems can provide various supports for depression prevention, diagnosis, therapy, care and recovery.

Depressive symptoms are characterized not only by negative thought, mood, and behavior but also by specific changes in bodily functions (for example, crying spells, body aches, low energy or libido, as well as problems with eating, weight, or sleeping). Neuroimaging studies [9, 25, 49] also found that the abnormal activity for depressed patients in brain regions including prefrontal, limbic, cinguale, subthalamus, hippocampus, amygdala, as well as globus pallidus. Depression is usually first identified in a primary-care setting, not in a mental health practitioner's office. Moreover, it often assumes various disguises, which cause depression to be frequently underdiagnosed.

Although clear research evidences and clinical guidelines have been found, treating depression is still a long-term and hardy process which cannot be completed only depending on hospitals, physicians and nurses. The depression prevention, diagnosis, therapy, care and recovery need the support of ubiquitous computing and wireless communication technologies. This research field has received increasing attention.

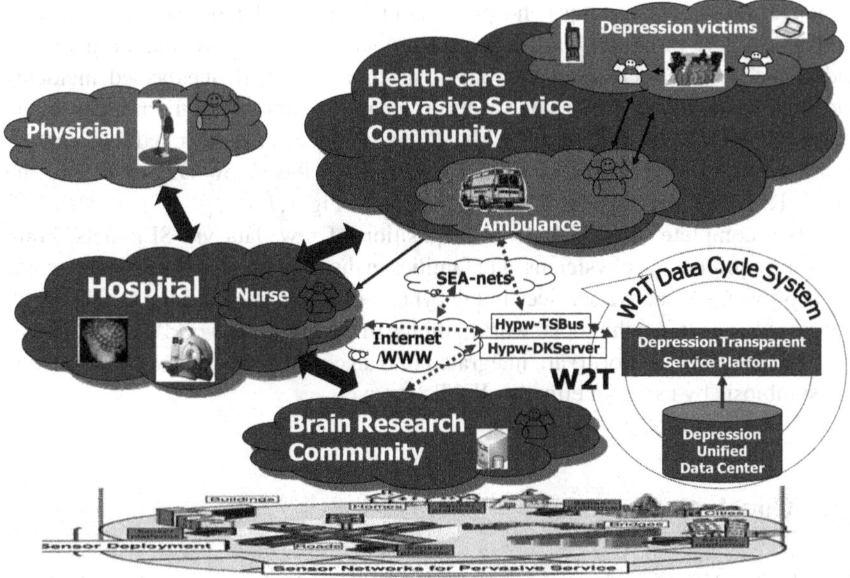

Fig. 1.7 The W2T based depression data center and diagnosis-recovery platform

Based on related research results, we will develop a W2T based depression data center and diagnosis-recovery platform, as shown in Fig. 1.7, which can be briefly described as follows.

Treating depression needs the cooperation among hospitals, brain research institutions, families and society. The first step is to timely gather multi-aspect data of depressed patients or latent patients, including medical data obtained by hospitals, brain activity data obtained by the brain research community, and other health-related data, such as mood, behavior, physical symptoms, recorded by sensors or people around patients in the health-care pervasive service community. As shown in Fig. 1.7, these data are transferred via the Internet/WWW and SEA-nets to the Depression Unified Data Center.

Multiple types of databases are included in this data center. Some stored data are with a well-organized data structure and implicit or explicit relationships. Others are multimedia data and stream data with semantic and well-organized metadata. The derived multi-granularity information and knowledge are also organized and stored in this data center.

The processes from gathered data, information and knowledge to the provision of transparent and active services are diversiform because of different requirements of depression prevention, diagnosis, therapy, care and recovery. For monitoring latent patients, their behavior modes are extracted from data to find physical symptoms and to provide active reminding services by SEA-nets. For diagnoses of depressed patients, intelligent data query services are provided to integrate multi-aspect information, including mood, behavior, brain activities, and present/history medical treatments, for assisting diagnoses in hospitals. For treatments of depressed patients, mild patients can join the health-care pervasive service community to obtain transparent and active treatment/care services out of hospitals. Even if unexpected incidents happen on patients, physicians on vacation can give treatment programs and provide treatment services by ambulances. All of these services are integrated in a depression transparent service platform and published by the Hypw-DKServer and the Hypw-TSBus on the top of IoT/WoT, as shown in Fig. 1.7.

It is a complete data cycle from acquisition of raw data via SEA-nets, brain detecting equipments, physicians, and families in the physical world and social world to the provision of active services in the cyber world to patients in the social world. Depressed patients (in the social world), things (in the physical world), and computer systems (in the cyber world) are integrated into an entity to realize their harmonious and symbiosis by using an effective W2T data cycle.

1.6 Conclusions

With the development of advanced information technologies, especially IoT related technologies, a hyper world, which integrates the social, physical and cyber worlds, is emerging. Data will be the vital ingredients of the hyper world. Although the WoT constructed on the IoT, data "run" in the hyper world with multiple formats, including information and knowledge, to tightly connect humans, computers and things, which are dispersed in the social, physical and cyber worlds.

The existing intelligence technologies for the Web and ubiquitous computing have focused on the conversion and utilization of data to provide more intelligent services on the Internet/Web or SEA-nets. However, these studies are limited in specific technologies, applications, data, and data conversions. Only using these technologies cannot fully utilize the enormous data and realize holistic intelligence for the harmonious symbiosis of humans, computers and things in the hyper world.

Integrating the existing studies of intelligent information technologies, this chapter proposed the W2T as a holistic intelligence methodology in the hyper world. A W2T data cycle system is designed to drive the cycle, namely "from things to data, information, knowledge, wisdom, services, humans, and then back to things" for realizing the W2T. This is a practically technological way to realize the harmonious symbiosis of humans, computers and things in the emerging hyper world.

Acknowledgments The work is partially supported by the National Natural Science Foundation of China (Number: 60905027), Beijing Natural Science Foundation (4102007), China Scholarship Council (CSC) (File No. 2009654018), Open Foundation of Key Laboratory of Multimedia and Intelligent Software (Beijing University of Technology), Beijing, Support Center for Advanced Telecommunications Technology Research, Foundation (SCAT), Japan, and JSPS Grants-in-Aid for Scientific Research (No.21500081), Japan.

References

1. Australian EEG Database. http://eeg.newcastle.edu.au/inquiry/
2. M. Armbrust, A. Fox, R. Griffith, A. Joseph, R.H. Katz, A. Konwinski, G. Lee, D.A. Patterson, A. Rabkin, I. Stoica, M. Zaharia, *Above the Clouds: A Berkeley View of Cloud Computing* (Technical report, EECS Department, University of California, Berkeley, 2009)
3. T. Berners-Lee, J. Hendler, O. Lassila, The semantic web. Sci. Am. **284**(5), 34–43 (2001)
4. R. Casas, R.B. Marin, A. Robinet, A.R. Delgado, A.R. Yarza, J. McGinn, R. Picking, V. Grout, User modelling in ambient intelligence for elderly and disabled people, in *Proceedings of the 11th International Conference on Computers Helping People with Special Needs (ICCHP 2008)* (2008), pp. 114–122
5. H. Chaouchi, *The Internet of Things-Connecting Objects to the Web* (ISTE Ltd., Wiley, 2010)
6. J.H. Chen, N. Zhong, Data-brain modeling based on brain informatics methodology, in *Proceedings of the 2008 IEEE/WIC/ACM International Conference on Web Intelligence (WI'08)* (2008), pp. 41–47
7. J.H. Chen, N. Zhong, Data-brain modeling for systematic brain informatics, in *Proceedings of the 2009 International Conference on Brain Informatics (BI 2009)* (2009), pp. 182–193
8. J.H. Chen, N. Zhong, R.H. Huang, Towards Systematic human brain data management using a data-brain based GLS-BI system, in *Proceedings of the 2010 International Conference on Brain Informatics (BI 2010)* (2010), pp. 365–376
9. R.J. Davidson, W. Irwin, M.J. Anderle, N.H. Kalin, The neural substrates of affective processing in depressed patients treated with venlafaxine. Am. J. Psychiatry. **160**(1), 64–75 (2003)
10. T. Dillon, A. Talevski, V. Potdar, E. Chang. Web of things as a framework for ubiquitous intelligence and computing, in *Proceedings of the 6th International Conference on Ubiquitous Intelligence and Computing* (2009), pp. 1–10
11. D. Fensel, F. van Harmelen, Unifying reasoning and search to web scale. IEEE Internet Comput. **11**(2), 96, 94–95 (2007)
12. D. Fensel, F. van Harmelen, B. Andersson, P. Brennan, H. Cunningham, E.D. Valle, F. Fischer, Z.S. Huang, A. Kiryakov, T.K. Lee, L. Schooler, V. Tresp, S. Wesner, M. Witbrock, N. Zhong, Towards LarKC: a platform for web-scale reasoning, in *Proceedings of the 2008 IEEE International Conference on Semantic Computing* (2008), pp. 524–529
13. I. Foster, C. Kesselman, The grid: blueprint for a new computing infrastructure (Morgan Kaufmann, 1999)
14. I. Foster, C. Kesselman, The grid 2: blueprint for a new computing infrastructure (Morgan Kaufmann, 2003)
15. fMRI Data Center. http://www.fmridc.org/f/fmridc
16. M.X. Gao, C.N. Liu, A constraints-based semantic mapping method from natural language questions to OWL. Acta Electronica Sinica **35**(8), 1598–1602 (2007)
17. B. Hayes, Cloud computing. Commun. ACM **7**, 9–11 (2008)
18. D. Heckmann. Ubiquitous user modeling for situated interaction, in *Proceedings of the 8th International Conference on User Modeling* (Springer LNCS 2109, Sonthofen, Germany, 2001), pp. 280–282
19. D. Heckmann, A. Krueger, A User modeling Markup Language (UserML) for ubiquitous computing, in *Proceedings of the 9th International Conference on User Modeling*, Johnstown, Pennsylvania, USA (2003), pp. 393–397
20. J. Hendler, Web 3.0: chicken farms on the semantic web. Computer **41**(1), 106–108 (2008)
21. K. Henricksen, J. Indulska, A. Rakotonirainy, Modeling context information in pervasive computing systems, in *Proceedings of the 1st International Conference on Pervasive Computing*, Springer LNCS 2414, Zurich, Switzerland (2002), pp. 167–180
22. J. Hu, N. Zhong, Organizing multiple data sources for developing intelligent e-business portals. Data Min. Knowl. Discov. **12**(2–3), 127–150 (2006). Springer
23. R.H. Huang, J.H. Ma, Homelog based kid's activity awareness, in *Proceedings of the 2009 Computation World: Future Computing, Service Computation, Cognitive, Adaptive, Content, Patterns*, Athens, Greece (2009), pp. 591–596

24. IBM (2010) Smarter Planet. http://www.ibm.com/smarterplanet/us/en/overview/ideas/index.html
25. W. Irwin, M.J. Anderle, H.C. Abererombie, M.S. Stacey, N.H. Kalin, R.J. Davidson, Amygdalar interhemispheric functional connectivity differs between the non-depressed and depressed human brain. NeuroImage **21**(2), 674–86 (2004)
26. E. Kim, J. Choi. An ontology-based context model in a smart home, in *Proceedings of the 2006 International Conference on Computational Science and Its Applications (ICCSA 2006)* (2006), pp. 11–20
27. E.J. Ko, H.J. Lee, J.W. Lee, Ontology-based context modeling and reasoning for U-healthCare. IEICE Trans. Inf. Syst. **E90–D(8)**, 1262–1270 (2007)
28. T.L. Kunii, J.H. Ma, R.H. Huang, Hyperworld modeling, in *Proceedings of the International Conference on Visual Information Systems (VIS'96)* (1996), pp. 1—8
29. C.E. Landwehr, Green computing. IEEE Secur. Priv. **3**(6), 3 (2005)
30. O. Lassila, J. Hendler, Embracing "Web 3.0". IEEE Internet Comput. **11**(3), 90–93 (2007)
31. W.B. Li, N. Zhong, Y.Y. Yao, J.M. Liu, An operable email based intelligent personal assistant. World Wide Web **12**(2), 125–147 (2009). Springer
32. P.P. Liang, Y.H. Yang, S.F. Lu, K.C. Li, N. Zhong, The role of the DLPFC in inductive reasoning of MCI patient and normal aging: an fMRI study. Sci. China Ser. C Life Sci. **39**(7), 711–716 (2009)
33. P.P. Liang, N. Zhong, S.F. Lu, J.M. Liu, ERP characteristics of sentential inductive reasoning in time and frequency domains. Cogn. Syst. Res. **11**(1), 67–73 (2010)
34. J.M. Liu, N. Zhong, Y.Y. Yao, Z.W. Ras, The wisdom web: new challenges for Web intelligence (WI). J. Intell. Inf. Syst. **20**(1), 5–9 (2003)
35. J.M. Liu, Web Intelligence (WI): what makes wisdom web?, in *Proceedings of Eighteenth International Joint Conference on Artificial Intelligence (IJCAI'03)* (2003), pp. 1596–1601
36. J.M. Liu, X. Jin, K.C. Tsui, *Autonomy Oriented Computing: From Problem Solving to Complex Systems Modeling* (Springer, 2005)
37. J.H. Ma, R.H. Huang, Improving human interaction with a hyperworld, in *Proceedings of the Pacific Workshop on Distributed Multimedia Systems (DMS'96)* (1996), pp. 46–50
38. J.H. Ma, Smart u-Things-challenging real world complexity. IPSJ Symp. Ser. **2005**(19), 146–150 (2005)
39. J.H. Ma, L.T. Yang, B.O. Apduhan, R.H. Huang, L. Barolli, M. Takizawa, Towards a smart world and ubiquitous intelligence: a walkthrough from smart things to smart hyperspaces and UbicKids. Int. J. Pervasive Comput. Commun. **1**(1), 53–68 (2005)
40. J.H. Ma, Smart u-Things and ubiquitous intelligence, in *Proceedings of the 2nd International Conference on Embedded Software and Systems (ICESS 2005)* (2005), p. 776
41. J.H. Ma, Q.F. Zhao, V. Chaudhary, J.D. Cheng, L.T. Yang, R.H. Huang, Q. Jin, Ubisafe computing: vision and challenges (I), in *Proceedings of the 3rd International Conference on Autonomic and Trusted Computing (ATC 2006)* (2006), pp. 386–397
42. J.H. Ma. Spacelog concept and issues for novel u-Services in smart spaces, in *Proceedings of the 2nd International Conference on Future Generation Communication and Networking Symposia* (2008), pp. 89–92
43. C.J.L. Murray, A.D. Lopez, *The Global Burden of Disease: A Comprehensive Assessment of Cambridge (USA)* (Harvard University Press, 1996), pp. 412–417, 445–448, 553–556, 808–811
44. Neocortical Microcircuit Database. http://microcircuit.epfl.ch
45. R. Ogle, *Smart World: Breakthrough Creativity and the New Science of Ideas* (Harvard Business School Press, Boston, MA, 2007)
46. Olfactory Receptor Database. http://senselab.med.yale.edu/ORDB/default.asp
47. T. O'Reilly. What is Web 2.0. http://www.oreilly.com/pub/a/oreilly/tim/news/2005/09/30/what-is-web-20.html (2005)
48. T. O'Reilly. What is Web 2.0: design patterns and business models for the next generation of software. Commun. Strateg. **1**, 17–37 (2007)
49. S. Posse, D. Fitzgerald, K. Gao, U. Habel, D. Rosenberg, G.J. Moore, F. Schneider, Real-time fMRI of temporolimbic regions detects amygdala activation during single-trial self-induced sadness. NeuroImage **18**(3), 760–768 (2003)

50. H. Seiho, A couple responding to children's problems. Child Psychol. **805** (2004)
51. M.P. Singh, M.N. Huhns, *Service-Oriented Computing* (Wiley, 2005)
52. V. Stirbu, Towards a RESTful plug and play experience in the Web of things, in *Proceedings of the 2008 IEEE International Conference on Semantic Computing* (2008), pp. 512–517
53. Y.L. Su, L. Zheng, N. Zhong, C.N. Liu, J.M. Liu, Distributed reasoning based on Problem Solver Markup Language (PSML)—a demonstration through extended OWL, in *Proceedings of the 2005 IEEE International Conference on e-Technology, e-Commerce and e-Service (EEE'05)* (2005), pp. 208–213
54. K. Takata, J.H. Ma, B.O. Apduhan, A dangerous location aware system for assisting kids safety care, in *Proceedings of the 20th International Conference on Advanced Information Networking and Applications (AINA'06)* (2006), pp. 657–662
55. P.W. Tian, Y.X. Zhang, Y.Z. Zhou, L.T. Yang, M. Zhong, L.K. Weng, L. Wei, A novel service evolution approach for active services in ubiquitous computing. Int. J. Commun. Syst. **22**(9), 1123–1151 (2009)
56. E. Vildjiounaite, O. Kocsis, V. Kyllonen, B. Kladis. Context-dependent user modelling for smart homes, in *Proceedings of the 11th International Conference on User Modeling (UM 2007)* (2007), pp. 345–349
57. X. Wang, G. Chen, Complex network: small-world, scale-free and beyond. IEEE Circ. Syst. Mag. **3**(2), 6–20 (2003)
58. X.H. Wang, D.Q. Zhang, T. Gu, H.K. Pung, Ontology based context modeling and reasoning using OWL, in *Proceedings of the 2nd IEEE Annual Conference on Pervasive Computing and Communications Workshops*, IEEE CS Press, Orlando, Florida, USA (2004), pp. 18–22
59. P.W. Warren, From ubiquitous computing to ubiquitous intelligence. BT Technol. J. **22**(2), 28–38 (2004)
60. M. Weiser, The computer for the 21st century. Sci. Am. **265**(3), 66–75 (1991)
61. M. Weiser, Some computer science issues in ubiquitous computing. Commun. ACM **36**(7), 75–84 (1993)
62. E. Welbourne, L. Battle, G. Cole, K. Gould, K. Rector, S. Raymer, M. Balazinska, G. Borriello, Building the internet of things using RFID. IEEE Internet Comput. **33**(3), 48–55 (2009)
63. J. Wen, K. Ming, F.R. Wang, B.X. Huang, J.H. Ma, Cyber-I: vision of the individual's counterpart on cyberspace, in *Proceedings of the 8th IEEE International Conference on Dependable, Autonomic and Secure Computing* (2009), pp. 295–302
64. J. Williams, L. Curtis, Green: the new computing coat of arms. IT Prof. **10**(1), 12–16 (2008)
65. W.J. Xu, *New Approaches in Epidemiology and Treatment of Depression: With a Case Report* (The medicine of Zhejinag University (Psychiatry), 2007)
66. Y.Y. Yao, Granular computing: basic issues and possible solutions, in *Proceedings of the 5th Joint Conference on Information Sciences* (1999), pp. 186–189
67. Y.Y. Yao, N. Zhong, J.M. Liu, S. Ohsuga, Web Intelligence (WI): research challenges and trends in the new information age, in N. Zhong, Y.Y. Yao, J. Liu, S. Ohsuga (eds.), *Web Intelligence: Research and Development*, Springer, LNAI 2198 (2001)
68. Y.Y. Yao, N. Zhong, Granular computing. Encycl. Comput. Sci. Eng. **3**, 1446–1453 (2009). Wiley
69. Y. Zeng, Y. Wang, Z.S. Huang, N. Zhong, Unifying Web-scale search and reasoning from the viewpoint of granularity, in *Proceedings of the 2009 International Conference on Active Media Technology*, Springer, LNCS 5820 (2009), pp. 418–429
70. Y. Zeng, N. Zhong, Y. Wang, Y.L. Qin, Z.S. Huang, H.Y. Zhou, Y.Y. Yao, F. von. Harmelen, User-centric query refinement and processing using granularity based strategies. Knowl. Inf. Syst. (2010) (in press, Springer)
71. Y.X. Zhang, C.H. Fang, *Actives Services: Concepts, Architecture and Implementation* (Thomson Learning Press, Washington, 2005)
72. Y.X. Zhang, Y.Z. Zhou, Transparent computing: a new paradigm for pervasive computing, in *Proceedings of the 3rd International Conference on Ubiquitous Intelligence and Computing (UIC 2006)* (2006), pp. 1–11

73. Y.X. Zhang, L.T. Yang, Y.Z. Zhou, W.Y. Kuang, Information security underlying transparent computing: impacts, visions and challenges. Web Intell. Agent Syst. **8**(2), 203–217 (2010). IOS Press
74. N. Zhong, J.M. Liu, Y.Y. Yao, S. Ohsuga. Web Intelligence (WI), in *Proceedings of the 24th IEEE Computer Society International Computer Software and Applications Conference (COMPSAC 2000)* (2000), pp. 469–470
75. N. Zhong, J.M. Liu, Y.Y. Yao, In search of the Wisdom Web. IEEE Comput. **35**(11), 27–31 (2002)
76. N. Zhong, J.M. Liu, Y.Y. Yao, Web Intelligence (WI): a new paradigm for developing the Wisdom Web and social network intelligence, in *Web Intelligence* (Springer, 2003), pp. 1–16
77. N. Zhong, J.M. Liu, Y.Y. Yao, *Web Intelligence* (Springer, 2003)
78. N. Zhong. Building a brain-informatics portal on the wisdom web with a multi-layer grid: a new challenge for web intelligence research, in V. Torra, Y. Narukawa, S. Miyamoto (eds.) *Modeling Decisions for Artificial Intelligence* (Springer, LNAI 3558, 2005), pp. 24–35
79. N. Zhong, Impending brain informatics research from web intelligence perspective. Int. J. Inf. Technol. Decis. Mak. **5**(4), 713–727 (2006). World Scientific
80. N. Zhong, J.M. Liu, Y.Y. Yao, J.L. Wu, S.F. Lu, Y.L. Qin, K.C. Li, B. Wah, Web intelligence meets brain informatics, in N. Zhong et al. (eds.), *Web Intelligence Meets Brain Informatics* (Springer LNCS 4845, Sate-of-the-Art Survey, 2006), pp. 1–31
81. N. Zhong, J.M. Liu, Y.Y. Yao, Envisioning intelligent information technologies through the prism of web intelligence. Commun. ACM **50**(3), 89–94 (2007)
82. N. Zhong, Ways to develop human-level web intelligence: a brain informatics perspective, in E. Franconi, M. Kifer, W. May (eds.), *The Semantic Web: Research and Applications* (Springer LNCS 4519, 2007), pp. 27–36
83. N. Zhong J.M. Liu, Y.Y. Yao, Web Intelligence (WI). Encycl. Comput. Sci. Eng. **5**, 3062–3072 (2009, Wiley)
84. N. Zhong, P.P. Liang, Y.Y. Qin, S.F. Lu, Y.H. Yang, K.C. Li, Neural substrates of data-driven scientific discovery: an fMRI study during performance of number series completion task. Sci. China Ser. C Life Sci. **39**(3), 1–8 (2009)
85. Y.Z. Zhou, Y.X. Zhang, *Transparent Computing: Concepts, Architecture, and Implementation* (Cengage Learning, 2010)

Chapter 2
WaaS—Wisdom as a Service

Jianhui Chen, Jianhua Ma, Ning Zhong, Yiyu Yao, Jiming Liu, Runhe Huang, Wenbin Li, Zhisheng Huang and Yang Gao

Abstract An emerging hyper-world encompasses all human activities in a social-cyber-physical space. Its power derives from the Wisdom Web of Things (W2T) cycle, namely, "from things to data, information, knowledge, wisdom, services, humans, and then back to things." The W2T cycle leads to a harmonious symbiosis among humans, computers and things, which can be constructed by large-scale converging of intelligent information technology applications with an open and interoperable architecture. The recent advances in cloud computing, the Internet/Web of Things, big data and other research fields have provided just such an open system architecture with resource sharing/services. The next step is therefore to develop an open and interoperable content architecture with intelligence sharing/services for the

J. Chen
Department of Computer Science and Technology, Tsinghua University,
Beijing 100084, China
e-mail: chenjhnh@mail.tsinghua.edu.cn

J. Ma
Faculty of Computer and Information Sciences, Hosei University,
Tokyo 184-8584, Japan
e-mail: jianhua@hosei.ac.jp

N. Zhong (✉)
Department of Life Science and Informatics, Maebashi Institute of Technology,
Maebashi-city 371-0816, China
e-mail: zhong@maebashi-it.ac.jp; zhongn@bjut.edu.cn

N. Zhong
Beijing Advanced Innovation Center for Future Internet Technology,
The International WIC Institute, Beijing University of Technology,
Beijing, China

Y. Yao · J. Liu · Z. Huang
International WIC Institute, Beijing University of Technology,
Beijing 100124, China

Y. Yao
Department of Computer Science, University of Regina,
Regina, SK S4S 0A2, Canada
e-mail: yyao@cs.uregina.ca

N. Zhong et al. (eds.), *Wisdom Web of Things*, Web Information
Systems Engineering and Internet Technologies Book Series,
DOI 10.1007/978-3-319-44198-6_2

organization and transformation in the "data, information, knowledge and wisdom (DIKW)" hierarchy. This chapter introduces Wisdom as a Service (WaaS) as a content architecture based on the "paying only for what you use" IT business trend. The WaaS infrastructure, WaaS economics, and the main challenges in WaaS research and applications are discussed. A case study is described to demonstrate the usefulness and significance of WaaS. Relying on the clouds (cloud computing), things (Internet of Things) and big data, WaaS provides a practical approach to realize the W2T cycle in the hyper-world for the coming age of ubiquitous intelligent IT applications.

2.1 An Emerging Hyper-World

According to estimates by the International Telecommunication Union (ITU) (February 2013) [1], global Internet users and mobile Internet (MI) users will reach 2.7 billion and 2.1 billion, respectively, in 2013. A huge number of sensors, embedded appliances, and actuators have been deployed in almost every part of cities. The Internet, MI, Internet of Things (IoT) and Web of Things (WoT) [2] connect humans, computers and things to form an immense network, by which various information technologies (IT) and their applications are permeating into every aspect of our daily lives. The continuously extending IT applications have resulted in a *hyper-world*, consisting of the social, cyber, and physical worlds, and using data as a bridge to connect humans, computers, and things [3, 4].

In the hyper-world, the most important changes and characteristics include the following two aspects:

J. Liu
Department of Computer Science, Hong Kong Baptist University,
Kowloon Tong, Hong Kong SAR
e-mail: jiming@comp.hkbu.edu.hk

R. Huang
Faculty of Computer and Information Sciences,
Hosei University, Tokyo 184-8584, Japan
e-mail: rhuang@hosei.ac.jp

W. Li
Department of Computer Science, Shijiazhuang University of Economics,
Shijiazhuang 050031, China
e-mail: liwenbin@fireflymobile.cn

Z. Huang
Department of Computer Science, Vrije University Amsterdam, Amsterdam, The Netherlands
e-mail: huang@cs.vu.nl; z.huang@vu.nl; huang.zhisheng.nl@gmail.com

Y. Gao
Department of Computer Science, Nanjing University, Nanjing 210046, China
e-mail: gaoy@nju.edu.cn

- The first is the change of the human-computer relationship. In the past, we lived separately from the cyber world and accessed computers and networks only when we needed IT services. There was a loose coupling between humans and computers. The appearance of the hyper-world changes this kind of loose coupling. Owing to the fusion of the social, cyber, and physical worlds, today we live within a huge network of numerous computing devices, storage devices, and u-Things, where the real physical things are attached, embedded, or blended with computers, networks, and/or some other devices such as sensors, actors, e-tags and so on [5]. Adapting and utilizing this kind of new human-computer relationship is an urgent task for the development of IT applications.
- The second is the emerging big data. The extension of the Internet, IoT and MI greatly accelerates the production of data. IDC (a technology research firm) estimates that data has been constantly growing at a 50 % increase each year, or more than doubling every 2 years. Big data [6] becomes an important characteristic of the hyper-world in terms of four measures: volume, variety, velocity, and value. How to effectively manage, mine and utilize big data to improve the ability and quality of IT applications also becomes an urgent task and is attracting more and more attention [7, 8].

These changes have led to the appearance of many new phenomena and research issues. For example, in China, there is a phenomenon called Human Flesh Search Engine (HFSE), in which a large number of Web users voluntarily gathered together to collaborate and conduct truth-finding tasks, mostly without money reward. The organizational structure of people collaboration and the incentives that motivate people to contribute shed light on the intrinsic understanding the voluntary large-scale crowdsourcing and how the collective intelligence is fulfilled with the help of the Internet [9, 10]. The hyper world is bringing profound influences in both work and life to the whole human society. How to realize the organic amalgamation and harmonious symbiosis among humans, computers, and things in the hyper-world by using the network (consisting of numerous computing devices, storage devices and u-Things) and big data becomes a significant scientific and social issue.

2.2 From Wisdom Web to Wisdom Web of Things

Web Intelligence (WI) [11–15] may be viewed as an enhancement or an extension of Artificial Intelligence (AI) and Information Technology (IT) on the Web. One of its goals can be defined as the development of the Wisdom Web with top 10 problems [16, 17].

In the hyper-world age, this goal is extended to the development of Wisdom Web of Things (W2T) [4], where the "Wisdom" means that each of things in IoT/WoT is aware of both itself and others to provide the *right service* for the *right object* at a *right time* and *context*. W2T is a WI solution to the harmonious symbiosis of humans, computers, and things in the hyper-world. Its core concept is a processing cycle,

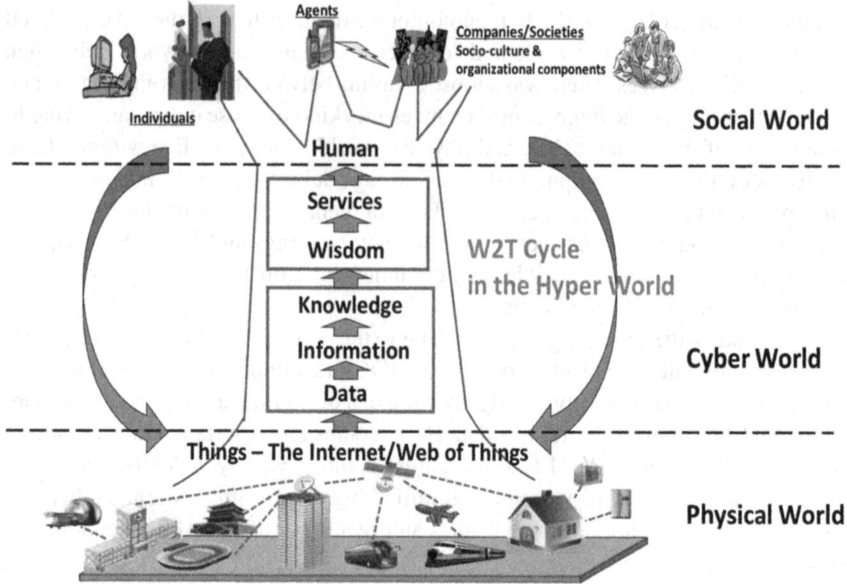

Fig. 2.1 A W2T cycle in the hyper-world

namely "from things to data, information, knowledge, wisdom, services, humans, and then back to things" (the W2T cycle, for short), as shown in Fig. 2.1. Similar to the real world material cycle that ensures the harmonious symbiosis of animal, plant, and microbe, the W2T cycle realizes the harmonious symbiosis of humans, computers and things in the hyper-world.

Constructing the W2T cycle relies on the large-scale converging of intelligent IT applications with an open and interoperable architecture. In recent years, two significant innovations have appeared in the IT field for meeting such a challenge:

- **Web of Things (WoT)** [18] focuses on the application layer and is to build an open and interoperable architecture on IoT by adapting technologies and patterns commonly used for traditional Web contents. By such an architecture, the Web is extended from the cyber world into the physical world. Various u-Things can be integrated into a common platform with traditional software for different applications in the hyper-world.
- **Cloud computing** [19] is a new trend in IT industry with the potential to realize a pay-as-you-go manner. From the viewpoint of IT technology, it also provides an open and service-oriented architecture for the converging of IT applications. On the one hand, by such an architecture, all IT applications can be deployed on a uniform platform and organized flexibly for varied applications. On the other hand, the enormous storage and computing resources needed by big data can be obtained by each IT application for improving its ability and quality.

However, both WoT and cloud computing mainly focus on the system resource service architecture of IT applications, i.e., infrastructures, platforms and software (developing and scheduling abilities). For the large-scale converging of intelligent IT applications, it is necessary to develop an open and interoperable intelligence service architecture for the contents of IT applications, i.e., data, information, knowledge, and wisdom (DIKW). The hyper-world with its W2T cycle will serve this purpose.

2.3 From Data to Wisdom

"Where is the life we have lost in living?"
"Where is the wisdom we have lost in knowledge?"
"Where is the knowledge we have lost in information?"
– T.S. Eliot, "The Rock", Faber and Faber 1934.

For developing a content architecture of IT applications, the first step is to investigate the relationships among the DIKW hierarchy. As suggested by T.S. Eliots poetic lines, a common understanding is the DIKW hierarchy [20] with the following four levels:

- Data are the un-interpreted, raw quantities, characters, or symbols collected, stored and transmitted.
- Information is a collection of interpreted, structured or organized data that is meaningful and useful for certain applications.
- Knowledge is acquaintance or familiarity about facts, truths, or principles, gained through study or investigation.
- Wisdom is sagacity, discernment, or insight to know what is true or right for making correct judgments, decisions and actions.

Each level in this hierarchy can affect the other and be changed into another: Data comes from the study or investigation about fact and truth; information can be obtained from data by data structuring, relational connection, distillation or pattern recognition; knowledge can be refined by collecting and understanding the information; and wisdom can be realized by transforming outside knowledge to the inner and judicious application of knowledge. Such creation, organization and transformation are the essence of the DIKW hierarchy and a core research issue of intelligent IT technologies. Because of the fusion of humans, computers, and things in the hyper-world, developing human-level intelligence becomes a tangible goal of the DIKW related research. Realizing it will depend on a holistic intelligence research [4], a joint effort of researchers and practitioners from diverse fields in exploring the key research problems of the interplay between the studies of human brain and informatics [21].

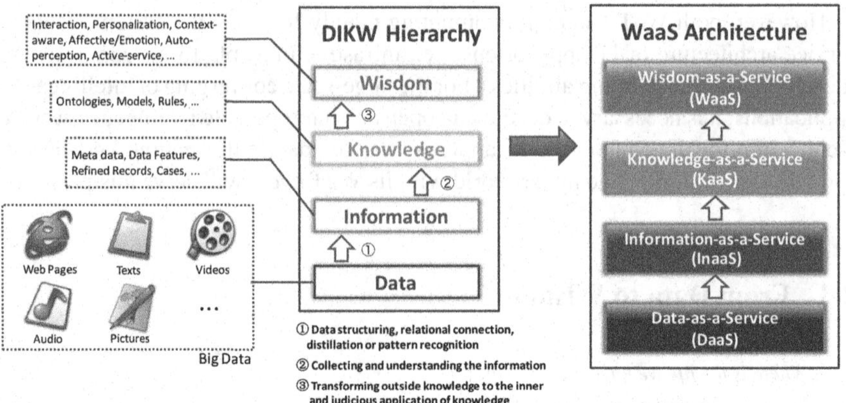

Fig. 2.2 From the DIKW hierarchy to WaaS

2.4 WaaS: Wisdom as a Service

2.4.1 What Is WaaS?

Based on the DIKW hierarchy, we propose "Wisdom as a Service" (WaaS) as a content architecture for intelligence services to IT applications shown in Fig. 2.2. WaaS is open and interoperable and constructed from a service-oriented viewpoint. It integrates many fields of research related to the DIKW-like service hierarchy, including the following four service categories:

- **Data as a Service (DaaS)** is to provide services based on both already-created and will-created raw data. Providing already-created data is just the data sharing service which is realized by all scientific databases, such as fMRIDC [22]. In order to realize data sharing, the data collection service is also necessary for finding and integrating dispersive data into a unified database. Providing will-created data is the data production service which obtains data according to users demands. For example, various experimental studies of Brain Informatics [21] can become a kind of data production service which designs and performs experiments to product brain data for the intelligence study and industry.
- **Information as a Service (InaaS)** is to provide services by using both already-created and will-created information. Providing already-created information is the activity of obtaining needed information from diversified information resources. Information retrieval is typical one. Providing will-created information is to extract information from data for users demands. Related services include data mining services and data curation services [7].
- **Knowledge as a Service (KaaS)** is to provide services with respect to existing and will-refined knowledge. The knowledge includes implicit knowledge and explicit knowledge. Knowledge stated in KaaS contains only explicit knowledge,

such as formal ontologies, user models, etc. Providing existing knowledge is just knowledge query services. Providing will-refined knowledge is to refine knowledge according tousers demands. Related work is concerned with knowledge retrieval [23], the development and management of knowledge base, etc. The model is a core issue in the W2T research. From this viewpoint, the KaaS can be specialized as the Model as a Service (MaaS) [24] which involves many interesting and important research issues and challenges.

- **Wisdom as a Service (WaaS)** is to provide various intelligent IT applications, including software and u-Things, as "Wisdom" services. Intelligent technologies are core of WaaS and involved with personalization, context-aware, affective/emotion, interaction, auto-perception, active services, and so on. By using these intelligent technologies on data, information and knowledge, those software and u-Things can make correct judgments, decisions and actions to provide the *right service* for the *right object* at a *right time* and *context*.

In the Internet protocol model, TCP/IP denotes both the whole protocol stack and two important protocols in this stack. Similarly, WaaS also includes two levels of meanings. Strictly speaking, WaaS is an intelligent service layer which includes various intelligent IT applications. Broadly speaking, WaaS is a service hierarchy, including the DaaS, InaaS, KaaS and WaaS, just like a Web hierarchy model [25].

2.4.2 *WaaS Standard and Service Platform*

A WaaS standard and service platform should be constructed as the infrastructure of WaaS. It integrates W2T-cycle-related theories and technologies. Figure 2.3 gives its architecture, with four components according to the four service categories. Each component includes a software platform and a standard system, which provide a practical and propagable approach for realizing all services in the corresponding service category. The software platform is an open portal on which different service modules can be deployed to provide various services of the corresponding service category. The standard system is a group of standards and specifications which describe the requirements and methods for developing and using service modules on the software platform. All of software platforms and standard systems can be described as follows:

- **The DaaS platform** includes the data collection module, data cleaning module, data management module, and data query module to support the three types of DaaS services. The core is the data collection module consisting of many data collection interfaces for "reading" data from the Web, information systems, deploying sensors, embedded chips, experimental devices, etc.
- **The DaaS standard system** consists of four types of standards, i.e., data collection interface standards, data transmission protocols, data content and format standards, and data accessing standards. These standards or protocols are based

on applications and can be classified into different types according to different data sources, application environments and application purposes. For example, different data transmission protocols should be designed and used in the Internet and MI.

- **The InaaS platform** includes the information retrieval module, data mining module, information management module and data curation module to support the three types of InaaS services. The data curation focuses on information organization, including metadata construction and case creation. Because the hyper-world includes mutable data, computing, and network environments, it is necessary to perform the off-line information extraction and organization before services are requested.
- **The InaaS standard system** consists of four types of standards, i.e., information-retrieval-related standards, data-mining-related standards, metadata standards, and information accessing standards. Information-retrieval-related standards mainly focus on application service definition and protocol specification. Data-mining-related standards are involved with mining languages, result representation languages, mining system architectures, etc. Metadata standards are classified and defined according to application domains. Information accessing standards are

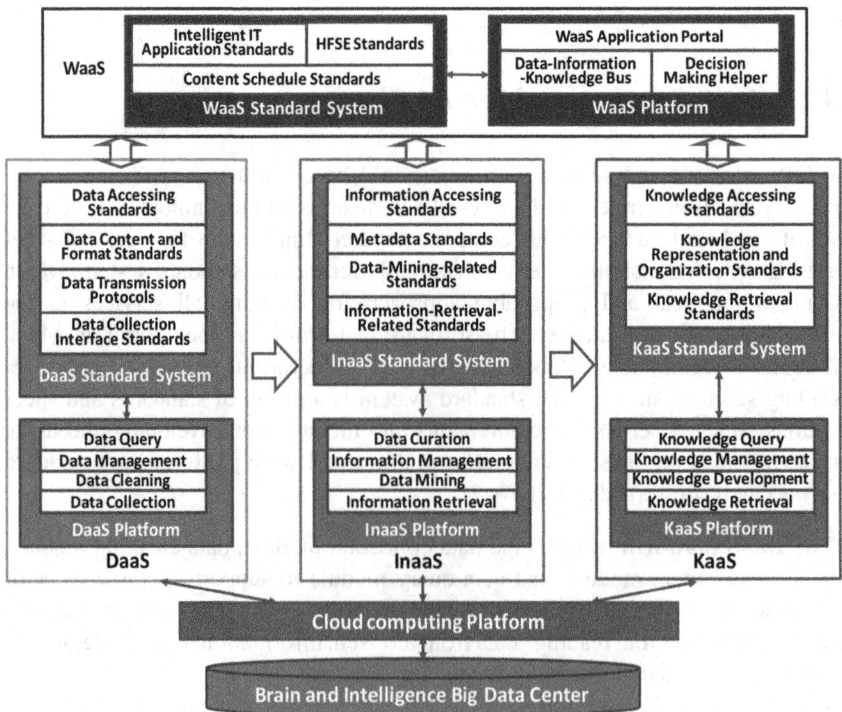

Fig. 2.3 The architecture of WaaS standard and service platform

used to define accessing interfaces and transmission protocols of InaaS service modules on the InaaS platform.

- **The KaaS platform** includes the knowledge retrieval module, knowledge development module, knowledge management module and knowledge query component for various KaaS services. The knowledge retrieval module is developed based on the WI-specific technology that extracts knowledge from enormous information sources. The knowledge development module provides various tools for the development of ontologies, models, as well as other types of formal knowledge. The knowledge management module and knowledge query module are used to manage formal knowledge and provide knowledge sharing services, respectively.
- **The KaaS standard system** consists of knowledge-retrieval-related standards, knowledge representation and organization standards, and knowledge accessing standards. The knowledge-retrieval-related standards are mainly used to define application services and protocols. The knowledge representation and organization standards focus on knowledge representation languages, for example, the cyber-individual (Cyber-I) representation language [26]. Knowledge accessing standards mainly involve knowledge query languages, knowledge accessing interfaces, knowledge system architectures, knowledge transmission protocols, and so on.
- **The WaaS platform** includes the data-information-knowledge bus, decision making helper and WaaS application portal. The data-information-knowledge bus is a special Enterprise Service Bus (ESB) for discovery and integration of DaaS services, InaaS services and KaaS services. The decision making helper is used to assist judgments and decisions. Based on them, various intelligent IT applications can be deployed on the WaaS application portal to make correct actions, namely, provide intelligent services. Furthermore, HFSE can also be regarded as a kind of special intelligent applications.
- **The WaaS standard system** consists of content (data, information and knowledge) schedule standards, intelligent IT application standards and HFSE standards. They concern content schedule languages, application interfaces, application wrappings, application communications, as well as HFSE related technical standards and laws.

As shown in Fig. 2.3, all platforms are constructed on a cloud computing platform and a brain and intelligence big data center. These platforms are open. Based on the standards and protocols in the four standard systems, any third party can develop and plug in their service modules on platforms. These platforms are also interoperable. Because of adopting the same standards and protocols, different service modules on platforms can effectively communicate and cooperate with each other for providing various services in the DIKW hierarchy. Furthermore, other systems and platforms can also access service modules on platforms by using those public standards and protocols in the standard systems, for realizing complex intelligent IT applications. Such open and interoperable platforms make it possible to converge all technologies and resources in the intelligence study and industry into a unifying framework for realizing a W2T cycle.

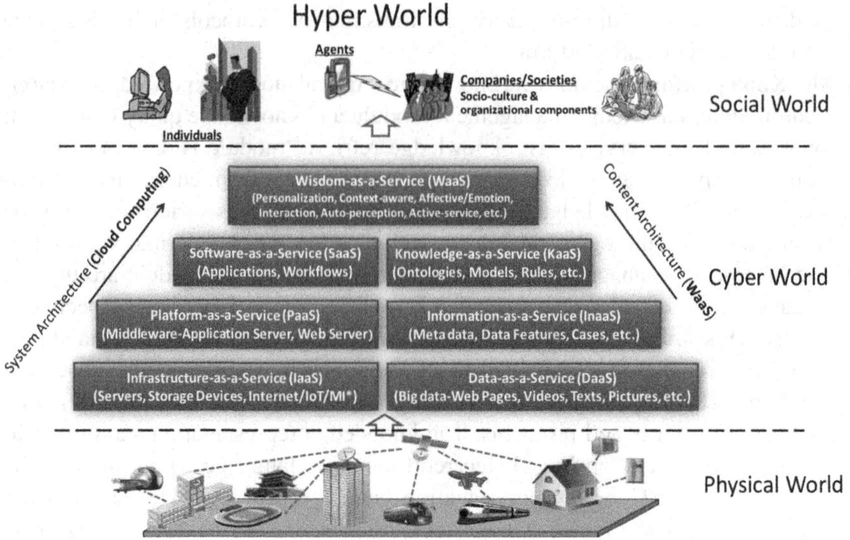

Fig. 2.4 An open and interoperable architecture of IT applications for W2T

2.4.3 *An Open and Interoperable Architecture of IT Applications: Binding WaaS with Cloud Computing*

The development of intelligent IT applications needs to meet various demands, not only system-level demands but also content-level demands. The system-level demands are related to infrastructures (network, storage and computing resources), running platforms and software (developing and scheduling abilities). The content-level demands are related to big data and their processing.

Figure 2.4 shows an open and interoperable architecture of IT applications by binding WaaS and cloud computing. It meets two types of demands in a unified and pay-as-you-go manner. As shown in Fig. 2.4, cloud computing provides an open IT architecture for sharing system resources, including infrastructures, platform and software, by means of IaaS, PaaS and SaaS. Paralleling to the cloud model, WaaS is for sharing content resources and processing utilities and closely related to big data and their processing through DaaS, InaaS and KaaS. By these layers of "as a service", six factors, i.e., infrastructures, platforms, software (developing and scheduling abilities), data, information, and knowledge, will converge into an open and interoperable uniform platform, on which all factors can be effectively utilized by various intelligent technologies to form an intelligent service layer, i.e., the WaaS layer. A large number of intelligent IT applications will converge into the WaaS layer towards a W2T cycle.

Based on the successful practices on existing cloud computing platforms, it would be reasonable to expect that the large-scale converge of intelligent IT applications can be realized by such IT architecture, towards a W2T cycle for realizing the harmonious symbiosis of humans, computers, and things in the hyper-world.

2.5 A Case Study: The Portable Brain and Mental Health Monitoring System Based on Peculiarity-Oriented Mining of EEG Data

With the accelerating process of urbanization, brain and mental health has become a huge public-health problem. According to a survey in 2011 [27], mental disorders affect more than 160 million Europeans—38 % of the population. Mental disorders also make up China's largest disease burden—20 % of total burden of disease—in 2011. It is necessary to strengthen the monitoring of brain and mental disorders for diagnosing and treatment as soon as possible. However, only depending on doctors and nurses to complete the monitoring is unpractical because of the giant susceptible population. Using information technologies to support the monitoring of brain and mental disorders becomes a promising approach.

We have developed a prototype of the portable brain and mental health monitoring system (brain monitoring system, for short) whose technological framework is shown in Fig. 2.5. It adopts the architecture integrating cloud computing and WaaS to meet system-level and content-level demands in developing IT applications:

- **Cloud computing** (including IaaS, PaaS, SaaS) is adopted to meet system-level demands of the brain monitoring system based on the "anything as a service" paradigm. As a cross-platform and data-intensive intelligent system, the brain

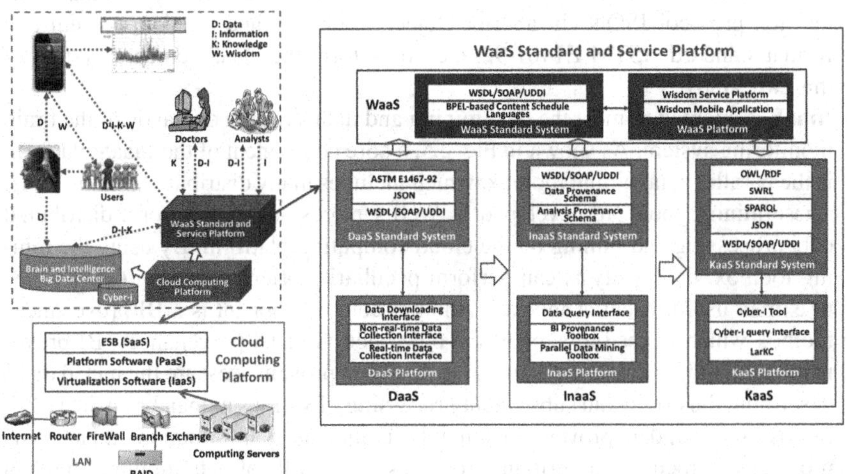

Fig. 2.5 The technological framework of the portable brain and mental health monitoring system

monitoring system needs credible infrastructures (network, storage and computing resources), an open running platform and an extensible developing and scheduling mode. We construct a private cloud having a group of servers and a redundant array of independent disk (RAID) for meeting these demands. As shown in Fig. 2.5, servers, RAID, mobile phones, the local area network, the Internet and MI form a powerful infrastructure, on which virtualization software is stepped up to dynamically provide needed infrastructure resources as services for the brain monitoring system based on the IaaS mode. Furthermore, open platform software, e.g., Web application server software, is used to provide the needed running platform as a service based on the PaaS mode, and Web service technologies are adopted to develop all functional components and software systems as services on the ESB based on the SaaS mode.

- **DaaS** is adopted to meet the data demands of the brain monitoring system. As shown in Fig. 2.5, it is realized by the DaaS platform. Data collection interfaces and a data downloading interface are developed as Web services and deployed on the DaaS platform for the data production service. They collect users' EEG (Electroencephalogram) data for data analysts. Data collection interfaces include a real-time interface and a non-real-time interface. The real-time interface is deployed on mobile phones, which is regarded as an extending part of DaaS platform, to collect patients EEG data continuously. The non-real-time interface is deployed on the server part of DaaS platform to collect EEG data stored in mobile phones periodically and sent them to the brain and health big data center. In addition to the collection of EEG data, other non-real-time data, such as users information, are collected. If the data come from other information systems, the corresponding data collection interfaces are developed and deployed on the DaaS platform. Such a DaaS platform is based on the data collection and accessing interface standards WSDL (Web Services Description Language)/SOAP (Simple Object Access Protocol)/UDDI (Universal Description, Discovery, and Integration), the data transmission protocol JSON (JavaScript Object Notation), and the data content and format standard ASTM E1467-92, etc.; they form the DaaS standard system of this case study.
- **InaaS** is adopted to meet the data mining and data curation demands of the brain monitoring system. As shown in Fig. 2.5, a core component of the InaaS platform is the parallel data mining toolbox, which includes many distributed mining tools. These mining tools are developed as Web services and can perform distributed data processing and mining on the cloud computing platform. By using the mining toolbox, data analysts can perform peculiarity-oriented mining (POM) [28] to extract useful peculiar indexes. Another core component is a BI provenances toolbox which is used to support the construction of BI provenances. BI provenances, including data provenances and analysis provenances, are the metadata of describing the origin and subsequent processing of various human brain data [29]. In this use case, data provenances mainly include users information and analysis provenances focus on describing processes and results of data mining. The data query interface based on BI provenances is also an important component of the InaaS platform. All modules are developed as Web services. As metadata stan-

dards, mining language and result representation language, the schemata of data and analysis provenances are major contents of the InaaS standard system.

- **KaaS** is adopted to meet the knowledge extraction, management and query demands of the brain monitoring system. As shown in Fig. 2.5, its realization depends on the KaaS platform developed on the LarKC (Large Knowledge Collider, a cloud platform for massive distributed incomplete reasoning) [30]. Because the management and query services of knowledge can be realized by the LarKC, the core of the KaaS platform is the Cyber-I tool, which provides Web services of knowledge extraction and the construction of diagnosis models. The knowledge extraction service can extract individualized rules from domain ontologies and BI provenances through reasoning and mining on the LarKC. The rules can be used to identify users brain risk states. Integrating them and POM-centric arithmetic modules, individualized diagnosis models can be constructed as a kind of special Cyber-I. Furthermore, in order to effectively utilize these models, a Cyber-I query interface was also constructed on the KaaS platform. The KaaS standard system includes the ontological language OWL (Web Ontology Language) and RDF (Resource Description Framework), rule language SWRL (Semantic Web Rule Language), knowledge query language SPARQL (Simple Protocol and RDF Query Language), model transmission language JSON and knowledge accessing interface standards WSDL/SOAP/UDDI. The KaaS platform is developed based on these standards.
- **WaaS** is adopted to organize and deploy the brain monitoring system as a kind of wisdom service for the monitoring of brain and mental health. It is realized by a wisdom service platform and a wisdom mobile application. The wisdom service platform is a Web service deployed on the WaaS application portal, providing various remote monitoring functions, such as data collection, data mining, model publishing, domain knowledge publishing, risk state discovery, message sending to the third parties, etc. All these functions are realized by using the data, information and knowledge buses to call the corresponding DaaS, InaaS and KaaS. The wisdom mobile application provides various local monitoring functions, including data collection, data mining and result display, risk state discovery and reminding. Various intelligent technologies, including personalization, context-aware, auto-perception and active services, need to be applied on the service platform and the mobile application to provide right service for the right object at a right time and context. Related standards include intelligent IT application standards WSDL/SOAP/UDDI and BPEL (Business Process Execution Language) based content schedule languages.

The brain monitoring system can provide a smart monitoring service for suspected/mildbrain and mental patients. For example, Bob is a suspected epilepsy patient and needs some reliable evidences to persuade himself to receive a comprehensive physical examination. This can be realized by using the brain monitoring system. The whole process integrates services in the DIKW hierarchy and is involved with users, analysts and doctors as explained in the following:

- The DaaS services: before Bob gets the system, a large number of EEG data have to been collected from mild epilepsy patients and normal subjects, and provided to analysts. This DaaS service is realized by the above DaaS platform. All of EEG data are collected into the brain and intelligence big data center by the real-time and non-real-time data collection interfaces, and analysts obtain fit EEG data by the data downloading interface.
- The InaaS services: Dr. Motomura is a senior analyst of EEG data. He is both user and provider of InaaS services. On the one hand, he uses the data-related information retrieval service provided by the data query interface to find fit EEG data. On the other hand, he provides a data mining service to extract peculiar indexes of patients EEG databy using the mining toolbox. Finally, obtained indexes and other related information are integrated into BI provenances and provided to doctors by the data query interface.
- The KaaS services: Dr. Wang is a doctor which has rich experiences on the diagnosis and treatment of epilepsy disorder. He provides a knowledge service to construct individualized epilepsy diagnosis models based on domain knowledge, obtained peculiar indexes, patients information and other related information. Such a KaaS service is realized by using the Cyber-I tool.
- The WaaS services: Bob can get needed diagnosis evidences by the WaaS service provided by the brain monitoring system. He only needs to download the wisdom mobile application from the WaaS platform. When he wears the custom portal EEG device, the mobile application will collect his EEG data continuously and identify epilepsy-like peculiar indexes based on his individual diagnosis model. These indexes are just the needed evidences and will be provided to Bob by an easy-to-understand mode.

Generally speaking, an open and interoperable platform can be built by adopting the architecture with binding WaaS and cloud computing. It can meet all system-level and content-level demands of the brain monitoring system. Furthermore, other intelligent IT applications can also be realized on this platform. Such a uniform platform will effectively support the large-scale convergence of intelligent IT applications to realize the W2T cycle for the harmonious symbiosis of humans, computers, and things in the hyper-world.

2.6 WaaS Economics

WaaS will bring the "paying only for what you use" mode for intelligence IT industry, one of the most important IT business trends with a huge economic value. This section discusses WaaS economics from three different aspects.

2.6.1 *Reducing the Risk*

Although the economic appeal of cloud computing is often described as "converting capital expenses to operating expenses" (CapEx to OpEx) for reducing the cost, the purchase mode "paying only for what you use" does not mean an absolutely low price. Hence, it may not be able to ensure that WaaS can reduce users cost by providing cheap DIKW services.

WaaS is an effective approach to reduce the risk for each member of the intelligence industry, including research institutions and manufacturers. From data to wisdom, the development of smart software and u-Things needs large numbers of input. Each member in the intelligence industry has to face high capital, time and human resource risk. By realizing WaaS on cloud computing, IoT/WoT and big data, the achievements in each stage of the development of intelligent IT applications can be shared quickly and multi-level global cooperation will be possible. Various risks will be balanced in the whole intelligence industry and ensure that both large-sized and medium/small-sized research institutions/manufacturers are able to participate in the research and development of intelligent IT applications.

2.6.2 *Enlarging the Value*

From data to wisdom, the development of each intelligent IT application needs a large number of efforts and produces a lot of intermediate achievements, such as experimental data, analytical methods/experiences, domain ontologies, and so on. These intermediate achievements are often important for other similar research and development. At present, the sharing of these achievements is limited within a research group or small-scale cooperative members.

The hyper-world requires human-levels intelligent IT applications, which are based on an understanding of not only IT technologies but also mechanisms of human intelligence. For developing an intelligent IT application, its direct research and commercial value may be lower than the input. The existing small-scale sharing of achievements cannot effectively solve this problem. Large-scale sharing is necessary for intelligence IT industry in the age of the hyper-world.

WaaS provides an open mode to share at each stage of achievements in the research and development. The value can be enlarged to ensure a reasonable input-output ratio. It is very important for realizing W2T, which needs not only small-scale research but also the large-scale development and converging of intelligent IT applications.

2.6.3 Building the Intelligence Industry Chain

The large-scale development of intelligent IT applications needs a complete intelligence industry chain to integrate various abilities and resources. The core issue is to develop an effective distribution mode for transferring industrial value among all the chain nodes. Furthermore, the W2T cycle shows that the intelligence industry has a long industry chain. An effective value distribution mode is especially important, because it is difficult to complete all steps on such a long chain based only on individual enterprises or institutions.

WaaS is an open and interoperable content architecture of IT applications for the hyper-world. By WaaS, large-scale sharing and cooperation can be realized on a uniform platform during the DIKW organization and transformation. An effective distribution will be created to transmit industrial value from the sell node, namely "Service to Human", to other industrial nodes, namely "Data to Information, Knowledge, Wisdom, and Services", towards a complete W2T cycle.

2.7 Perspectives of Challenges and Issues on WaaS

WaaS is a multidisciplinary and interdisciplinary research field for the open intelligence service architecture, and also a business mode for the intelligence service industry in the era of IoT and big data. It requires cooperative efforts from science, technology and industry, and presents new challenges and issues from the scientific, technological, social and business perspectives.

2.7.1 Scientific Perspective

WaaS focuses on the DIKW organization and transformation, whose core is human brain intelligence. As one of the most important scientific issues in the 21st century, the study of human brain intelligence involves many challenges, such as:

- How to investigate human brain intelligence, including individual human differences and similarities, by means of the research on holistic intelligence?
- How to obtain sufficient brain intelligence big data through powerful equipments?
- How to manage and mining the huge volume of brain intelligence big data to gain a systematic investigation and understanding of human intelligence?

Brain Informatics (BI) [21, 31, 32] provides a systematic methodology for dealing with these challenges and many problems must be addressed.

How to develop brain intelligence inspired information technologies for realizing the DIKW organization and transformation is another core scientific issue in the WaaS research and industry. An important aspect is the cyber-individual (Cyber-I) which is a comprehensive digital description of individual humans as a counterpart in the cyber world [26]. In order to develop a "telepathic partner" for the real-individual at all times and contexts, the creation of Cyber-I brings many scientific challenges and issues, including the study of individual human differences, individual human modeling, and CI-Mind [26].

2.7.2 Technological Perspective

WaaS is an open and interoperable content architecture of IT applications for supporting large-scale sharing and cooperation on the DIKW hierarchy. It is important to have an open, flexible and friendly platform, for example, the web-scale knowledge integration and reasoning platforms (e.g., the LarKC), for any third party to develop and plug in its WaaS applications.

The WaaS applications include various kinds of software and u-Things and will be involved in a sustainable development process. Hence, another basic technological challenge is how to design a scalable and sharable system architecture based on cloud computing platforms, allowing the maximum utilization of limited resources.

A conflict often exists between a systems openness and security. The security and privacy protection is an important challenge for the open WaaS. The technological architecture of security and privacy protection should be fit for different application environments, including not only the Internet but also IoT and MI.

2.7.3 Social Perspective

WaaS will impel a global cooperation in research and in industry and might cause potential socio-economical issues, such as:

- How to create an effective incentive mechanism to accelerate the concentration of DIKW resources from different government departments, research/social institutions and enterprises? It could involve such problems as related to DIKW right, protection, management, evaluation, value distribution, and so on.
- How to build a high-efficiency identification and arbitration mechanism to quickly identify responsibilities and solve dissensions? Are the existing laws and regulations perfect enough for supporting such a mechanism?

2.7.4 Business Perspective

At present, cloud computing has great effects on intelligence industry and causes a platform-leading value distribution mode. The providers of software or hardware platforms, such as Internet service providers and manufacturers of operating systems, play a leading role in the value distribution. The DIKW hierarchy and the W2T cycle have revealed that the content of IT applications is another core issue for the development of intelligent IT applications in the hyper-world age. A huge business challenge brought by WaaS is to transform the value distribution from the existing platform-leading one to the platform-and-content-leading one. It is necessary to let the market and capital know the importance of resources and technologies with respect to the DIKW hierarchy. It is also necessary to develop an effective business model for these resources and technologies, including evaluation mechanism, transaction mode, pricing/payment methods, and so on.

2.8 Conclusion

Recent advances in cloud computing, IoT, WoT, big data, W2T and other research fields have created a great opportunity to study and realize WaaS based on achievements and accumulations of intelligence science, BI and other intelligent computing technologies. We have presented the basic concepts, infrastructure and applications of WaaS, as well as the first step toward the final goal of constructing the W2T cycle to realize the harmonious symbiosis of humans, computers and things in the hyper-world. As a demonstration, we discussed the development of portable brain and mental health monitoring system. The WaaS standard and service platform will be fine-tuned continuously as a core infrastructure for intelligence industry and smart city to support the development of various intelligent IT applications. WaaS will be the core architecture of IT applications in the coming age of the hyper-world. It will bring a huge economic value for intelligence IT industry by realizing the pay-as-you-go manner.

Acknowledgments The work is supported by National Key Basic Research Program of China (2014CB744605), China Postdoctoral Science Foundation (2013M540096), International Science & Technology Cooperation Program of China (2013DFA32180), National Natural Science Foundation of China (61272345), Research Supported by the CAS/SAFEA International Partnership Program for Creative Research Teams, the Japan Society for the Promotion of Science Grants-in-Aid for Scientific Research (25330270).

References

1. International Telecommunication Union (ITU), The World in 2013: ICT Facts and Figures, http://www.itu.int/ITU-D/ict/facts/material/ICTFactsFigures2013.pdf. Accessed 27 Feb 2013
2. L. Atzori, A. Iera, G. Morabito, The internet of things: a survey. Comput. Netw. **54**, 27872805 (2010)
3. J.H. Ma, R.H. Huang, Improving human interaction with a hyperworld, in *Proceedings of the Pacific Workshop on Distributed Multimedia Systems (DMS96)* (1996), pp. 46–50

4. N. Zhong, J.H. Ma, R.H. Huang, J.M. Liu, Y.Y. Yao, Y.X. Zhang, J.H. Chen, Research challenges and perspectives on wisdom web of things (W2T). J. Supercomput. **64**(3), 862882 (2013)
5. J.H. Ma, Smart u-things challenging real world complexity, in *IPSJ Symposium Series* (2005), pp. 146–150
6. S. Lohr, *The age of big data* (New York Times, 2012)
7. D. Howe, M. Costanzo, P. Fey, T. Gojobori, L. Hannick, W. Hide, D.P. Hill, R. Kania, M. Schaeffer, S. St. Pierre, S. Twigger, O. White, S.Y. Rhee, Big data: the future of biocuration. Nature **455**, 4750 (2008)
8. N.B. Turk-Browne, Functional interactions as big data in the human brain. Science **342**(6158), 580–584 (2013)
9. Q.P. Zhang, Z. Feng, F.Y. Wang, D. Zeng, Modeling cyber-enabled crowd-powered search, in *The Second Chinese Conference on Social Computing*, Beijing (2010)
10. Q.P. Zhang, F.Y. Wang, D. Zeng, T. Wang, Understanding crowd-powered search groups: a social network perspective. PLoS ONE **7**(6), e39749 (2012). doi:10.1371/journal.pone.0039749
11. N. Zhong, J.M. Liu, Y.Y. Yao, S. Ohsuga, Web intelligence (WI), in *Proceedings of the 24th IEEE Computer Society International Computer Software and Applications Conference (COMPSAC 2000)* (2000), pp. 469–470
12. N. Zhong, J.M. Liu, Y.Y. Yao, In search of the wisdom web. IEEE Comput. **35**(11), 27–31 (2002)
13. N. Zhong, Towards web intelligence, in E. Menasalvas Ruiz, J. Segovia, P.S. Szczepaniak (eds.), *Advances in Web Intelligence*, LNAI 2663 (Springer, 2003), pp. 1–14
14. N. Zhong, J. Liu, Y.Y. Yao, Envisioning intelligent information technologies through the prism of web intelligence. Commun. ACM **50**(3), 8994 (2007)
15. N. Zhong, J.M. Liu, Y.Y. Yao, Web intelligence (WI), in *The Encyclopedia of Computer Science and Engineering*, vol. 5 (Wiley, 2009), pp. 3062–3072
16. J.M. Liu, Web intelligence (WI): what makes wisdom web? in *Proceedings the 18th International Joint Conference on Artificial Intelligence (IJCAI'03)* (2003), pp. 1596–1601
17. J.M. Liu, N. Zhong, Y.Y. Yao, Z.W. Ras, The wisdom web: new challenges for web intelligence (WI). J. Intell. Inf. Syst. **20**(1), 59 (2003)
18. D. Guinard, V. Trifa, F. Mattern, E. Wilde, From the internet of things to the web of things: resource-oriented architecture and best practices, in *Architecting the Internet of Things* (Springer, 2011), pp. 97–129
19. M. Armbrust, A. Fox, R. Griffith, A.D. Joseph, R. Katz, A. Konwinski, G. Lee, D. Patterson, A. Rabkin, I. Stoica, M. Zaharia, A view of cloud computing. Commun. ACM **53**(4), 5058 (2010)
20. R.L. Ackoff, From data to wisdom. J. Appl. Syst. Anal. **16**, 39 (1989)
21. N. Zhong, J.M. Liu, Y.Y. Yao, J.L. Wu, S.F. Lu (eds.) *Web Intelligence Meets Brain Informatics, State-of-the-Art-Survey* (Springer LNCS 4845, 2007)
22. http://www.fmridc.org/f/fmridc
23. Y.Y. Yao, Y. Zeng, N. Zhong, X.J. Huang, Knowledge retrieval (KR), in *Proceedings of the 2007 IEEE/WIC/ACM International Conference on Web Intelligence (WI'07)* (2007), pp. 729–735
24. G.B. Zou, B.F. Zhang, J.X. Zheng, Y.S. Li, J.H. Ma, MaaS: model as a service in cloud computing and cyber-I space, in *Proceedings of the 12th IEEE International Conference on Computer and Information Technology (CIT2012)* (2012), pp. 1125–1130
25. Y.Y. Yao, Web intelligence: new frontiers of exploration, in *Proceedings of 2005 International Conference on Active Media Technology (AMT 2005)* (2005), pp. 3–8
26. J.H. Ma, J. Wen, R.H. Huang, B.X. Huang, Cyber-individual meets brain informatics. IEEE Intell. Syst. **26**(5), 3037 (2011)
27. H.U. Wittchen, F. Jacobi, J. Rehm, A. Gustavsson, M. Svensson, B. Jansson, J. Olesen, C. Allgulander, J. Alonso, C. Faravelli, L. Fratiglioni, P. Jennum, R. Lieb, A. Maercker, J. van Os, M. Preisig, L. Salvador-Carulla, R. Simon, H.-C. Steinhausen, The size and burden of mental disorders and other disorders of the brain in Europe 2010. Eur. Neuropsychopharm. **21**(9), 655679 (2011)

28. N. Zhong, S. Motomura, Agent-enriched data mining: a case study in brain informatics. IEEE Intell. Syst. **24**(3), 3845 (2009)
29. J.H. Chen, N. Zhong, Toward the data-brain driven systematic brain data analysis. IEEE Trans. Syst. Man Cybernet. Syst. **43**(1), 222228 (2013)
30. D. Fensel, F. van Harmelen, B. Andersson, P. Brennan, H. Cunningham, E. Della Valle, F. Fischer, Z.S. Huang, A. Kiryakov, T.K.-i. Lee, L. Schooler, V. Tresp, S. Wesner, M. Witbrock, N. Zhong, Towards LarKC: a platform for web-scale reasoning, in *Proceedings of the 2nd IEEE International Conference on Semantic Computing (ICSC08)* (2008), pp. 524–529
31. N. Zhong, J.M. Bradshaw, J.M. Liu, J.G. Taylor, Brain informatics, Special Issue on Brain Informatics. IEEE Intell. Syst. **26**(5), 16–21 (2011)
32. N. Zhong, J.H. Chen, Constructing a new-style conceptual model of brain data for systematic brain informatics. IEEE Trans. Knowl. Data Eng. **24**(12), 21272142 (2011)

Chapter 3
Towards W2T Foundations: Interactive Granular Computing and Adaptive Judgement

Andrzej Skowron and Andrzej Jankowski

[Hyper world] consists of the cyber, social, and physical worlds, [...] [Wisdom Web of Things] focuses on the data cycle, namely "from things to data, information, knowledge, wisdom, services, humans, and then back to things."A W2T data cycle system is designed to implement such a cycle, which is, technologically speaking, a practical way to realize the harmonious symbiosis of humans, computers, and things in the emerging hyper world.
– Ning Zhong et al. [53]

Abstract Development of methods for Wisdom Web of Things (W2T) should be based on foundations of computations performed in the complex environments of W2T. We discuss some characteristic features of decision making processes over W2T. First of all the decisions in W2T are very often made by different agents on the basis of complex vague concepts and relations among them (creating domain ontology) which are semantically *far away* from dynamically changing and huge raw data. Methods for approximation of such vague concepts based on information granulation are needed. It is also important to note that the abstract objects represented by different agents are dynamically linked by them with some physical objects and the aim is very often to control performance of computations in the physical world for achieving the target goals. Moreover, the decision making by different agents working in the W2T environment requires mechanisms for understanding (to a satisfactory degree) reasoning performed in natural language on concepts and relations from

A. Skowron (✉)
Institute of Mathematics, Warsaw University, Banacha 2, 02-097 Warsaw, Poland
e-mail: skowron@mimuw.edu.pl

A. Skowron
Systems Research Institute, Polish Academy of Sciences, Newelska 6, 01-447 Warsaw, Poland

A. Jankowski
The Dziubanski Foundation of Knowledge Technology, Nowogrodzka 31, 00-511 Warsaw, Poland
e-mail: andrzej.adgam@gmail.com

N. Zhong et al. (eds.), *Wisdom Web of Things*, Web Information Systems Engineering and Internet Technologies Book Series,
DOI 10.1007/978-3-319-44198-6_3

the domain ontology. We discuss a new computation model, where computations are progressing due to interactions of complex granules (c-granules) linked with the physical objects. C-granules are defined relative to a given agent. We extend the existing Granular Computing (GrC) approach by introducing *complex granules* (c-granules, for short) making it possible to model interactive computations of agents in complex systems over W2T. One of the challenges in the approach is to develop methods and strategies for adaptive reasoning, called *adaptive judgement*, e.g., for adaptive control of computations. In particular, adaptive judgement is required in the risk/efficiency management by agents supported by W2T. The discussed approach is a step toward realization of the Wisdom Technology (WisTech) program. The approach was developed over years of work on different real-life projects.

3.1 Introduction

Problems related to Interactive Intelligent Systems (IIS) based on Wisdom Web of Things (W2T) technology are often of complex nature with many heterogeneous agents involved and linked by complex interactions of different nature [53]. There are numerous hierarchical levels of agents responsible, in particular, for linking them with the physical world. In [53] the ideas of hyper world and W2T are explained (see motto of this chapter).

Cyber-Physical Systems (CPSs) belong to another emerging domain related to W2T. In [17] they are characterized in the following way:

> A cyber-physical system (CPS) is a system of collaborating computational elements controlling physical entities.

There are huge expectations for applications of CPSs [17]:

> Cyber-Physical Systems will transform how we interact with the physical world just as the Internet transformed how we interact with one another. [...] *Applications with enormous societal impact and economic benefit will be created.*

Nowadays, many problems related to CSPs and W2T are challenging. Some of them are well expressed in [17]:

> The design of such systems requires understanding the joint dynamics of computers, software, networks, physical, chemical and biological processes and humans in the loop. It is this study of joint dynamics that sets this discipline apart. Increasingly, CPSs are autonomous or semiautonomous and cannot be designed as closed systems that operate in isolation; rather, the interaction and potential interference among smart components, among CPSs, and among CPSs and humans, requires coordinated, controlled, and cooperative behaviour.

> [...] the size of cyber-physical systems of systems and their multimodality or hybrid nature consisting of physical elements as well as quasicontinuous and discrete controls, communication channels, and local and system-wide optimization algorithms and management systems, implies that hierarchical and multi-domain approaches to their simulation, analysis and design are needed. These methods are currently not available.

Further development of methods for W2T (and CPSs) requires solid foundations for computations performed in the complex environments.

Let us consider some characteristic features of decision making processes realized by IIS based on W2T technology.

First of all the decisions in such IIS are very often made by different agents on the basis of complex vague concepts and relations between them (creating domain ontology) which are semantically *far away* from dynamically changing huge raw data. New methods for approximation of such vague concepts based on information granulation are needed. Usually, it is not possible to approximate these vague concepts directly from the data (or, in other words, to induce their models directly from such data). Hence, we need new methods for hierarchical learning based on objects with structures and features discovered on different levels of hierarchy in cooperation with domain experts.

It is also important to note that the abstract objects represented by different agents from W2T are linked with the physical objects and the aim is very often to control performance of computations in the physical world for achieving the target goals. Hence, in developing of our computation model we should take into account opinions expressed by physicists [4]:

> It seems that we have no choice but to recognize the dependence of our mathematical knowledge (...) on physics, and that being so, it is time to abandon the class independent of that of computation as a physical process.

Computations in the physical world are progressing through complex interactions among physical objects. Some results of such interactions can be perceived by agents.

Moreover, the decision making by agents requires mechanisms for understanding (to a satisfactory degree) reasoning performed in natural language fragments on concepts and relations from the domain ontology. This is related to Computing With Words Paradigm (CWP) proposed by Professor Lotfi Zadeh some years ago (see, e.g., [19, 47, 49–52] and also http://www.cs.berkeley.edu/~zadeh/presentations.html):

> Manipulation of perceptions plays a key role in human recognition, decision and execution processes. As a methodology, computing with words provides a foundation for a computational theory of perceptions—a theory which may have an important bearing on how humans make—and machines might make—perception-based rational decisions in an environment of imprecision, uncertainty and partial truth. [...] computing with words, or CW for short, is a methodology in which the objects of computation are words and propositions drawn from a natural language.

or recently to the challenge formulated by Judea Pearl [27]:

> Traditional statistics is strong in devising ways of describing data and inferring distributional parameters from sample. Causal inference requires two additional ingredients: a science-friendly language for articulating causal knowledge, and a mathematical machinery for processing that knowledge, combining it with data and drawing new causal conclusions about a phenomenon.

Information granules (infogranules, for short) are widely discussed in the literature (see, e.g., [28, 37, 48]). In particular, let us mention here the rough granular computing approach based on the rough set approach and its combination with other approaches to soft computing (e.g., with fuzzy sets). However, the issues related to interactions of infogranules with the physical world and to perception of interactions in the physical world represented by infogranules are not well elaborated yet. On the other hand the understanding of interactions is the critical issue of complex systems [7] in which computations are progressing by interactions among information granules and physical objects.

We extend the existing approach to GrC by introducing *complex granules* (c-*granules*, for short) [9] making it possible to model interactive computations performed by agents in W2T. Any agent operates in a local world of c-granules. The agent control is aiming to control computations performed on c-granules from this local world for achieving the target goals.

The proposed model of computations in W2T is based on c-granules. The risk management and cost/benefit analysis [9] in W2T are of the great importance for the success of behaviors of individuals, groups and societies of agents. The risk management and cost/benefit analysis tasks are considered as control tasks aiming at achieving the high quality performance of (societies of) agents. The novelty of the proposed approach is the use of complex vague concepts as the guards of control actions. These vague concepts are represented, e.g., using domain ontologies. The rough set approach in combination with other soft computing approaches is used for approximation of the vague concepts relative to attributes (features) appearing in risk management and cost/benefit analysis.

One of the challenges in the approach is to develop methods and strategies for adaptive reasoning, called *adaptive judgement*, e.g., for adaptive control of computations. In particular, adaptive judgement is very much needed in the risk/efficiency management and cost/benefit analysis. They require access to approximate reasoning schemes (ARS) (over domain ontologies) [3, 22, 37] approximating, in a sense, reasoning expressed in relevant fragments of simplified natural language. Methods for inducing of ARS are under further development. The decision systems are enriched not only by approximations of concepts and relations from ontologies but also by ARS.

The developed model of interactive computations on c-granules, different from the Turing model (see also, e.g., ecorithms[1] discussed by Leslie Valiant in [46]), seems to have some importance for different areas such as Robotics, Natural Computing, CPSs or W2T. In particular, interactive computations on c-granules may be used for modeling computations in Natural Computing [5, 16, 33].

The discussed approach is a step toward realization of the Wisdom Technology (WisTech) program. The approach was developed over years of work on different real-life projects.

This chapter is organized as follows. Some basic postulates concerning agents and the physical world in which the agents are operating are included in Sect. 3.2.

---

[1] *Unlike most algorithms, they can run in environments unknown to the designer, and they learn by interacting with the environment how to act effectively in it. After sufficient interaction they will have expertise not provided by the designer, but extracted from the environment* [46].

In Sect. 3.3, an introduction to Interactive Rough Granular Computing (IRGC) is presented. Issues related to reasoning based on adaptive judgement are included in Sect. 3.4. In Sect. 3.5, the relationships of complex granules with the satisfiability relations are outlined. Agent computability issues in the framework of interactive computations on complex granules are outlined in Sect. 3.6. The approach to risk management based on IRGC is discussed in Sect. 3.7. Comments on dialogues of Agents in W2T are presented in Sect. 3.8. Section 3.9 concludes the chapter.

This chapter covers some issues presented in the plenary talk at the 5th International Conference on Pattern Recognition and Machine Intelligence (PReMi 2013), December 10–14, 3013, Kolkata, India and is a summarization and an extension of [12–14, 36].

3.2 Postulates About Physical World and Agents

One of the main objectives of the WisTech [9] is to provide some conceptual tools supporting (i) constructions of models of complex adaptive interactive systems (in particular for Complex Systems Engineering projects implementation and/or for development of AI technologies), which aggregate many local models interacting in an open environment and (ii) development of techniques for reasoning about the behavior of such models. One of the basic task on the way to achieve the WisTech goals is related to construction of an ontological base for WisTech. In this section, we only outline some basic postulates concerning agents and the physical world in which the agents are operating. Agents are partially perceiving the physical world and they are interacting with this world. The first group of postulates is about the physical world and the second one about the agents. The postulates are specifying some basic concepts which are important for discussed here interactive computations on complex granules realized by agents for achieving their goals. The reader will find more detailed elaboration of these postulates in [9] aiming at describing a very complex ontological base of WisTech necessary for dealing with complex adaptive interactive systems.

Physical World Postulates

1. *Physical world* consists of (spatio-temporal) *physical beings*.
2. Physical beings may *interact*.
3. *Interactions* are satisfying some *cause-effect relationships* following from the physical world laws concerning interactions.

Agent Postulates

1. Agent is a *physical being*.
2. Agent can *perceive* and *record* some interaction results. Due to uncertainty only some interaction results may be partially recorded and perceived by agents. Agent has only a partial knowledge about cause-effect relationships as well as about physical laws.
3. Agent is equipped with some private *clocks*.

4. *Agent control* consists of physical beings for realization of some cause-effect relationships. The agent control may activate realization of cause-effect relationships. This leads to creating of structures of physical beings activating interactions. The agent control may try to predict the results of these interactions.
5. *Agent control* has some skills for perceiving some physical beings and their interactions. More precisely, the agent control has some skills for perceiving and recording some properties of physical beings and results of their interactions. This is realized by perceiving, recording and verifying by agent control the results of interactions of the agent control with those physical beings which are in interactions with each other.
6. *Agent control* has some skills for perceiving of physical beings and/or their interactions in a specific space consisting of potentially perceivable by the agent physical beings. This space is called the *agent activity environment*. The physical beings perceived in the agent activity environment are called *hunks*.
7. At any moment *t* in the agent time, the agent perceives the physical world using *complex granules* (c-*granules*, for short) generated by the agent control. By employing c -granules the agent is developing such skills as

   a. initialization, storing and judgment of interaction results over hunks accessible by c-granules,
   b. aggregation and decomposition of c-granules.

8. Perception of the physical world by agents is based on construction of c-granules used for representation of *models of interactions and their results*. Agent is using these models for construction of *interaction plans*, their implementation, judgment, adaptation and learning of strategies for efficient construction of new c-granules.
9. Agent has a distinguished class of c-granules representing the *actual hierarchy of the agent needs* and related to this class another class representing construction techniques of *the interaction plans for satisfying the agent priority needs*.
10. *The agent main task* consists of construction, implementation, judgment and adaptation of the agent interaction plans enabling the agent in the best way: (i) to discover (learn) the adaptively changing agent priority needs and also (ii) to provide that they can be satisfied in the most efficient way.

3.3 Interactive Rough Granular Computing (IRGC)

The essence of the proposed approach is the use of IIS implemented on the basis of IRGC [9, 11, 36, 38–40]. In this sense IRGC creates the basis for the W2T technology. The approach is based on foundations for modeling of IRGC relevant for IIS in which computations are progressing through interactions [7]. In IRGC interactive computations are performed on objects called *complex granules* (*c-granules*, for short) linking information granules [28] (or infogranules, for short) with physical objects called hunks [8, 9].

Infogranules are widely discussed in the literature. They can be treated as specifications of compound objects (such as complex hierarchically defined attributes) together with scenarios of their implementations. Such granules are obtained as the result of information granulation [52]:

> Information granulation can be viewed as a human way of achieving data compression and it plays a key role in implementation of the strategy of divide-and-conquer in human problem-solving.

Infogranules belong to the concepts playing the main role in developing foundations for AI, data mining and text mining [28]. They grew up as some generalizations from fuzzy sets [48, 50, 52], rough set theory and interval analysis [28]. The rough set approach is crucial because of necessity to deal with approximations of inforgranules, e.g., in inducing classifiers for complex vague concepts. The IRGC is based on the rough set approach in combination with other approaches to soft computing (such as fuzzy sets). However, the issues related to interactions of infogranules with the physical world and their relationship to perception of interactions in the physical world are not well elaborated yet [7, 45]. On the other hand the understanding of interactions is the critical issue of complex systems [21]:

> [...] interaction is a critical issue in the understanding of complex systems of any sorts: as such, it has emerged in several well-established scientific areas other than computer science, like biology, physics, social and organizational sciences.

We propose to model complex systems by societies of agents. Computations in the IIS based on societies of agents have roots in c-granules [9]. Any c-granule consists of three components, namely soft_suit, link_suit and hard_suit. These components are making it possible to deal with such abstract objects from soft_suit as infogranules as well as with physical objects from hard_suit. The link_suit of a given c-granule is used as a kind of c-granule interface for handling interaction between soft_suit and and hard_suit.

Calculi of c-granules are defined by elementary c-granules (corresponding to, e.g., reading or storing measured values, simple sensory measurements, indiscernibility or similarity classes) and more compound c-granules constructed from already defined c-granules. Any compound c-granule is defined using networks of already defined c-granules corresponding to soft_suit, link_suit and hard_suit of the new constructed c-granule. These networks are properly linked for enabling transmission of interactions from the hard_suit network through the link_suit network to the sof_link network, where the interaction properties are recorded.

The hierarchy of c-granules is illustrated in Fig. 3.1. It is worthwhile mentioning that c-granules create also the basis for the agent (communication) language construction and the language evolution.

Any agent operates in a local world of c-granules. The agent control is aiming at controlling computations performed on c-granules from this local world for achieving the target goals. Actions (sensors or plans) represented by c-granules are used by the agent control in exploration and/or exploitation of the environment on the way to achieve their targets. C-granules are also used for representation of perception by

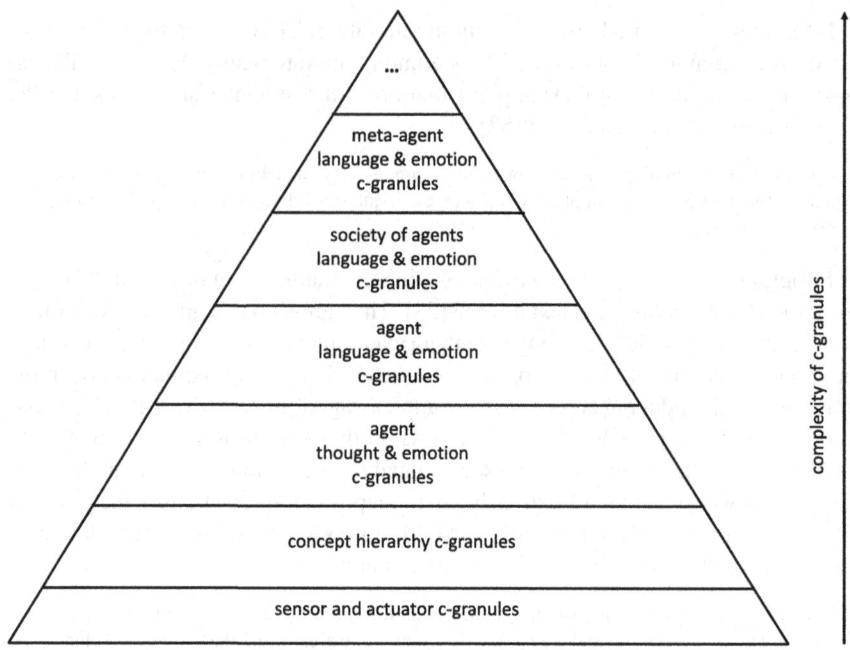

Fig. 3.1 Hierarchy of c-granules

agents concerning of interactions in the physical world. Due to the bounds of the agent perception abilities usually only a partial information about the interactions from physical world may be available for agents. Hence, in particular the results of performed actions by agents can not be predicted with certainty. For more details on IRGC based on c-granules the reader is referred to [9].

One of the key issues of the approach to c-granules presented in [9] is some kind of integration of investigation of physical and mental phenomena. The integration follows from suggestions presented by many scientists. For illustration let us consider the following two quotations:

> As far as the laws of mathematics refer to reality, they are not certain; and as far as they are certain, they do not refer to reality.
>
> – *Albert Einstein* [6]

> Constructing the physical part of the theory and unifying it with the mathematical part should be considered as one of the main goals of statistical learning theory.
>
> – *Vladimir Vapnik* ([45], p. 721)

A special role in IRGC play information (decision) systems from the rough set approach [23–25, 42]. They are used to record processes of interacting configurations of hunks. In order to represent interactive computations (used, e.g., in searching for new features) information systems of a new type, namely interactive information systems, are needed [9, 39, 40].

3.4 Adaptive Judgement

The reasoning making it possible to derive relevant information granules for solutions of the target tasks is called *adaptive judgment*. *Intuitive judgment* and *rational judgment* are distinguished as different kinds of judgment [15]. Among the tasks for adaptive judgement following are the ones supporting reasoning towards:

- inducing relevant classifiers, e.g.,
  - searching for relevant approximation spaces,
  - discovery of new features,
  - selection of relevant features (attributes),
  - rule induction,
  - discovery of inclusion measures,
  - strategies for conflict resolution,
  - adaptation of measures based on the minimum description length principle,
- prediction of changes,
- initiation of relevant actions or plans,
- discovery of relevant contexts,
- adaptation of different sorts of strategies e.g., for
  - existing data models,
  - quality measure over computations realized by agents,
  - objects structures,
  - knowledge representation and interaction with knowledge bases,
  - ontology acquisition and approximation,
  - hierarchy of needs, or for identifying problems to be solved according to priority,
- learning the measures of inclusion between granules from sources using different languages (e.g., the formal language of the system and the user natural language) through dialogue,
- strategies for development and evolution of communication language among agents in distributed environments, and
- strategies for efficiency management in distributed computational systems.

Adaptive judgement in IIS is a mixture of reasoning based on deduction, abduction, induction, case based or analogy based reasoning, experience, observed changes in the environment, meta-heuristics from natural computing. Let us also note the following remark [44]:

> Practical judgment is not algebraic calculation. Prior to any deductive or inductive reckoning, the judge is involved in selecting objects and relationships for attention and assessing their interactions. Identifying things of importance from a potentially endless pool of candidates, assessing their relative significance, and evaluating their relationships is well beyond the jurisdiction of reason.

We would like to stress that still much more work should be done to develop approximate reasoning methods about complex vague concepts for making progress

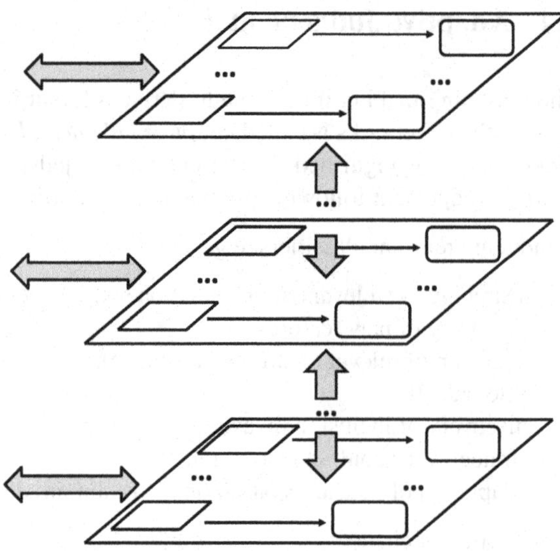

Fig. 3.2 Interactive hierarchical structures (*gray arrows* show interactions between hierarchical levels and the environment, *arrows* at hierarchical levels point from information (decision) systems representing partial specifications of satisfiability relations to induced from them theories consisting of rule sets)

in development of IIS, in particular for the risk management and cost/benefit analysis in IIS. This idea was very well expressed by Leslie Valiant[2]:

> A fundamental question for artificial intelligence is to characterize the computational building blocks that are necessary for cognition. A specific challenge is to build on the success of machine learning so as to cover broader issues in intelligence. [...] This requires, in particular a reconciliation between two contradictory characteristics—the apparent logical nature of reasoning and the statistical nature of learning.

It is worthwhile to mention here again two more views by Lotfi A. Zadeh and Judea Pearl, already cited in this chapter (see Sect. 3.1).

The question arises about the logic relevant for the above discussed tasks. Let us observe that the satisfiability relations in the IRGC framework can be treated as tools for constructing new information granules. If fact, for a given satisfiability relation, the semantics of formulas relative to this relation is defined. In this way the candidates for new relevant information granules are obtained. We would like to emphasize a very important feature. The relevant satisfiability relation for the considered problems is not given but it should be induced (discovered) on the basis of a partial information encoded in information (decision) systems. For real-life problems, it is often necessary to discover a hierarchy of satisfiability relations before we obtain the relevant target level. Information granules constructed at different levels of this hierarchy finally lead to relevant ones for approximation of complex vague concepts related to complex information granules expressed in natural language (see Fig. 3.2).

[2]see, e.g., http://en.wikipedia.org/wiki/Vagueness, http://people.seas.harvard.edu/~valiant/research interests.htm, [46].

3.5 Complex Granules and Satisfiability

In this section, we discuss some examples of c-granules constructed over a family of satisfiability relations being at the disposal of a given agent. This discussion has some roots in intuitionism (see, e.g., [18]). Let us consider a remark made by Per Martin-Löf in [18] about judgment presented in Fig. 3.3.

In the approach based on c-granules, the judgment for checking values of descriptors (or more compound formulas) pointed by links from simple c-granules is based on interactions of some physical parts considered over time and/or space (called hunks) and pointed by links of c-granules. The judgment for the more compound c-granules is defined by a relevant family of procedures also realized by means of interactions of physical parts.

Let us explain in more detail the above claims.

Let assume that a given agent ag has at the disposal a family of satisfiability relations

$$\{\models_i\}_{i \in I}, \tag{3.1}$$

where $\models_i \subseteq Tok(i) \times Typ(i)$, $Tok(i)$ is a set of tokens and $Type(i)$ is a set of types, respectively (using the terminology from [2]). The indices of satisfiability relations are vectors of parameters related, e.g., to time, space, spatio-temporal features of physical parts represented by hunks or actions (plans) to be realized in the physical world.

In the discussed example of elementary c-granules, $Tok(i)$ is a set of hunks and $Type(i)$ is a set of descriptors (elementary infogranules), respectively, pointed by link represented by $\models_i$. The procedure for computing the value of $h \models_i \alpha$, where h is a hunk and α is an infogranule (e.g., descriptor or formula constructed over descriptors) is based on interaction of α with the physical world represented by hunk h.

The agent control can aggregate some simple c-granules into more compound c-granules, e.g., by selecting some constraints on subsets of I making it possible to select relevant sets of simple c-granules and consider them as a new more compound c-granule. In constraints also values in descriptors pointed by links in elementary c-granules can be taken into account and sets of such more compound c-granules can be aggregated into new c-granules. Values of new descriptors pointed by links of these more compound granules are computed by new procedures. The computation process again is realized by interaction of the physical parts represented by hunks pointed by links of elementary c-granules included in the considered more compound c-granule as well as by using the procedure for computing of values of more com-

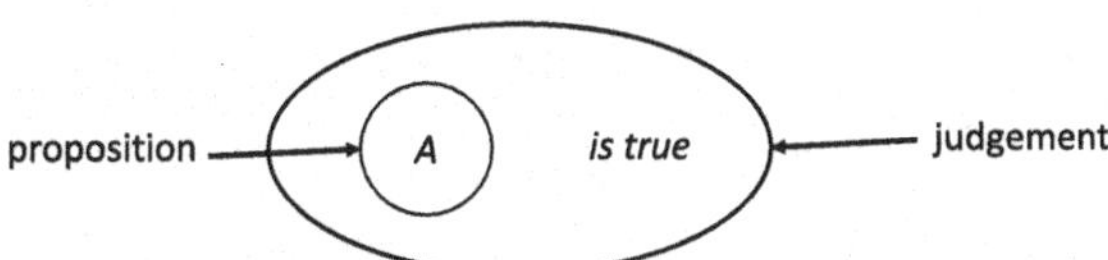

Fig. 3.3 When we hold a proposition to be true, then we make a judgment [18]

pound descriptors from values of descriptors included in elementary c-granules of the considered more compound c-granule. Note that this procedure is also realized in the physical world thanks to relevant interactions.

In hierarchical modeling aiming at inducing of relevant c-granules (e.g., for approximation of complex vague concepts), one can consider so far constructed c-granules as tokens. For example, they can be used to define structured objects representing corresponding hunks and link them using new satisfiability relations (from a given family) to relevant higher order descriptors together with the appropriate procedures (realized by interactions of hunks) for computing values of these descriptors. This approach generalizes hierarchical modeling developed for infogranules (see, e.g., [3, 20]) to hierarchical modeling of c-granules which is important for many real-life projects.

We have assumed before that the agent *ag* is equipped with a family of satisfiability relations. However, in real-life projects the situation is more complicated. The agent *ag* should have strategies for discovery of new relevant satisfiability relations on the way of searching for solutions of target goals (problems). This is related to a question about the adaptive judgment relevant for agents performing computations based on configurations of c-granules. In the framework of granular computing based on c-granules, satisfiability relations are tools for constructing new c-granules. In fact, for a given satisfiability relation, the semantics of descriptors (and more compound formulas) relative to this relation can be defined. In this way candidates for new relevant c-granules are obtained. Hence, here arises a very important issue. The relevant satisfiability relations for the agent *ag* searching for solutions of problems are not given but they should be induced (discovered) on the basis of a partial information encoded in information (decision) systems including results of measurements of interaction of parts of physical world pointed by links of elementary c-granules as well as on the basis of c-granules representing domain knowledge. This problem is strongly related to reasoning from sensory measurement to perception [50, 52]. For real-life problems, it is often necessary to discover a hierarchy of satisfiability relations before the relevant target level will be obtained (see Fig. 3.2) [12]. C-granules constructed at different levels of this hierarchy finally lead to relevant c-granules (e.g., for approximation of complex vague concepts) expressed very often in natural language. This is illustrated in Figs. 3.4 and 3.5, where the complex vague concepts *safe driving* and *similarity in respiratory failure* are represented, respectively, together with concepts and relations from fragments of domain ontologies used as hints in searching for relevant attributes (features) on different levels of the hierarchy. For details, the reader is referred to [3, 20].

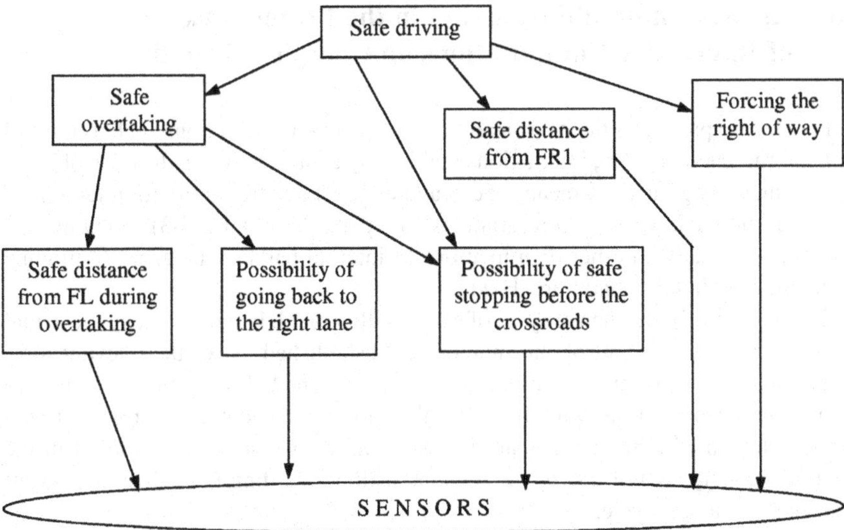

Fig. 3.4 Fragment of ontology used for approximation of the vague concept *safe driving* for decision support in traffic control

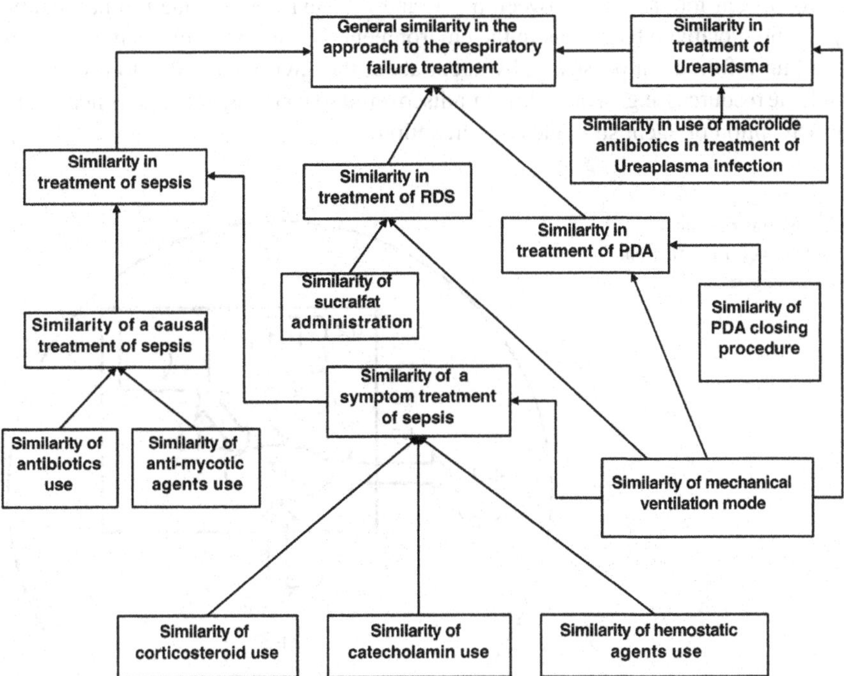

Fig. 3.5 Fragment of ontology used for approximation of the vague concept *similarity* in decision support for respiratory failure

3.6 Agent Computability Issues in the Framework of Interactive Computations on Complex Granules

In Fig. 3.6 are presented the basic agent components for interactions such as control (C), internal memory (M), interactions realized by control between the control granule and memory granule by means of c-granules generated by control for interactions with the external environment (c-granules with parts: M, link l-2 (l-3) and hunk H-2 (H-3)) as well as with other than memory M internal parts of the agent (c-granule with parts: M, link l-1, and hunk H-1).

In Fig. 3.7 the basic control cycle of agent is illustrated. In the first stage the actual interactions between control and memory are established. Next, the relevant for a given moment of (agent) time c-granules are established. The agent is planning to using hem for interactions with the external environment and with the agent internal parts. After this the interactions are initiated and their results are recorded in the internal memory (M) of the agent. As soon as the recording is finalized the agent control starts a new cycle.

It is worthwhile mentioning that contrary to the existing computation models realized by Turing machine the results of interactions can be only predicted by the agent control but the results of this prediction can be in general different from the results of real interactions between agent and the environment due to uncertainty, e.g., unpredictable interactions in the environment. In particular, this is the result of uncertain information possessed by agent about the environment due to bounds on available resources, e.g., available (or undiscovered so far) by agent sensors necessary for perception or agent strategies of perception.

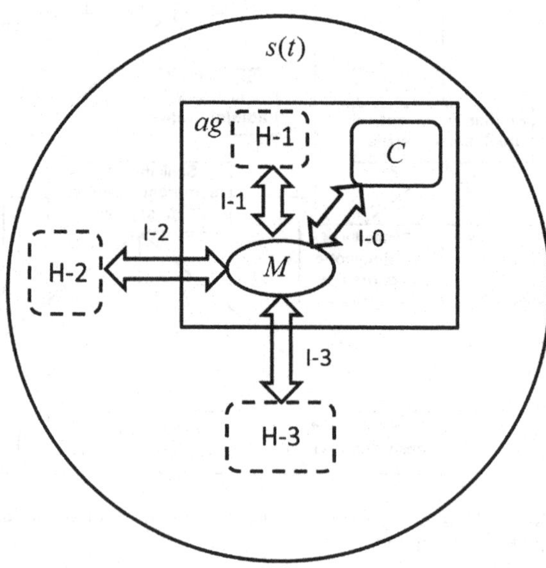

Fig. 3.6 Basic agent components for interactions

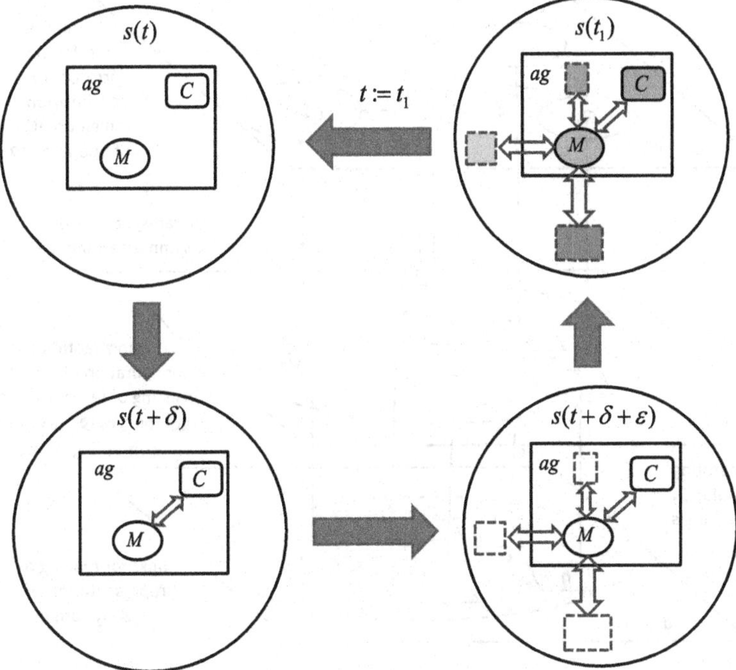

Fig. 3.7 Basic control cycle of agent

In Fig. 3.8, we illustrate how the abstract definition of operation from soft_suit interacts with other suits of c-granule. It is necessary to distinguish two cases. In the first case, the results of operation realized by interaction of hunks are consistent with the specification in the link_suit. In the second case, the result specified in the soft suit can be treated only as an estimation of the real one which may be different due to the unpredictable interactions in the hard_suit.

The point of view that the interactive computations on complex granules are progressing due to interactions with the physical world is important for Natural Computing [33] too. The agent-observer trying to understand such computations in dependent on the physical world (see the already cited sentence from [4] (p. 268)).

The agent hypotheses about the models of computations can be verified only through interactions within the physical world. These models should be adaptively adjusted when deviations of the predicted from the perceived real trajectories of computations are becoming significant (see Fig. 3.9).

The issue discussed in this section are raising a question about the control of interactive granular computations. In the next section we emphasize importance of the risk management and cost/benefit analysis by the agent control.

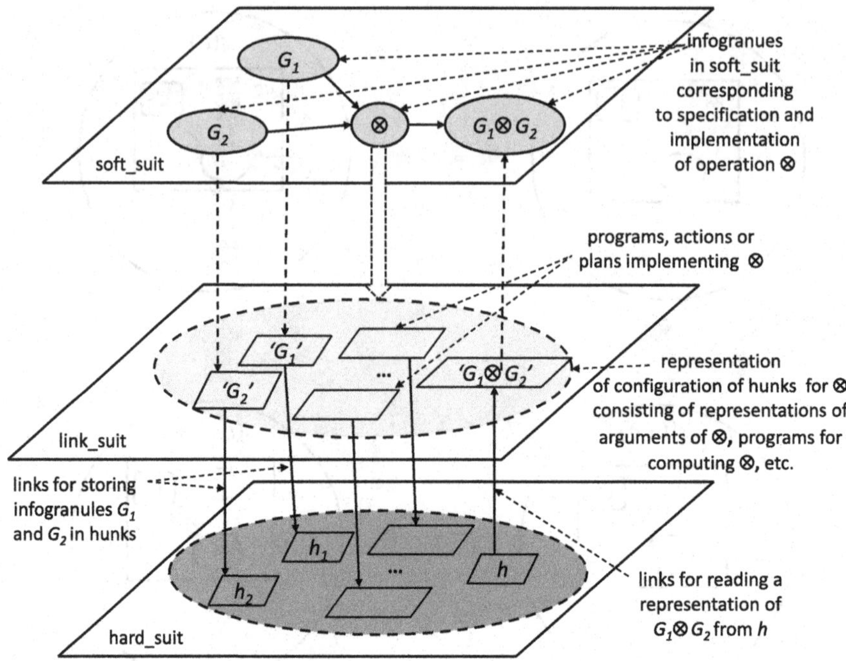

Fig. 3.8 Explanation of roles of different suits of a c-granule for operation ⊗

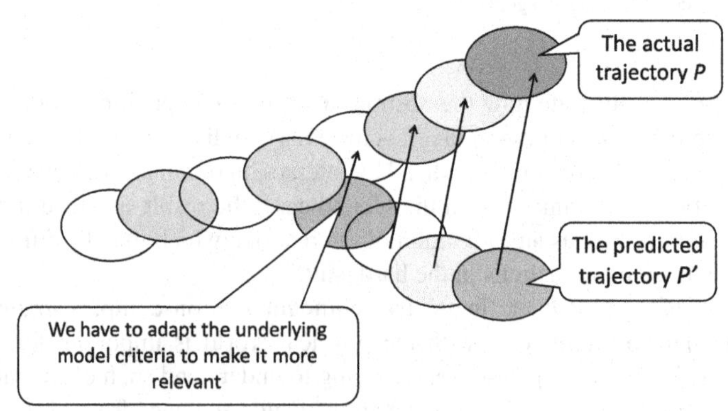

Fig. 3.9 Adaptation of trajectory approximations

3.7 Risk Management and Cost/Benefit Analysis by Agents in W2T Technology

The meaning of practical judgment goes beyond typical tools for reasoning based on deduction or induction. Our understanding of (practical) judgement can be related to the cited already intuition from [44]. For example, a particular question for the agent control arises about learning strategies for inducing models of dynamic changes of the agent attention. This may be related, e.g., to inducing changes in the relevant context necessary for judgment.

Practical judgment is involved in risk management and cost/benefit analysis [9]. Let us concentrate on some comments about risk management.

Risk may be understood as interaction with uncertainty. Risk perception is the subjective judgment people make about the severity and/or probability of a risk, and may vary person to person. Any human endeavor carries some risk, but some are much riskier than others (The Stanford Encyclopedia of Philosophy: http://plato.stanford.edu/archives/spr2014/entries/risk/).

Since the very beginning, all human activities were done at risk of failure. Recent years have shown the low quality of risk management in areas such as finance, economics, and many others. In this context, improvement in the risk management has a particular importance for the further development of complex systems. The importance of risk management illustrates the following example from financial sector. Many of financial risk management experts consider Basel II rules[3] as a causal factor in the credit bubble prior to the 2007–8 collapse. Namely, in Basel II one of the principal factors of financial risk management was

> outsourced to companies that were not subject to supervision, credit rating agencies.

Of course, now we do have a new "improved" version of Basel II, called Basel III. However, according to an OECD[4] *the medium-term impact of Basel III implementation on GDP growth is negative and estimated in the range of* −0.05 *to* −0.15 % *per year* (see also [41]).

On the basis of experience in many areas, we have now many valuable studies on different approaches to risk management. Currently, the dominant terminology is determined by the standards of ISO 31K [1]. However, the logic of inferences in risk management is dominated by the statistical paradigms, especially by Bayesian data analysis initiated about 300 years ago by Bayes, and regression data analysis initiated by about 200 years ago by Legendre and Gauss. On this basis, resulted many detailed methodologies specific for different fields. A classic example is the risk management methodology in the banking sector, based on the recommendations of Basel II standards for risk management mathematical models [35]. The current dominant statistical approach is not satisfactory because it does not give effective tools for inferences about the vague concepts and relations between them (see the included before sentences by Valiant).

---

[3] see http://en.wikipedia.org/wiki/Basel_Committee_on_Banking_Supervision.

[4] see http://en.wikipedia.org/wiki/Basel_III.

A particularly important example of the risk management vague concept relation is the relation of a cause-effect relationships between various events. It should be noted that the concept of risk in ISO 31K is defined as *the effect of uncertainty on objectives*. Thus, by definition, the vagueness is also an essential part of the risk concept.

To paraphrase the motto of this study by Judea Pearl, we can say that traditional statistical approach to risk management inference *is strong in devising ways of describing data and inferring distributional parameters from sample*. However, in practice risk management inference requires two additional ingredients (see the citation of Pearl sentences in this chapter):

- *a science-friendly language for articulating risk management knowledge*, and
- *a mathematical machinery for processing that knowledge, combining it with data and drawing new risk management conclusions about a phenomenon.*

Adding both mentioned above components is an extremely difficult task and binds to the core of AI research very accurately specified by the Turing test. With regard to our applications, properly adapted version of the test boils down to the fact that on the basis of a "conversation" with a hidden risk management expert and a hidden machine one will not be able to distinguish who is the man and who is the machine.

We propose to extend the statistical paradigm by adding the two discussed components for designing of the high quality risk management systems supported by IIS.

For the risk management in IIS one of the most important task is to develop strategies for inducing approximations of the vague complex concepts involved in the risk management. The approximations are making it possible to check their satisfiability (to a degree). A typical example of such vague concept is the statement of the form: "now we do have very risky situation". Among such concepts especially important are vague complex playing the role of guards on which is based activation of actions performed by agents.

These vague complex concepts are represented by the agent hierarchy of needs. In risk management one should consider a variety of complex vague concepts and relations between them as well as reasoning schemes related, e.g., to the bow-tie diagram (see Fig. 3.10).

Let us explain the bow-tie diagram using the chess game. Of course the chess game is a very simple example. In practice the game could be much more complex. The bow-tie diagram has 3 basic parts:

1. concepts from risk sources,
2. current situation description represented by a hierarchy of concepts defined by the input sensors and context data,
3. concepts from risk consequences.

To make the next move in chess game the player should understood the current situation. To do this, he or she should use the domain knowledge representation (especially, related to the domain of risk management) and apply the relevant inference rules to the current situation description (see parts 1 and 2) enriched by knowledge

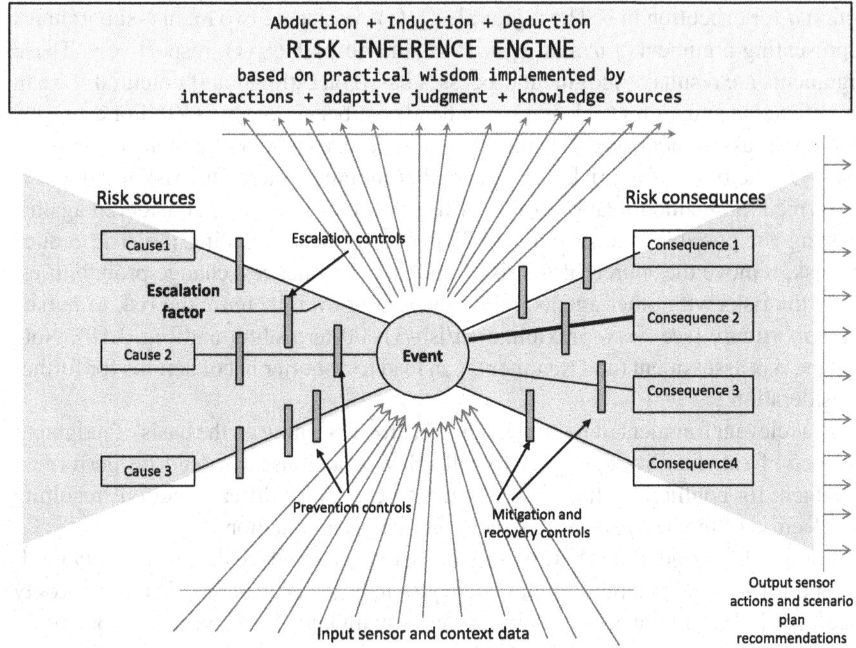

Fig. 3.10 Bow-tie diagram

about the history of moves. Based on the knowledge about possible sources of risk (expressed in part 1) and features of moves history, one should identify the prioritized list of hypotheses about the opposite player strategy. If the opposite player strategy is identified then it is much easier to win. This kind of inference leading to a list of the most likely to be true hypotheses for the opposite player strategy, is called abduction. This *is a form of logical inference that goes from observation to a hypothesis that accounts for the reliable data (observation) and seeks to explain relevant evidence* (by Wikipedia http://en.wikipedia.org/wiki/Abductive_reasoning). In the following step, the best possible next move should be proposed on the basis of the list of hypotheses for the opposite player strategy. For the chess game, one can generate the tree of all possible n-moves and propose the best next move using some well known algorithms (such as $minimax$, *alpha-beta*, *A-star* [26, 34]). In real life applications, such trees theoretically could be generated using the part of risk ontology related to consequences (part 3). If these trees are becoming huge then using relevant abduction inference one can try to identify constraints helping to make searching for the best next move in such trees feasible.

Agents are realizing their goals performing actions. Hence, it is very important to discover measures evaluating the correctness of a given action selection in a given situation. One can consider for each action a a complex vague concept Q_a representing such a measure. For a given situation s, the value of $Q_a(s)$ is a c-granule representing the degree to which $Q_a(s)$ is satisfied at s, *i.e.*, the correctness degree of selection the action a for execution in s. The c-granule $Q_a(s)$ consists of two main c-subgranules representing arguments *for* and *against* satisfiability of $Q_a(s)$, respectively. These arguments are results of judgment processes based on estimation if potentially a can be initiated in situation s, risk assessment and cost/benefit analysis [9]. For example, in the risk assessment (see [1]) the goal of judgment is identification of the main risks. On the basis of the risk degrees another judgment called the risk treatment is performed. Some modifications of controls (or new controls) are considered against existing (or possible) vulnerabilities. This can result in avoiding the risk, reduce the risk, remove the source of the risk, modify consequences, change probabilities, share the risks with other agents, retain the risk or even increase the risk to pursue the opportunity (see www.praxiom.com/iso-31000-terms.htm and Fig. 3.10). Note that the risk assessment (and treatment) can lead to a shorter list of actions for further consideration.

In a relevant fragment of natural language, after assigning on the basis of judgment degrees of satisfiability of $Q_a(s)$ for all relevant actions, it should be performed judgment for conflict resolution among these degrees for different actions resulting in selection of the best action for execution in a given situation.

For real-life projects it is hardly possible to expect to induce the high quality models of the discussed complex vagues concepts on the basis of automatic methods only (see, e.g., [43]) without acquiring by agents domain knowledge through cooperation with domain experts.

One can consider the mentioned above tasks of approximation of complex vague concepts related to actions as the complex game discovery task (see Fig. 3.11) from data and domain knowledge.

The discovery process of complex games, in particular embedded in them complex vague concepts, often is based on hierarchical learning supported by domain knowledge [3, 9]. It is also worthwhile mentioning that these games are evolving in time (drifting in time) together with data and knowledge about the approximated concepts and the relevant strategies for adaptation of games used by agents are required.

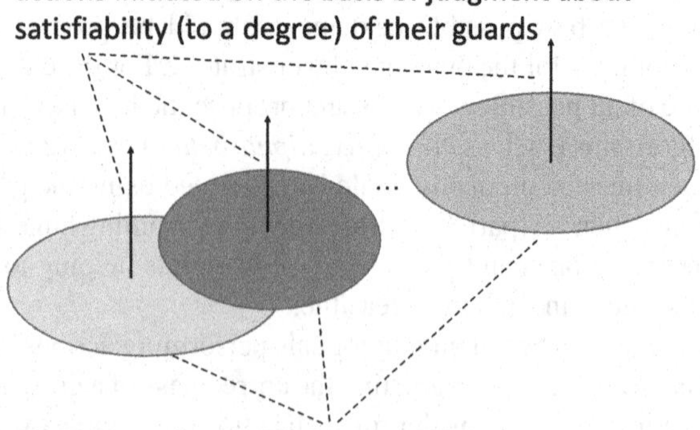
actions initiated on the basis of judgment about
satisfiability (to a degree) of their guards
...
action guards: complex vague concepts

Fig. 3.11 Games based on complex vague concepts

These adaptive strategies are used by agents to control their behavior on the way toward achieving by them the targets. Note that also these strategies should be learned from available uncertain data and domain knowledge.

3.8 Comments on Dialogues of Agents in W2T

In this section, we present some preliminary comments on dialogues among agents. Dialogues of agents from a given team of agents can lead e.g., to a common understanding of problems to be solved by the team and next to common problem solving by this team. The issues related to reasoning based on dialogues are not trivial especially when one would like to base their treatment on dominating paradigms for reasoning in logic. This point of view is well expressed by Johan van Benthem in [32] (see Foreword, p. viii):

> I see two main paradigms from Antiquity that come together in the modern study of argumentation: Platos Dialogues as the paradigm of intelligent interaction, and Euclids Elements as the model of rigour. Of course, some people also think that formal mathematical proof is itself the ultimate ideal of reasoning—but you may want to change your mind about reasonings peak experiences when you see top mathematicians argue interactively at a seminar.

Dialogues enable the agents to search (efficiently) for solutions. Very often queries formulated in W2T technology by agents are represented by vague concepts in natural language (e.g., in dialogue based search engines). Agents are expecting to receive c-granules satisfying their specifications to satisfactory degrees. The meaning of *satisfiability to a degree* should be learned on the basis of dialogue of agents embedded in the W2T. Satisfiability to a degree gives some flexibility in searching for solutions. The solutions do nod need to be *exact*. This makes the process of searching for constructions of such c-granules feasible. Usually such constructions should be robust relative to some deviations of components. The interested reader may find more details on these issues in (see, e.g., [29–31]), where the approach is based on the rough mereological approach.

Through dialogues agents may try to recognize the meaning of c-granules received from other agents. They can do this by learning approximations of received c-granules in their own languages. A given agent may acquire the concept ontology used by another agent. However, usually a given agent can only acquire approximation of concept ontology possessed by another agent. This knowledge transfer may be very useful in solving problems by the agent (see e.g., [3, 20]). Let us observe that the ontology approximation may also be used in efficient searching for relevant contexts of queries received by agents from other agents.

One of the challenges for adaptive judgment performed by a given agent ag is a learning task of *approximation of derivations* performed by another agent ag', assuming that the concept ontology of ag' was already approximated by ag. Approximation by ag of derivations performed by ag' may be understood as approximation (to satisfactory degree) by ag of solution constructions delivered by ag'.

3.9 Conclusions

The approach for modeling interactive computations based on c-granules was presented and its importance for the risk management and cost/benefit analysis in W2T was outlined.

The discussed concepts such as interactive computation and adaptive judgment are among the basic ingredient elements in the Wisdom Technology (WisTech) [9, 10]. Let us mention here the WisTech meta-equation:

$$\begin{aligned} \text{WISDOM} = \; & \\ & \text{INTERACTIONS} + \\ & \text{ADAPTIVE JUDGEMENT} + \\ & \text{KNOWLEDGE} . \end{aligned} \tag{3.2}$$

The discussed c-granules may represent complex objects. For example, Fig. 3.12 presents some guidelines for implementation of AI projects in the form of a cooperation scheme of agents responsible for relevant cooperation areas [9]. This cooperation scheme may be treated as a higher level c-granule.

The presented approach seems also to be of some importance for developing computing models in different areas such as natural computing (e.g., computing models for meta-heuristics or computations models for complex processes in

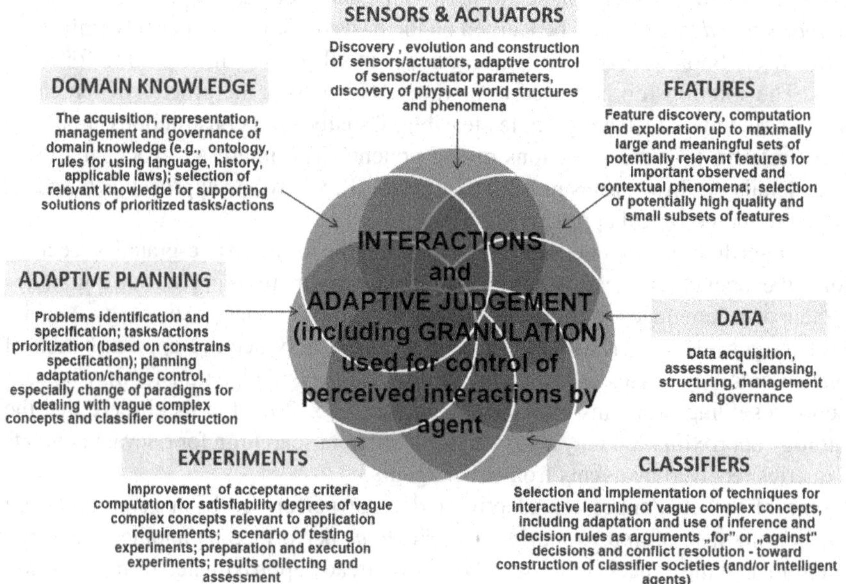

Fig. 3.12 Cooperation scheme of agents responsible for relevant competence area

molecular biology), computing in distributed environments under uncertainty realized by multi-agent systems (e.g., in social computing), modeling of computations for feature extraction (constructive induction) used for approximation of complex vague concepts, hierarchical learning, discovery of planning strategies or strategies for coalition formation by agents as well as for approximate reasoning about interactive computations based on such computing models. All these areas are strongly related to the W2T technology.

In our research, we plan to further develop the foundations of interactive computations based on c-granules toward tools for modeling and analysis of computations in Natural Computing [33], Wisdom Web of Things [53] or Cyber-Physical Systems [17].

Acknowledgments This work was partially supported by the Polish National Science Centre (NCN) grants DEC-2011/01/D/ST6/06981, DEC-2013/09/B/ST6/01568 as well as by the Polish National Centre for Research and Development (NCBiR) under the grant DZP/RID-I-44/8/NCBR/2016.

References

1. ISO 31000 standard, http://webstore.ansi.org/
2. J. Barwise, J. Seligman, *Information Flow: The Logic of Distributed Systems* (Cambridge University Press, 1997)
3. J. Bazan, Hierarchical classifiers for complex spatio-temporal concepts. Trans. Rough Sets IX: J. Subline LNCS **5390**, 474–750 (2008)
4. D. Deutsch, A. Ekert, R. Lupacchini, Machines, logic and quantum physics. Bull. Symbol. Logic **6**, 265–283 (2000)
5. A. Ehrenfeucht, J. Kleijn, M. Koutny, G. Rozenberg, Reaction systems: a natural computing approach to the functioning of living cells, in *A Computable Universe, Understanding and Exploring Nature as Computation*, ed. by H. Zenil (World Scientific, Singapore, 2012), pp. 189–208
6. A. Einstein, *Geometrie und Erfahrung (Geometry and Experience)* (Julius Springer, Berlin, 1921)
7. D. Goldin, S. Smolka, P. Wegner (eds.), *Interactive Computation: The New Paradigm* (Springer, 2006)
8. M. Heller, *The Ontology of Physical Objects. Four Dimensional Hunks of Matter* (Cambridge Studies in Philosophy, Cambridge University Press, 1990)
9. A. Jankowski, *Complex Systems Engineering: Wisdom for Saving Billions Based on Interactive Granular Computing* (Springer, Heidelberg, 2016). (in preparation)
10. A. Jankowski, A. Skowron. A WisTech paradigm for intelligent systems. Trans. Rough Sets VI: J. Subline, 94–132
11. A. Jankowski, A. Skowron. Wisdom technology: a rough-granular approach, in M. Marciniak, A. Mykowiecka (eds.), *Bolc Festschrift*, Lectures Notes in Computer Science, vol. 5070, pp. 3–41 (Springer, Heidelberg, 2009)
12. A. Jankowski, A. Skowron, R.W. Swiniarski. Interactive computations: toward risk management in interactive intelligent systems, in P. Maji, A. Ghosh, M.N. Murty, K. Ghosh, S.K. Pal (eds.), *Pattern Recognition and Machine Intelligence—5th International Conference, PReMI 2013*, Kolkata, India, December 10–14, 2013. Proceedings. Lecture Notes in Computer Science, vol. 8251, pp. 1–12 (Springer, 2013)

13. A. Jankowski, A. Skowron, R.W. Swiniarski, Interactive complex granules. Fundamenta Informaticae **133**, 181–196 (2014)
14. A. Jankowski, A. Skowron, R.W. Swiniarski, Perspectives on uncertainty and risk in rough sets and interactive rough-granular computing. Fundamenta Informaticae **129**, 69–84 (2014)
15. D. Kahneman, Maps of bounded rationality: psychology for behavioral economics. Am. Econ. Rev. **93**, 1449–1475 (2002)
16. L. Kari, G. Rozenberg, The many facets of natural computing. Commun. ACM **51**, 72–83 (2008)
17. F. Lamnabhi-Lagarrigue, M.D. Di Benedetto, E. Schoitsch, Introduction to the special theme cyber-physical systems. Ercim News **94**, 6–7 (2014)
18. P. Martin-Löf, *Intuitionistic Type Theory (Notes by Giovanni Sambin of a series of lectures given in Padua, June 1980)* (Bibliopolis, Napoli, Italy, 1984)
19. J.M. Mendel, L.A. Zadeh, E. Trillas, R.Yager, J. Lawry, H. Hagras, S. Guadarrama, What computing with words means to me. IEEE Comput. Intell. Mag. pp. 20–26 (February 2010)
20. S.H. Nguyen, J. Bazan, A. Skowron, H.S. Nguyen, Layered learning for concept synthesis. Trans. Rough Sets I: J. Subline LNCS **3100**, 187–208 (2004)
21. A. Omicini, A. Ricci, M. Viroli. The multidisciplinary patterns of interaction from sciences to computer science, in Goldin et al. [7], pp. 395–414
22. S.K. Pal, L. Polkowski, A. Skowron (eds.), *Rough-Neural Computing: Techniques for Computing with Words* (Cognitive Technologies, Springer, Heidelberg, 2004)
23. Z. Pawlak, A. Skowron, Rudiments of rough sets. Inf. Sci. **177**(1), 3–27 (2007)
24. Z. Pawlak, Rough sets. Int. J. Comput. Inf. Sci. **11**, 341–356 (1982)
25. Z. Pawlak, *Rough Sets: Theoretical Aspects of Reasoning about Data, System Theory, Knowledge Engineering and Problem Solving*, vol. 9 (Kluwer Academic Publishers, Dordrecht, The Netherlands, 1991)
26. J. Pearl, *Heuristics: Intelligent Search Strategies for Computer Problem Solving* (The Addison Wesley, Moston, MA, 1984)
27. J. Pearl, Causal inference in statistics: an overview. Stat. Surv. **3**, 96–146 (2009)
28. W. Pedrycz, S. Skowron, V. Kreinovich (eds.), *Handbook of Granular Computing* (Wiley, Hoboken, NJ, 2008)
29. L. Polkowski, A. Skowron, Rough mereological approach to knowledge-based distributed ai, in J.K. Lee, J. Liebowitz, J.M. Chae (eds.), *Critical Technology, Proc, Third World Congress on Expert Systems, February 5–9, Soeul, Korea* (Cognizant Communication Corporation, New York, 1996), pp. 774–781
30. L. Polkowski, A. Skowron, Rough mereology: a new paradigm for approximate reasoning. Int. J. Approximate Reasoning **15**(4), 333–365 (1996)
31. L. Polkowski, A. Skowron, Rough mereological calculi of granules: a rough set approach to computation. Comput. Intell. Int. J. **17**(3), 472–492 (2001)
32. I. Rahwan, G.R. Simari, *Argumentation in Artificial Intelligence* (Springer, Berlin, 2009)
33. G. Rozenberg, T. Bäck, J. Kok (eds.), *Handbook of Natural Computing* (Springer, 2012)
34. L. Schäfers, *Parallel Monte-Carlo Tree Search for HPC Systems and its Application to Computer Go* (Logos Verlag, Berlin, 2014)
35. P. Shevchenko (ed.), *Modelling Operational Risk Using Bayesian Inference* (Springer, 2011)
36. A. Skowron, A. Jankowski, P. Wasilewski, Risk management and interactive computational systems. J. Adv. Math. Appl. **1**, 61–73 (2012)
37. A. Skowron, J. Stepaniuk. Information granules and rough-neural computing, in Pal et al. [22], pp. 43–84
38. A. Skowron, J. Stepaniuk, R. Swiniarski, Modeling rough granular computing based on approximation spaces. Inf. Sci. **184**, 20–43 (2012)
39. A. Skowron, P. Wasilewski, Information systems in modeling interactive computations on granules. Theor. Comput. Sci. **412**(42), 5939–5959 (2011)
40. A. Skowron, P. Wasilewski, Interactive information systems: toward perception based computing. Theor. Comput. Sci. **454**, 240–260 (2012)

41. P. Slovik, *Cournède: Macroeconomic Impact of Basel III, Working Papers*, vol. 844 (OECD Economics Publishing, OECD Economics Department, 2011) http://www.oecd.org/eco/Workingpapers
42. J. Stepaniuk, *Rough-Granular Computing in Knowledge Discovery and Data Mining* (Springer, Heidelberg, 2008)
43. R.S. Sutton, A.G. Barto, *Reinforcement Learning: An Introduction* (The MIT Press, 1998)
44. L.P. Thiele, *The Heart of Judgment: Practical Wisdom, Neuroscience, and Narrative* (Cambridge University Press, Cambridge, UK, 2010)
45. V. Vapnik, *Statistical Learning Theory* (Wiley, New York, NY, 1998)
46. L. Valiant, *Probably Approximately Correct. Nature's Algorithms for Learning and Prospering in a Complex World* (Basic Books, A Member of the Perseus Books Group, New York, 2013)
47. A. Zadeh, *Computing with Words: Principal Concepts and Ideas, Studies in Fuzziness and Soft Computing*, vol. 277 (Springer, Heidelberg, 2012)
48. L.A. Zadeh, Fuzzy sets and information granularity, in *Advances in Fuzzy Set Theory and Applications* (North-Holland, Amsterdam, 1979), pp. 3–18
49. L.A. Zadeh, Fuzzy Logic = Computing With Words. IEEE Trans. Fuzzy Syst. **4**, 103–111 (1996)
50. L.A. Zadeh, From computing with numbers to computing with words—from manipulation of measurements to manipulation of perceptions. IEEE Trans. Circuits Syst. **45**, 105–119 (1999)
51. L.A. Zadeh, *Foreword*, in Pal et al. [22], pp. IX–XI
52. L.A. Zadeh, A new direction in AI: toward a computational theory of perceptions. AI Mag. **22**(1), 73–84 (2001)
53. N. Zhong, J.H. Ma, R.H. Huang, J.M. Liu, Y.Y. Yao, Y.X. Zhang, J. Chen, Research challenges and perspectives on Wisdom Web of Things (W2T). J. Supercomput. **64**, 862–882 (2013)

Chapter 4
Towards a Situation-Aware Architecture for the Wisdom Web of Things

Akihiro Eguchi, Hung Nguyen, Craig Thompson and Wesley Deneke

Abstract Computers are getting smaller, cheaper, faster, with lower power requirements, more memory capacity, better connectivity, and are increasingly distributed. Accordingly, smartphones became more of a commodity worldwide, and the use of smartphones as a platform for ubiquitous computing is promising. Nevertheless, we still lack much of the architecture and service infrastructure we will need to transition computers to become situation aware to a similar extent that humans are. Our Everything is Alive (EiA) project illustrates an integrated approach to fill in the void with a broad scope of works encompassing Ubiquitous Intelligence (RFID, spatial searchbot, etc.), Cyber-Individual (virtual world, 3D modeling, etc.), Brain Informatics (psychological experiments, computational neuroscience, etc.), and Web Intelligence (ontology, workflow, etc.). In this chapter, we describe the vision and architecture for a future where smart real-world objects dynamically discover and interact with other real or virtual objects, humans or virtual humans. We also discuss how the vision in EiA fits into a seamless data cycle like the one proposed in the Wisdom Web of Things (W2T), where data circulate through things, data, information, knowledge, wisdom, services, and humans. Various open research issues related to internal computer representations needed to model real or virtual worlds are identified, and challenges of using those representations to generate visualizations in a virtual world and of "parsing" the real world to recognize and record these data structures are also discussed.

A. Eguchi
Oxford Centre for Theoretical Neuroscience and Artificial Intelligence,
University of Oxford, Oxford, UK
e-mail: akihiro.eguchi@psy.ox.ac.uk

H. Nguyen · C. Thompson (✉)
Department of Computer Science and Computer Engineering,
University of Arkansas, Fayetteville, AR, USA
e-mail: cwt@uark.edu

W. Deneke
Department of Computer Science and Industrial Technology,
Southeastern Louisiana University, Hammond, LA, USA
e-mail: wesley.deneke@selu.edu

N. Zhong et al. (eds.), *Wisdom Web of Things*, Web Information Systems Engineering and Internet Technologies Book Series,
DOI 10.1007/978-3-319-44198-6_4

4.1 Everything Is Alive

We know that computers are getting smaller, cheaper, faster, with lower power requirements, more memory capacity, better connectivity, and are increasingly distributed. Mainframes were bulky centralized computers; desktops distributed computing to the masses; and laptops began the portability revolution that resulted in today's smartphones which you can both talk into and compute with—they know where you are and help you connect to your 1000 closest friends as well as to "the cloud" which can provide a repository of relevant, accessible information, unlimited storage and global connectivity. What is the next paradigm shift in how computing will connect into our lives?

We observe that humans are situation aware. We use our built-in perceptual senses (sight, hearing, taste, smell, and touch) or augmented senses (telescopes, microscopes, remote controls, and many more) to sense, communicate with, and control our world. We can flip channels on the television and quickly identify the kind of show and whether we are interested. We know how to cross the street safely and may know how to cook broccoli casserole or perform a heart operation. We can use language to query, command, and control others. Also, we can quickly recognize common known situations and learn about new situations.

In contrast, until recently and with few exceptions, computers were context unaware and did what they were told. You could take your laptop to a ball game, and it might send and receive email or let you browse the web, but it was unaware of the no-hitter in progress. Similarly, observing a heart operation, a computer would not remind a physician that she left a sponge in the patient. Exceptions are when computers are used in combination with control systems to sense the water level at a dam and open a spillway, or recognize faces in videos, or identify that if you like that movie, you might like others. However, each of these is a brittle instance of being context-aware and is hard to generalize. One of the more important signs of the dawn of a more general kind of situation-aware computing is location awareness, which smartphones have by virtue of on-board GPS and the ability to connect to the cloud to download location-relevant information. Nevertheless, we are in the early stages of computers being able to sense their environment. We lack much of the architecture and service infrastructure we will need to transition computers to become situation aware to a similar extent that humans are.

Imagine if you could talk to any object in your house (e.g., TV, AC, a chair) as if they were alive. What would you like to ask? How would you like them to behave? Perhaps you ask the TV to auto-recommend channels to you after studying your preferences, or the AC to auto-adjust to maximize everyone's comfort in the room, or a chair to auto-configure itself to fit your body. The Everything is Alive (EiA) project at the University of Arkansas is exploring pervasive computing in a future smart, semantic world where every object can have identity and can communicate with humans and other smart objects. In that sense, all objects are context and situation-aware agents. The focus of the project is broad, including the fields of ontology, virtual worlds, smart objects, soft controllers, image recognition, mobile computing, mobile robots, and human workflows. In this chapter, we discuss how those technologies are architected to combine together to build up the future world of EiA.

As Thompson described EiA in 2004 [1], in ancient days, peoples' lives were surrounded by many "living things" including rocks and trees, and many natural "living phenomena" such as wind and rain; people believed spirits resided in things and influenced their life in various ways. Therefore, people tried to understand those "living things" and "living phenomena" and asked how to live with those to maximize the happiness of their lives. With the introduction of science, people developed technology as a means of conquering nature; as a result, we humans became self-centered believing that our intelligence distinguishes us from other things. It is true that peoples' lives became a lot more efficient and convenient. However, count how many physical objects you have in your room. If these were intelligent, imagine how many new services you could access. In EiA, we believe that any of those objects can be "living things" (dynamic, active objects) and any of those services are possibly "living phenomena," as we associate knowledge, action, and rules with those things or services in the world around us. The basic concept of the EiA project might be stated as make everything alive to make our lives richer. We are exploring the architecture to convert a world of ordinary objects into the world of smart semantic objects where everything is alive, can sense, act, think, feel, communicate, and maybe even move and reproduce [1].

Our work contains various aspects that are related to or categorized into Ubiquitous Intelligence, Cyber-Individual, Brain Informatics, and Web Intelligence which combine together to add Intelligence to the *hyper world* where the social world, the physical world, and the virtual world are mixed together [2] as shown in Table 4.1. Within the Ubiquitous Intelligence field of study, one focus of the EiA project is the smart object research that explores and identifies the way to make an object smart based on the protocols it obeys [3]. Similar to the concept of the Internet of Things, we assign unique identity to each object and develop a communicative structure with networking capability. Regarding Cyber-Individual, EiA emphasizes the use of 3D virtual worlds to represent real environments and our individual lives [1]. We build a realistic environment in a virtual world and use it as an environment to simulate and test architectures we developed for the future world of pervasive computing,

Table 4.1 Various aspects in EiA

Ubiquitous intelligence	Brain informatics
• Smart objects • RFID • Spatial searchbot	• Psychological experiment • Biologically-inspired simulation • Interdisciplinary study
Cyber individual	Web intelligence
• 3D modeling • Virtual world • Prototyping	• Ontology service • Dynamic API distribution • Workflow

which includes a spatial search bot [4], soft controllers [5], smart objects [3, 6], and autonomous floor mapping robots [7]. This is significantly different from 3D modeling in that we can include social interactions of people. This type of Cyber-Individual technology can help to develop the concepts and architecture of Ubiquitous Intelligence.

In addition, as a part of the Brain Informatics field of study, we also emphasize the importance of learning from human behavior to build more efficient models. We proposed a new model of object recognition, which was inspired by a study of child language acquisition in developmental psychology [8]. Also, based on a biologically-inspired genetic model of economics, we analyzed effective decision making strategies, which would be important to build up Web Intelligence to distribute services effectively [9]. As the development of Web Intelligence, in terms of the architecture of distribution of services, one of the main foci of EiA is modularity via plugins and services. i.e., the way any agent can dynamically extend or remove their capabilities depending on need [6, 10]. Therefore, our development of Web Intelligence is based on goal-oriented service distribution. Depending on need for a certain goal, Web Intelligence provides appropriate support to our world. This work includes the idea of a soft controller, dynamic interface loading, and ontology services. The challenge for our project is how to efficiently combine those four domains of studies to develop an ultimate architecture for realizing the world of EiA where people, things, and services are synthesized to provide benefits in our lives.

4.1.1 Ubiquitous Intelligence

4.1.1.1 Key Concepts

Ubiquitous Intelligence means that "intelligent things are everywhere" [2]. In other words, it also means "Everything is Alive." It happens when the world is transformed into a smart, semantic world with intelligent objects harmoniously coordinates with each other by utilizing omnipresent sensors. Key challenges include how things are aware of themselves, how to figure out user's need or context, and how to understand common knowledge [2].

Self-awareness is one important concept that makes objects behave more efficiently based on context understanding and on the way others perceive them. For replacement of human language communication, the objects may use a query language that can retrieve and manipulate data. The work of GS [11] divided the smart object as agents into three different levels: owner object, active object, and passive object. They used a refrigerator as an active object, which can read RFID information of objects inside of the refrigerator as passive objects. Both owner object and active object have sets of query languages, and depending on the query sent by the owner object, an active object can send a query to some passive object to meet the goal. This opens a new door to the way people interact with objects. We specify *what* rather than *how* things should be done to accomplish some goals, and the objects coordinate with each other to accomplish the stated goals. For example, people can be anywhere and tell objects in their house to take meat from a freezer to defrost before they get home and start cooking. The freezer figures out what types of meat are available and takes out an appropriate one. The smartphone, freezer, and meat act as owner, active, and passive objects, respectively.

4.1.1.2 Ubiquitous Intelligence in EiA

In our EiA project, one important question is what it is about objects that makes them smart and how we can create a world for them. In order to answer the question, we identified protocols that can be added to an ordinary object to transform it into a smart(er) object. Example protocols are explicit identity, message-based communication, API, plug-in behaviors, security, associated 3D models and ontologies, and others.

To demonstrate these ideas, Eguchi and Thompson [3] developed a demonstration in a virtual world, Second Life, on University of Arkansas island of a baby mannequin that nurses can use to learn how to help infants who need special care. Such babies stay in warming beds with several smart features. We visited our School of Nursing, modeled an infant bed, and created scripts to operate the bed (Fig. 4.1). By itself, that was not our main contribution, it just set the stage to understand smart objects. In order to understand how to create "smart objects," we associated application program interfaces (APIs) with objects and then added the ability to discover the API of smart objects nearby. Then, when a remote control device, which we term a soft controller since it is a programmable remote (e.g., a smartphone), is near those objects, it "discovers" the API and imports it to a display so that the object can be operated by remote control. This works with all objects that follow the API discovery protocol. We also identified several other protocols that make an object smart or rather smarter [3].

We described how to do this in the real world using RFID and smartphones but demonstrate this using 3D virtual worlds where an avatar passing by smart objects can

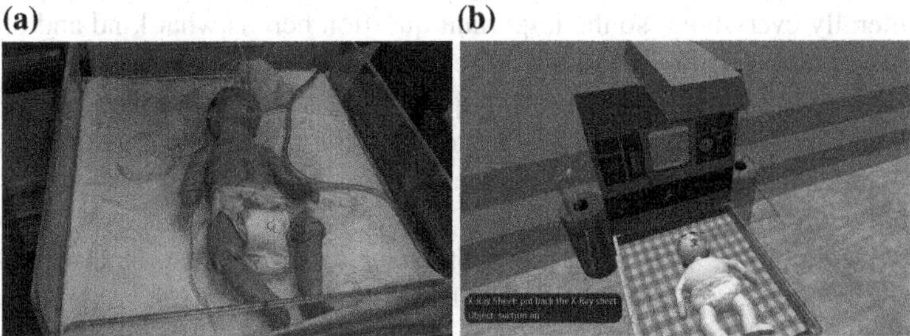

Fig. 4.1 **a** Baby mannequin in a bed that is actually used in a nursing school; **b** the model of the baby mannequin in Second Life

use a universal remote (which is a smartphone in the real world) to read an object's API and control the object. We first used 3D virtual worlds to demonstrate and explore such protocols [3], and then translated these protocols to the real world [6].

Our next challenge was to give stronger context inference ability based on relationships between other objects. Eno and Thompson [4, 12] built an avatarbot that autonomously roams around the virtual world to collect information of objects, similar to a searchbot in the web. Based on the spatial relationship and semantic relationship of meta-data retrieved, they successfully inferred names of unlabeled objects. We believe with the increasing number of smartphones, in the future, each person can be a "searchbot": by walking around the world with smartphones, everyone can contribute to gather the knowledge in Ubiquitous Intelligence via crowdsourcing and sharing the results.

In the EiA project, we first recognize that everything can be associated with intelligence by providing unique identity for each object and event. People can use the identity of an object of interest to retrieve associated knowledge or possible commands to control the object. In addition, our searchbot collects such identities distributed in a space. However, one important focus of W2T is a circular flow of data. Even though this architecture may satisfy people's intellectual curiosities by providing more knowledge about objects around in the world, the data flow eventually stops by achieving the goal.

4.1.2 Cyber-Individual

4.1.2.1 Key Concepts

Cyber-Individual is a term that refers to a real individual's counterpart in a virtual space. The main idea of this research is to virtually place humans in the center of the world with Ubiquitous Intelligence [13]. Using a user's preference list, Lertlakkhanakul and Choi [14] showed how to coordinate smart objects (e.g., AC, sofa, light, and TV) to make the environment most enjoyable for the user. Although Cyber-Individual ideally contains a full description of an individual, it is not possible to reflect literally everything, so the important question here is what kind and how to represent descriptions of individuals. Wen et al. [15] divided the set of descriptions of an individual into two: descriptions that require instant refresh such as psychological emotion and physical status, and descriptions that require gradual updates such as social relationships, experience, and personality. This kind of classification is important to build a realistic Cyber-individual. Commercial concerns make use of Cyber-individual technology: Acxiom Corporation collects information on individuals and uses a product called Personicx Lifetime [16, 17] that clusters U.S. households into one of 70 segments within 21 life-stage groups based on consumer-specific behavior and demographic characteristics.

Another area related to Cyber-Individual is mirror world research [18]. The concept of a mirror world is to synchronize any activity, environment, and interactions between the real and virtual worlds. Various types of sensing technology help to build models of the real world in a virtual world, and Ubiquitous Intelligence adds additional information of object, people, and places in the world. However, the other way around to reflect the change in the virtual world to the same change in a real world had been a big challenge. Fortunately, with recent technology of Augmented Reality, those two worlds are starting to be merged together [19].

Therefore, we can assume that a Cyber-Individual can represent an individual in a real world more accurately, both physically and socially. Based on the analysis over interactions in this virtual world, we may see similar results from what we expect in a real world. This field of study brought us a new means of freely simulating our life.

4.1.2.2 Cyber-Individual in EiA

EiA emphasizes the use of 3D virtual worlds as a mean of prototyping pervasive computing architectures, assuming the virtual world is a suitable surrogate representation of our physical and social world. Each person in the virtual world platform Second Life has an associated avatar. The avatar can interact with other objects: get information from and control other objects. One challenge in the past is how to link an individual in the real world with his/her counterpart in the virtual world. There are two problems to deal with: complexity and time consumption of life-like modeling of humans or things; and spatial, temporal, and social tracking of individuals.

Recent advances in research are promising keys to solving these two problems. With the creation of Microsoft Kinect, we now have easy access to real-time and life-like 3D modeling of objects in the real world [8] (Fig. 4.2a). Given the complexity of modeling objects in 3D and the diversity of objects surrounding us, this new technology enables a normal person to not only model nearby things but also the individual. Then, to link the 3D models with their counterparts in the real world, we can use RFID to tag and link objects between the two worlds. One disadvantage of this method is that we cannot track the objects in space or time. We can only identify the object. However, since most objects in the real world are static and

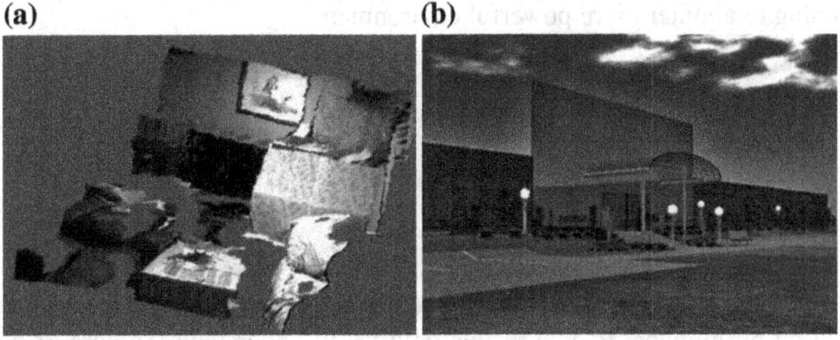

Fig. 4.2 **a** 3D reconfiguration with Kinect; **b** hospital in Second Life island of University of Arkansas

sometimes immovable: TV's, refrigerators, lights, etc., identities of the object are enough for us to interact intelligently with them [6]. As for human individuals, identity is not enough, especially if we want to model interactions between human and objects or even just between humans. Fortunately, with smartphones becoming a commodity, we can track individuals not only in space and time, but also their social interactions [20].

These leaps in technology enable us to view the real world as a very high definition 3D virtual world that can be modeled by 3D virtual worlds that strongly resemble the real world both graphically and socially (Fig. 4.2b). Nevertheless, we cannot represent everything in the virtual world, but we do not think that would be a problem. The question is what kind and how much information we need to make everyday decisions like making coffee, playing chess with friends, etc. We do not need molecular level precise replicas of our world, and the growing information we can extract from the real world with current technology is already sufficient to make an increasing number of decisions in our daily life.

Currently in the real world, most objects are passive and not very smart. However, in 3D virtual worlds, objects can have associated behaviors (scripts). A virtual world such as Second Life or Unity can be used to represent the semantics of the real world since all objects are provided with unique ID, i.e., every object has a built-in identity. Additionally, in virtual worlds, we can easily track xyz coordinates of every object, experience simple physics, and interact with other people as in a real world. Therefore, we see virtual worlds as a powerful environment to test new programs and architectures that will build Ubiquitous Intelligence. Thus, many of our results can be applied no matter whether we are connected to the real world or one of the virtual worlds. The Cyber-Individual concept is not just a suitable representation of our everyday life but also as a reasonable way to understand our own social interactions, both with other people and with objects surrounding us.

However, at the same time, Perkins [21] pointed out two areas for improvement in the current model of virtual worlds: the security issue of communication in the world and the need for better methods to communicate with external servers. Nguyen and Eguchi [6, 7] also discussed several problems with using Second Life in the development of autonomous floor mapping robot. However, these problems are specific only to the virtual world Second Life and can be solved by extending its capabilities or switching to another more powerful environment.

4.1.3 Brain Informatics

4.1.3.1 Key Concepts

Brain informatics is the interdisciplinary field of study that focuses on actual mechanisms used by humans. People in this field try to understand the core of human intelligence to offset the disadvantages of dependence upon logic-based inference by introducing many different perspectives such as biology, psychology, cognitive science, neuroscience, etc. [2, 22].

While object recognition is an actively investigated field of studies in computer science, physiological evidence show that the primate ventral visual pathway develops neurons that respond to particular objects or faces independently of their position, size or orientation, which seem to responsible for recognitions of transform-invariant visual objects and faces [23–25]. Over the past twenty years, Oxford Centre for Theoretical Neuroscience and Artificial Intelligence has investigated a range of problems in this field by developing a biologically plausible simulation model of the primate ventral visual pathway. This model has solved problems like invariant object recognition [26], segmentation of simultaneously presented objects [27], and human body segmentation based on motion [28]. Additionally, this model is able to learn separate representations of different visual spaces such as identity and expression from the same input [29].

In addition to the detailed investigations of actual mechanisms of our brains, Brain Informatics also includes human's behaviors, which are controlled by the brain. One interesting example is Roy's project [30] to solve the puzzle of children's language acquisition. He set video cameras on the ceilings of every room in his house and recorded two full years of his son's growth, which can be reconstructed with 3D models to later analyze any moment of time with video image and sound. Based on the detailed analysis of the data, his group found a tendency of caregivers to adjust the way they speak to a child, which resulted in a significant impact on his child's words learning process. This experiment provided not only keys to solve the word acquisition problem but also insights to many other related areas such as action segmentation [31] and social interaction [32].

Furthermore, the interdisciplinary field called neuro-economics has been growing recently [33]. In traditional economics, the researchers have often assumed that our behaviors of choices follow a simple principle of utility maximization, which assumes that our choices simply reflect the values assigned to different options [34]. In other words, they tended to think our choices and preferences are synonymous. However, as the preferences are in reality dynamic and flexible, this theory cannot oftentimes explain many of our decision making behaviors which are strongly influenced by other instances such as status quo bias and addiction. Accordingly, rather than exploring such hard-coded formula for our decision-making behaviors, it is more reasonable to investigate the black-box of which the decisions are made in our brain [35]. For example, decades of study on the brain region called Orbitofrontal cortex (OFC) have shown to encode reward value of stimuli [36, 37]. Interestingly, this representation is influenced not only by the value of stimuli itself but also by the context and other goal-oriented information, which makes the representation of preferences more flexible [38]. This physiological evidence should provide a better understanding of our brain to actually make decisions.

These works indicate that Brain Informatics can help solve current technical problems with insights to humans' behaviors, without which it might be prone to errors or impossible to solve.

4.1.3.2 Brain Informatics in EiA

One important characteristic of the EiA project is that the system includes not only smart objects but also humans or humans represented by their avatars in a virtual world. Therefore, in order to develop the communication between humans and objects, the field of Brain Informatics becomes important. One important fact that we cannot disregard is that the change in humans' psychological behavior in a computer mediated communication (CMC) setting. Experimental data collected by Eguchi and Bohannan [39] showed that Americans with their use of web-cam in CMC decreased both personal identity (self-perception of their uniqueness) and social identity (self-perception of their belongingness), which may be explained by a significantly increased feeling of anonymity. This study indicated that even if the Cyber-Individual accurately mirrors individuals, there will still remain strong psychological differences between communication in a real world and in a virtual world.

Brain Informatics can also enhance learning ability of computer program, specifically object recognition. A traditional object recognition model is usually focused on the shape of the objects, but it was challenging to distinguish two very different objects whose shapes are very similar to each other (deodorant spray can and insecticide spray can), or two differently shaped objects which perform essentially the same function (a normal chair and an oddly shaped chair). To solve this problem, Eguchi [8] focused on the mechanism that human children actually use to learn names of objects from the field of developmental psychology. Using Microsoft Kinect and machine learning techniques, he developed a new method to recognize an object based not only on its shape but also on its function in the same manner children actually do [40, 41] and showed how an insight into humans' mental capability helps improve current techniques which solely rely on machines (Fig. 4.3).

Furthermore, Eguchi and his colleagues have recently started developing biologically accurate computational models of early visual processing of primates' visual pathway [42–44]. This is a beginning of a step towards a convergence between the fields of computational neuroscience and artificial neural networks (ANNs). While computational neuroscience has traditionally attempted to understand neu-

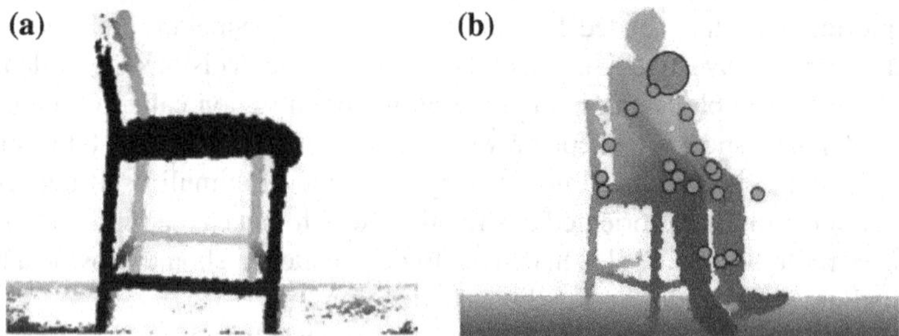

Fig. 4.3 Object recognition inspired by developmental psychology; **a** shape learning; **b** function learning

ronal dynamics by building models from the bottom-up, ANNs have stressed a goal-oriented top-down approach. In this way, we can investigate more efficient mechanisms.

Problems of the study in Brain Informatics, especially when focusing on functions of brain, is a need for the expensive facilities like fMRI and various issues to be addressed in order to use actual human subjects in the research. In the EiA project, we collaborate with researchers in the field of Psychology so that we can pursue our main goal of EiA which is to make everything alive to make our lives richer. Without a deeper understanding of ourselves, we may be able to make everything alive, but cannot *enrich* our lives. Our interdisciplinary study over humans provides a path to accomplish this.

4.1.4 Web Intelligence

4.1.4.1 Key Concepts

So far, this chapter has discussed the way to collect knowledge through Ubiquitous Intelligence, Cyber-Individual, and Brain Informatics to form the data cycle in W2T. Web Intelligence is the essential concept that provides the way to efficiently make use of the knowledge. Web Intelligence is the concept that focuses on the Artificial Intelligence and Information Technology aspect at the development of Web information systems [13]. Web Intelligence possibly realizes self-organizing servers to automatically and efficiently match up individual needs and services. The server can be seen as an agent that can dynamically adjust the behavior. Additionally, based on various streams of knowledge fed into the database, Web Intelligence is eventually able to provide people wisdom [45]. This research focuses on the new Web-based technology to process vast amount of information available in our world to provide people a better way of living, working, and learning. The challenges include design of goal-directed service, personalization feature, semantics, and feedback [2].

One example is the automated renewable home energy management system [46]. The system monitors daily energy consumption of a house and provides helpful recommendations to the owner via Internet. The provided information includes early warnings of low energy, task rescheduling suggestions, and tips for energy conservation that minimally affect our lives.

Based on data collected, Web Intelligence extracts knowledge and refines it to wisdom, and people will benefit from the services providing this new wisdom.

4.1.4.2 Web Intelligence in EiA

One of our main foci in Web intelligence is the ontology problem. Humans can tell the difference between a door and a castle; however, real world objects are not labeled with explicit identities, types, locations, or ownership [47]. 3D virtual worlds provide explicit identities, locations, and ownership, but names for object types are often not provided based on the analysis of collected data [4]. To build a smart, semantic world where every object is labeled and associated with knowledge, we need some way of associating information.

Like the semantic web [48], semantic worlds involve annotating things with metadata (types, super-types, API, attributes, costs, owners, locations, etc.). In the EiA project, Eno and Thompson [4] developed two ontology services, one that takes Second Life labels, looks them up in the WordNet ontology, and then overlays them with metadata from WordNet [49]. The other is an annotation service that depends on crowd sourcing so that any user can add metadata to any object. This service provides the computer a way to infer the type of an object even if that object is not labeled explicitly with identity. This information would help the unknown object to be aware of its identity or role based on the environment it is in and would also help other objects to establish appropriate relationship with the unknown object. This ontology service could operate platform-agnostic, no matter whether it is connected to the real or any particular virtual world. Even though their implementation operates in Second Life environment, with RFID and smartphones, we can do this in the real world in the same manner. This ontology service is a step towards context-aware applications.

Suppose we can correctly identify each object by the use of some means like RFID, object recognition, and ontology service; then the next challenge is how to distribute goal-directed services. This is where the smart objects and soft controller architecture discussed in Ubiquitous Intelligence plays a role [3, 5]. Whenever an active smart object like a controller detects identity of other smart object, it sends a query against a remote database, probably located in "the cloud," to see if any related information is available. The information can be the history of the object, API to control the object, owner information, and so on. An actual implementation of this architecture in the real world is presented in [6]. The model we developed can deal with the plural reference problem; i.e., differentiation between the command to turn off a single light and a command to turn off all the lights in this room. Future work will deal with business rules of smart objects like how an iPod and a speaker can be used together based on logic inference.

Additionally, Eguchi and Nguyen [9] discovered a challenge in the development of a Web Intelligence service based on centralized cloud knowledge. If people are trying to maximize their profits among limited resources, there are always winners and losers, the consequence of the zero-sum game. In the extreme case, the seemingly best choice based on shared knowledge actually becomes the worst since it will be used most often. Suppose there is a web service to provide traffic information based on users' report. If many people use the web service and choose the same least crowded route at the same time, that route suddenly becomes overcrowded, and the route Web Intelligence provided becomes worthless. Using a biologically-inspired genetic algorithm in a context of minority game, we determined the pattern of cooperation over limited resources. The result indicated that people's accuracy of the report to build the centralized knowledge and the tendency of users to follow the centralized knowledge may play key roles in the context. Therefore, it is important to take those findings into account to build a future Web Intelligence.

4.2 Implementing the Wisdom Web of Things

The challenge of our EiA project is how the various architectures we developed will be integrated into one unified concept of EiA. Zhong et al. [2] describe the data cycle for Wisdom Web of Things as composed of the following steps:

- Things to data
- Data to information
- Information to knowledge
- Knowledge to wisdom
- Wisdom to services
- Services to humans
- Humans to things

shown graphically in Fig. 4.4.

In this section, we describe how to realize the data cycle with the current technology discussed in the previous section; and we identify open research issues related to internal computer representations needed to model real or virtual worlds. We also consider how we can use those representations to generate visualizations in a virtual

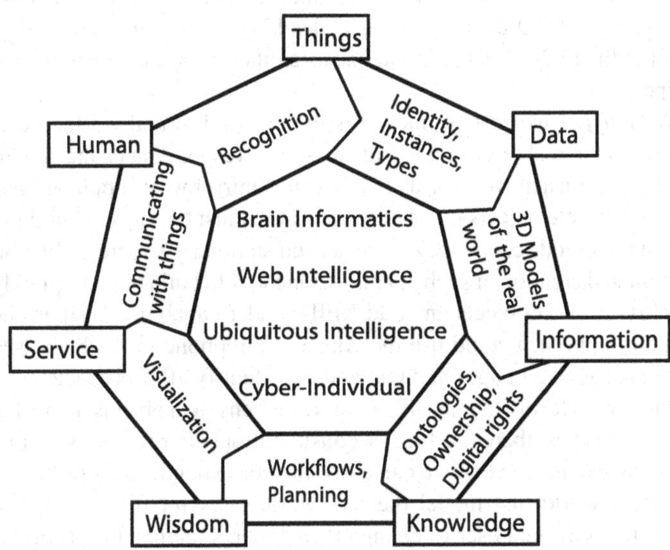

Fig. 4.4 Data cycle in EiA and W2T

world and also how we can “parse” the real world to recognize and record these data structures.

4.2.1 From Things to Data: Identity, Instances, Types

How can we associate symbolic names with subkinds of physical objects? Entity identity is at the heart of identity management technologies [50] that are used in the real world to track humans, animals, products, medical supplies, inventory, and other “things” throughout their supply chain or life cycle [5]. Virtual worlds like Second Life and Unity provide ways to create virtual instances of things from a prototype. For example, a virtual world user can design a Maserati and then create (by copying the model) as many instances as they wish. The Maserati and the behavioral scripts that implement its function in the model can be separately owned by the model’s creator and granted to third parties by a variant of digital rights management that enables granting rights to create, modify, or copy objects. However, a challenge is that in the real worlds, chairs are not labeled with the type chair and the same is true in virtual worlds. Although it is possible to label objects in these virtual worlds with text strings like “chair,” most users do not bother to do so. As yet, there is no real notion of strong typing in either real or virtual worlds.

Instead, in both, users use their brain’s ability to recognize objects in order to recognize and name them. Earlier, we indicated we’d developed an annotation mechanism so that third parties in a virtual world could identify or provide explicit associations of types for objects. In the real world, one way to do this is to attach identifiers to each thing, e.g., RFID tags [3] or bar codes [51]. Identifying objects by type is useful in either the real or virtual world because other information can be associated with the type.

In the W2T *hyper world* that integrates the real and virtual world, we can then make changes in the real or virtual world and see corresponding changes in the other world, which we term a mirror world [18]. For such mirror world applications, having 3D models of concrete objects is not enough. There must be ways to build models of places. Manual methods can work for places and stationary structures like buildings through automated creation of such 3D maps. One way to build models quickly would be to put RFID tags on objects and add RFID reader capability to smartphones. A complementary approach could use the Amazon Firephone [52] which uses image processing to recognize images and text and can identify 70M products.

Above the lowest level of being able to represent physical objects in virtual worlds via graphics and types, there are further considerations. For real-world objects like thermostats that can have APIs, we can associate corresponding script-based behaviors in a virtual world that model the real world behavior [6]. Smartphone apps already exist that enable a user to change their home’s temperature from any location. Such mirror world mappings can be sparse or dense depending on the ability to connect updates in one world to the other. Still, even passive objects can have APIs which could enable querying objects for information, e.g., *chair: tell me your color or how to repair you*. It also appears that physical objects can have associated plug-in behaviors like a history plug-in that records state changes in an object's history (*thermostat: what was the temperature on June 10, 2013 at 9am?*) or a scheduling plug-in that schedules the thermostat for different temperature ranges on different days and times of day. Many kinds of objects could have history, scheduling, or other kinds of plug-in behaviors.

In a world of smart objects (smart networked devices) as described above, there is a need for inter-object communication. Objects can send each other messages in a direct analog to object-oriented programming except that all the devices are distributed in a wide area network and may become unavailable (e.g., out of range). However, there is also a need to specify rules that control suites of objects as if they are one object. A familiar case is home entertainment components that can be controlled by today's programmable Harmony remotes [53]. A generalization would allow a user to build a condition-action rule like: *IF (the yard sensor indicates 'dry') AND (the web weather service indicates 'no rain'*) *THEN (turn on the yard's sprinkler system*). Similarly, it will be convenient to use plurals in rules like: Turn off the lights in the living room.

In short, in the phase of things to data, various data are collected from the real world using sensors [2]. An object in the real world is represented by its unique ID in the virtual world. This ID can be given to the objects using RFID tags by their manufacturers (or by other means, e.g., biometric, visual). In addition, the shapes of objects and their locations can be updated using both GPS and RFID tags. Societal higher level issues remain ahead, especially those dealing with security, e.g., who has access to your home's virtual model and how can you protect it from intruders? Security and privacy are covered in more detail below.

4.2.2 From Data to Information: 3D Models of the Real World

Then, data collected undergoes "cleaning, integration, and storage" [2]. For location and distance, the data can be a 3D vector describing the translation of object in 3D from some origin, either globally across different environments and domains or locally within a specific environment such as the coordinate system in Second Life. Data collected by sensors like mouse and IR sensor build a map of the environment [7].

Following the previous step discussed in Sect. 2.1, every smartphone user becomes a search spider with a record of what objects their phone identified at what locations. Crowd sourcing (since most people have a smartphone) can then keep the "map" of the objects in the world up to date. However, the issue is that RFID alone does not provide precise locations so this would provide a useful but coarse map. Also, GPS works out of doors but other means like Real Time Location Services [54] or image understanding would be needed for interior spaces.

In our autonomous floor mapping robot project, more accurate 2D maps were generated by an autonomous robot that was embedded with a computer mouse to track a floor and an IR sensor to recognize shapes of the surrounding environment [7]. The project utilized two virtual environments, Simbad and Second Life, and a real robot to develop a new algorithm for floor mapping. This abstraction of software and hardware sped up the development. The abstraction of software simulator and hardware implementation can be regarded as the abstraction of the virtual and real worlds. Thus, the technique can also be applied to the development process of W2T [6].

First, the distance data between the robot and any obstacle in the environment is collected by an IR sensor. This data is then integrated into a map stored in memory, which is expanded as the robot acquires more data. Based on the knowledge from the partial map, the robot knows where it has already explored and determines where to map next. The map can be re-used by other autonomous agents to plan the most efficient path to reach a specific location in the map. Since the mapping robot can roam in an unknown environment, we can add an RFID reader located on top to discover objects' locations and label them in the map. Such a map can update the new location of mobile objects, for example, to help a nurse find a wheel chair in a hospital or to help find your glasses or car keys at home.

However, the question is how close we are to being able to build 3D (static) models of real world places and things? The macroscopic physical real world that humans inhabit can be statically represented as a collection of observables, concrete nouns representing terraformed terrain and objects. Populating the landscape are buildings, roads, rivers, vegetation, and man-made structures as well as vehicles, equipment, expendables like food, and also avatars. Interestingly, 3D virtual worlds and other 3D representations can reasonably represent these noun-ish things with at least cartoonish veracity so that a human can recognize the objects in a scene [55]. Tools like Second Life's prim representation, AutoCAD models, or standards like COLLADA can represent equipment with the precision needed to build the real-world equivalent. What that means is that we have sufficient 3D world representations to build a first approximation of the real world in virtual worlds. The field of graphics is rapidly providing improved realism via illumination models, etc. Similarly, the gaming industry is constantly providing better, more realistic physics models so that e.g., a non-player character's cloak moves naturally when she walks. Nonetheless, it is still difficult to combine graphics data from many data sources into a common 3D representation.

Williams [56] imported a 3D map into the game engine Unity, which provided a contour map and ground use coloration, so roads, buildings, and vegetation were visible. He added buildings as sugar cubes. However, all this was not trivial because representations of contour data, land use data, architectural models, equipment models and avatars often use incompatible representations. This seems an easy problem to fix, a small matter of getting many communities to rationalize graphics representations. In the ideal, it would then be easy to rapidly build representations of real-world places just by assembling existing model data from the various data sources. More work is needed in this area to make these various graphics representations compatible. Additional work is needed to scale representations to cover significant areas in the world, though models of cities now exist, some using the OpenGIS community's CityGML standard [57].

Consider just product data which would be needed to populate the interior of buildings. At present, every retail website commonly provides 2D images of products. However, they do not yet provide 3D models of data. If, when we purchased an item at a retailer, a compatible 3D model of the items was available for addition into our virtual model of our home, school, or office, then populating the 3D virtual model would become immediately more scalable, which would accelerate the technology of this step of data to information in W2T.

4.2.3 From Information to Knowledge: Ontologies, Ownership, and Digital Rights

The step of information to knowledge is to fit data into some known models in order to gain further insights [2]. For example, based on map and mouse tracking information, an object can locate itself [7]; furthermore, an ontology service can provide knowledge of the name of an object based on relational inference [4].

In artificial intelligence, the term ontology is used to describe a type-based classification system for a wide range of real world objects, e.g., kinds of amphibians. Functionally, an ontology is more than just standardized vocabulary but also includes interrelationships among concepts in a specific domain, providing a computational representation of domain knowledge. Ontologies are being used in business applications. For instance, in a "big data" industrial workflow, Phillips et al. [58] used ontologies to define a type system that was then used to recognize the format and content of files in a known domain but with unknown detailed structure and content to automatically determine a file's layout, which before required manual characterization by human operators. Similarly, Deneke [59] developed a declarative language to automate the composition of data processing workflows, making use of semantic annotations for expressing characteristics of the base workflow elements: data fields and operators. These annotations, drawn from a domain's ontology, provided the foundation of a domain-specific model that, once populated, establishes mappings between high-level business objectives and low-level workflow specifications.

In the context of widely used ontologies with broad coverage, DBpedia is a crowdsourced project aimed at extracting structured ontology information from Wikipedia [60]. *Linked data* is a mechanism for representing and publishing on the web the interlinkages between data from different data sources [61]. Also, as mentioned in Sect. 1.4.2, another widely used ontology is WordNet, which was developed at Princeton [49]. WordNet provides a word-concept ontology comparable to a dictionary. However, not covered by WordNet, humans can recognize and differentiate subtypes of objects below the level of word concepts, i.e., at the stock keeping unit

(SKU) level. Sangameswaran [62] used a specialized web search engine to build product ontologies for major retailers.

A virtual model of the world would require geographic and land use data, flora and fauna representations, building representations, but also representations of concrete nouns that represent commercial objects, e.g., products. For product data, one of the standards being developed is the universal Electronic Product Code (EPC). Similar to barcode, EPC enables product identification and naming among different vendors. Unlike barcode, EPC uses RFID tags to identify and track objects [63]. Nevertheless, EPC alone does not present an object's properties or its services or how to use them. However, if we combine EPC with OWL-S, which is "a standard ontology, consisting of a set of basic classes and properties, for declaring and describing services" which "enable[s] users and software agents to automatically discover, invoke, compose, and monitor Web resources offering services, under specified constraints" [64], we can have both a universal and easy way to identify smart objects, and the semantics necessary to describe them in such a way that an even smarter soft controller can automatically utilize.

EPC product data provides a way to uniquely identify individual kinds and instances of products but not product properties. A retailer like Wal-Mart might sell dozens of kinds of chairs, all with different technical specifications and prices and customers comment on these to provide various kinds of evaluations. As mentioned, we are currently investigating [47, 62] how to mine retail websites for descriptive product ontology information. It seems likely that different organizations could provide local ontologies so that, when you enter a store, you can access that store's ontology (inventory including location within the store). We believe ontology services that are situated "in the cloud" can contain most or all of the ontology content (as opposed to the things themselves providing that content). The ontology service(s) would combine with the 3D product models from the previous section to make it easier to populate 3D virtual worlds that model real places, real things, and open-ended content related to those things.

Ontology associations will also be useful to describe typical or expected elements related to a thing: a kitchen often contains a stove, refrigerator, range, sink, counter tops, and cupboards; an office contains desk, chair, white board, books, papers, and so on. These associations would help computers with default reasoning about human activities. Some of these kinds of associations can be recovered from nearness associations derived from virtual world data as described in [4, 12] and potentially also from Google-scale text analysis.

The Internet of (noun-ish) Things will eventually require ontologies (knowledge representations) that cover the types and instances of things that we want to communicate about. At the same time, humans use verbs to communicate about behaviors related to things so a behavioral ontology is as important as the noun-ish ontology. In cooking, boiling water and boiling an egg have related but differing workflows. Object-oriented representations treating boiling as a method for objects water and egg with a differing definition seem to be helpful in explaining this polymorphism.

Representations of objects and behaviors are not enough. We also need to overlay ownership concepts so we can identify digital rights related to who has the right to perform certain actions on certain things. Database systems already provide digital rights that enable specifications to the enable certain users to perform certain operations (e.g., create, insert, delete) on certain objects (e.g., tables, columns) and also a language for granting rights owned by one user to other users. Digital rights management extends this idea to arbitrary operations on typed objects. In addition to role-based access control (e.g., [65, 66]), there are several digital rights expression languages (e.g., XRML [67], ODML [68]).

The value of such access rights representations is the precise control of who can do what operations to what objects. Humans learn legal and politeness rules that prevent A from taking B's things. In the digital environment, in 3D virtual worlds, we come closest to seeing how rights management can work (and some of the associated problems). For instance, in Second Life, a popular 3D virtual world platform, each object or part of an object) can be acted on by scripts. Digital rights control granting rights on scripts to others. The rights to operate or copy a digital object are enforced by the virtual world system. While precise, the rights systems are not without some problems. Second Life users often build interesting objects and transfer them to others but fail to "unlock" some rights making the objects less useful to the receiving party.

Transferring this idea to the Internet of Things and the Wisdom Web of Things will create similar problems. A future smart gun might only fire if the owners biometric password is available, which is a good thing when protecting the gun from children or other unauthorized users but the gun might become unusable if the original owner never grants rights to successor owners or the context of use changes. More flexibility may be needed in future rights management schemes.

4.2.4 From Knowledge to Wisdom: Workflows and Planning

While concrete nouns and 3D models of things provide a static model of the world, that is not enough since the real world and 3D virtual worlds both change. Physical or virtual objects move from place to place; they receive and send communications and messages that change their internal, location, or ownership state. Therefore, it is important to investigate the concept of workflows and planning in order to turn the set of knowledge developed into wisdom.

In natural languages, action verbs are effectively operators that convey a command or description of a state change. More than that, an individual action is commonly part of a larger "workflow" or collection of actions, also associated with an action verb, and similarly the verb itself may be broken into finer grain actions. Thus, we can see getting dressed in the morning (called an "activity of daily living" by the healthcare community [58]) is part of a workflow that at a higher level involves getting ready for the day (which might have other steps like eating breakfast), and getting dressed is implemented by lower level actions like putting on your socks and shoes. WordNet ontologies provide word-concepts for action verbs, but in a similar way in which WordNet nouns like chair did not cover a retail store's SKU level of detail; action verbs record only one level of abstraction and do not provide enough information to recognize real world workflows. For example, in a recipe for mashed potatoes, the step of boiling the potatoes involves lower level steps of peeling the potatoes, filling a pan with water, putting them on the stove, turning on the burner, etc. For computers to gain an understanding of situations, they need to be able to observe detailed state changes and map those into higher level operations.

This kind of knowledge has not yet been collected or encoded in a general manner but there are important special cases that involving keeping a trace of events of certain types and analyzing them. For instance, logistics providers track locations of things like trucks or cargo and analyze the location log for opportunities to improve routes. Similarly, logs of household use of electricity can be analyzed and optimized. Other examples are budget logs, reviewing a stock portfolio, reviewing a patient's medical history, and the practice of keeping TO DO lists.

In the Artificial Intelligence community in the 1970s, Sacerdoti [69] recognized the hierarchical abstractions in workflows, and Schank and Abelson [70] explored scripts as a representation for common repeated connecting event sequences that make up much of our lives. Since that time, the concept of workflow has evolved and there are now standards that describe business process modeling (see the Workflow Reference Model by the Workflow Management Coalition [71], and later workflow standards BPEL [72] and XPDL [73]). While there is considerable work in using these workflow modeling languages to model certain business processes, there is little work in modeling everyday human workflows, e.g., getting ready for the day, driving to work, going shopping, cooking, dating, going to class, etc., the routine activities of life. That is, there is an open research area that involves collecting workflows that "cover" common human experiences. At present, we do not know how many workflows cover a kind of situation, how many situations cover a human life, or how to delimit, partition and compose workflows.

Nonetheless, workflows appear to be useful. Entity and workflow internal representations provide models of state and action. Internal representations of workflows can be used for several purposes:

- Internal representations can be used to record events in a log as a kind of memory of past states.
- The event log can be queried to recall specific events or mined to find patterns of behavior.
- A logged event in the interior of a workflow can be used to suggest and help recognize what large events it is part of and also to predict future events (e.g., you are eating a burger at a fast food restaurant and the workflow predicts you are expected to leave when you are done) [74]. In the same way, workflows can be used to fill in the gaps with default events that were not explicitly observed.
- Subevents in a workflow can be grouped together into high level events. For instance, putting on your socks and shoes is part of getting dressed is part of getting ready for the day which may also involve eating breakfast. Events above and below respectively provide the why and how for a give event.

- The event log may contain events that are not part of a given workflow because they are parts of other workflows and just happen to be interleaved with the present workflow. For instance, if a cardiologist discusses golf while operating on a patient, the golf discussion is unrelated to the patient operation workflow but is an interleaved event.

For instance, in one of our projects, we used kitchen recipes represented in XML as a simple internal representation. It is straightforward to represent a given recipe in XML Schema [75] and to represent several instances of using that recipe (and others) in a list of already executed recipes in XML. It is easy to find individual recipes using XQuery [76], to find lists of ingredients or all recipes that use chicken as an ingredient, or the sub-steps for boiling potatoes (putting water in a pan, peeling the potatoes, etc.). Recipe world is dense with thousands of workflows (recipes). Zeineldin [77] considered shopping and found that domain less complex, dependent on a path planner but fairly simple in the kinds of workflows involved (e.g., browsing for purchases; trying on clothing; waiting if the waiting room is occupied, carrying clothes to checkout; making the purchase, and leaving the store).

How we should represent human workflows is still an open research question. For instance, a physician learns the workflow to operate on a patient. All sorts of exceptional conditions can occur like cutting an artery or dropping the scalpel, and the physician must know how to handle these. Are these exceptions annotations on a workflow, other workflows, or rarely taken paths in a main workflow? Full-blown workflows are not the whole story: humans have to be able to learn new workflows that are already known by others; they need to be able to learn the variety of exceptions that can occur through experimentation; and they have to be able to evolve new workflows that never before existed. That is, beyond large learned workflows, humans have the ability to reason, infer, and plan. Planning involves searching a search space for solutions. The solutions are goal trees that solve problems; in short, they are new workflow instances. Therefore, it appears that humans can construct generalized workflows from previously successful workflow instances and can also modify workflows on the fly (that is, re-plan) when workflow exceptions occur, and we believe this is a key process required for the transition from knowledge to wisdom in W2T cycle.

4.2.5 From Wisdom to Service: Visualization

The W2T can "provide active, transparent, safe, and reliable services by synthetically utilizing the data, information, and knowledge in the data center" [2]. The wisdom synthesized from the previous phase can be converted or combined together into services readily available to whoever needs them. For example, house temperature sensors, AC/heaters, a person's temperature readings, his/her location, and perhaps his/her preference of temperature can be used to find the balance between a person's comfort and energy consumption. The wisdom of efficient decision making strategies

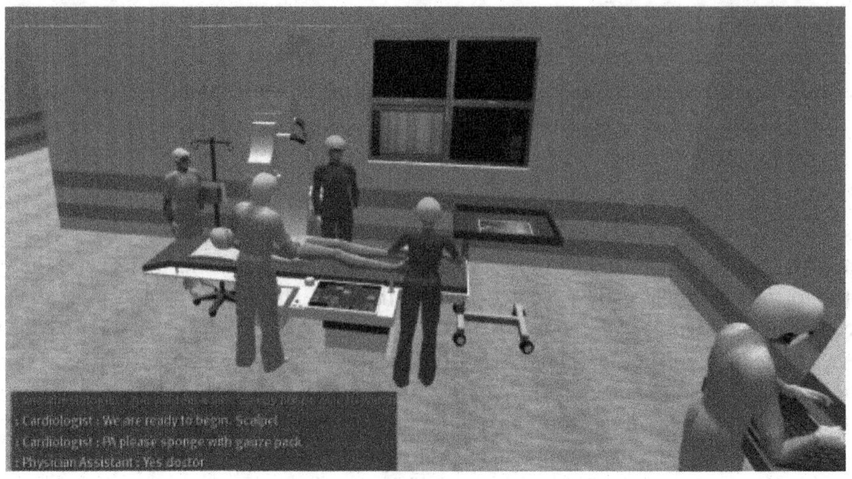
: Cardiologist : We are ready to begin. Scalpel
: Cardiologist : PA please sponge with gauze pack
: Physician Assistant : Yes doctor

Fig. 4.5 Heart catheterization operation demonstration

learned from human behavior will be an important key for developing the service as well [9].

Assuming we had a good representation for human workflows, another important use for the representation would be to visualize it. One way to do this is to graphically display the interplay of avatars and smart objects in a virtual world. Perkins [21, 78, 79] used a Petri Net representation of work flows internally and associated with every state transition a Lua script [80] to display a primitive action animation. A "Catheterization Lab Demo" [81] displays the result (see Figs. 4.5 and 4.6). Zeineldin [77] provided a similar workflow visualization for retail sales and others provided workflow visualizations of a restaurant and Shakespeare's Romeo and Juliet balcony scene. In each case, a scene was constructed in a virtual world, complete with scenery (topography, buildings) and props (objects) and avatar-bots (avatars controlled by a program) were programmed to execute the workflow steps. Primitive workflow steps included simple animations and chats (typed or spoken "strings" and various GO TO, PICK UP, and other events pre-programmed into the simulation. The workflow itself organized the steps into display order, providing a natural sequencing.

The Romeo and Juliet workflow was an interesting example where we can learn an important aspect of the development of services from workflow because Shakespeare provides his play as a sequence of chats (the script) and a few stage directions. It is the job of the director to visualize the script and guide development of the scene and the actors to fulfill that vision. That is, the script is one "trace" of the workflow containing mainly words spoken; and the play itself is a trace that contains visual as well as spoken information. In general, any system in operation might have many traces, each reflecting some projection of the simulation. Examples are logs of a person's heartbeat, their finances, their location track history, etc. These traces can be assembled, correlated, and analyzed to better understand the simulation or real world actions. One lesson we learned from Zeineldin's work was that, sometimes traces

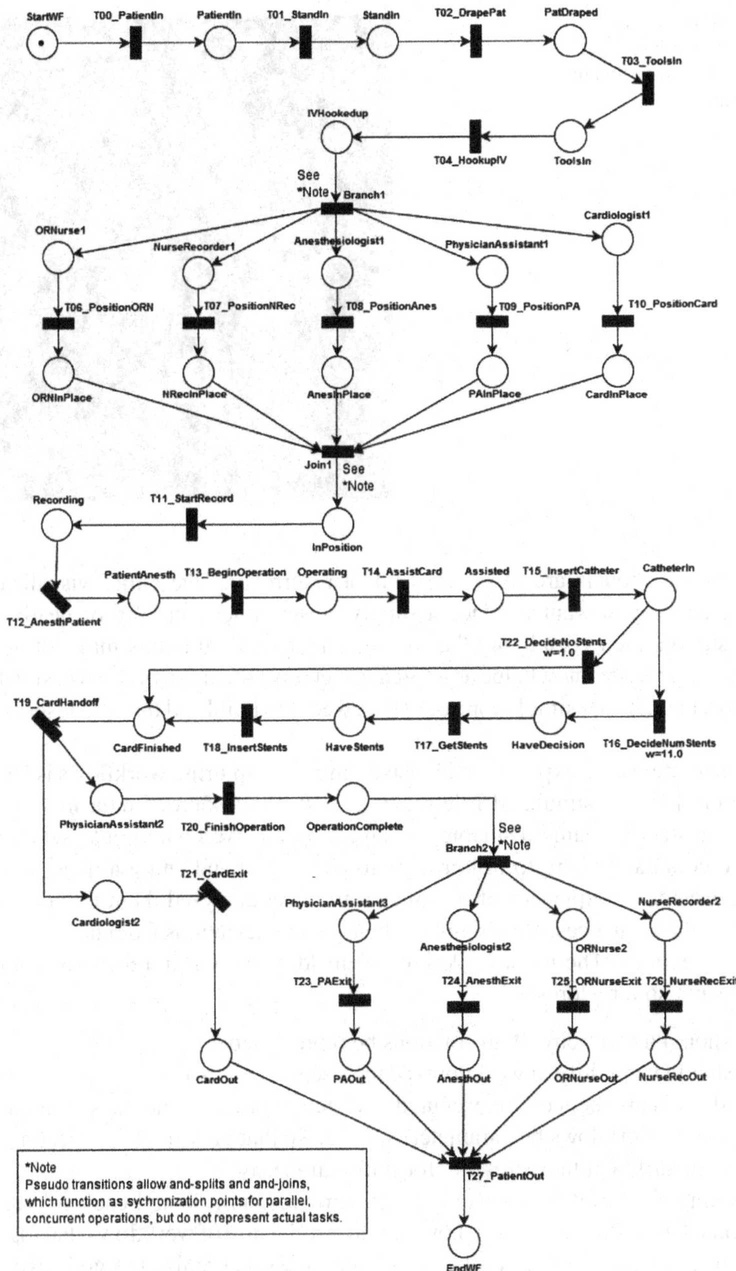

Fig. 4.6 Catheterization procedure workflow petri net

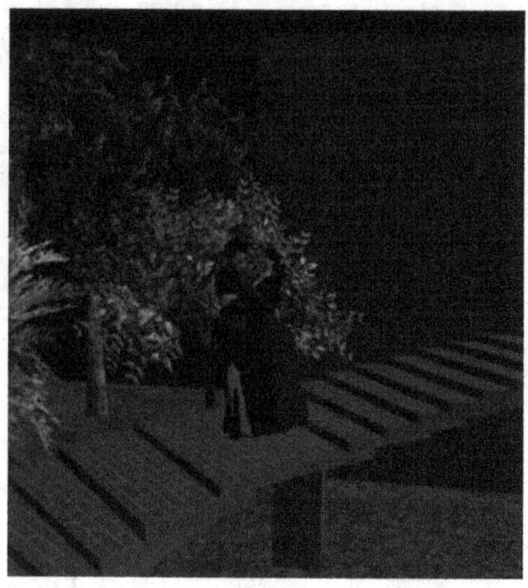

Fig. 4.7 Roboteo and Booliette avatarbots workflow demonstration in Second Life

and simplified models are more useful than resurrecting the entire visualization. For instance, if you want to place a supply closet either centrally or nearby to a nurses' station, then visualizing the two floor plan configurations may not give as much useful analytic knowledge as a spreadsheet representation of the two situations might provide. The 3D simulation could take weeks to build and the spreadsheet only hours.

Another interesting experiment in visualizing and capturing workflows is Orkin's dissertation [82] on simulated role-playing from crowdsourced data in which he created a restaurant game available to players on the Web who could select from a limited command menu to task avatars to order food and enjoy a meal. He captured thousands of sequences of commands and later analyzed them into dozens of workflow-like sequences. He did not explicitly view deviations from an ideal workflow as exceptions. The work of Perkins, Zeineldin, and Orkin raises several open questions not so far addressed:

- How should a hierarchy of abstractions be represented?
- How should variability of workflows be represented, e.g., so some steps take longer some days than others or are executed in different orders some days than others.
- How should workflows be parameterized, e.g., so that dressing for a meeting with the boss is different than dressing for informal Friday.
- Presuming each avatar in a workflow performs some role and each role has an associated workflow of its own, how should a collection of workflows that together make up a composite workflow be coordinated and synchronized. A gods-eye-view can act as a composite workflow that commands each individual avatar but that is not satisfying from the standpoint of modeling avatars with free will (Fig. 4.7).

4.2.6 From Service to Human: Communicating with Things

In this stage, services can be provided on-request or transparently to us humans [2]. We can ask the AC/heater to increase or decrease the temperature to our desire. A doctor can be notified of irregularities in a person's temperature and look for possible diseases that match the current set of sensory readings. Robots can be used to load or unload goods automatically using the 3D map, the RFID of the goods, and perhaps a protocol to realize where and how to load or unload between the robot and the smart vehicles.

Currently, computational objects talk to each other via messages and APIs (e.g., as web services using representations like XML or JSON and protocols like WSDL, SOAP and UDDI [83, 84]), essentially using remote procedure calls. In agent-based computing, speech acts divide between commands, requests, and queries. However, humans communicate with other humans using natural language. Language services like voice assistants Apple Siri or Google Search are impressive but do not query human workflows (yet). Menu-based natural language interfaces (MBNLI) [85–87] could be used as an alternative. In MBNLI, a domain-specific grammar mirrors the queries and commands that an object can understand (its methods). Cascaded menus predict all legal next phrases and display them on menus; the user selects menu phrases to build a sentence. All such sentences are guaranteed to be understood by the system in contrast to conventional natural language interfaces which may or often may not understand what the user wants to ask. For instance, a query like *find recipes which involve boiling potatoes* can result in XML Query commands to find a subset of recipes. Similarly, a command *boil the potatoes—for 5 min* can result in a workflow command to visualize an avatar showing off that next step in the recipe (which may involve sub-steps of putting water in the pan, carrying the pan to the stove, turning on the stove burner, bringing the water to a boil, adding the potatoes, and boiling for 25 min or until tender). Each of the command strings can have an associated translation as an XML Query command or an Avatarbot command such as [88].

The soft controller concept [3, 5] disassociates the physical interface of a physical object from its API so that the interface can be delivered instead or in addition on a smartphone or software controller, which becomes a truly universal remote, the ancestor to the Star Trek Communicator. This could mean that many ordinary everyday devices (like thermostats and car dashboards) are over-engineered and could be replaced by software interfaces. It also means that individuals can have custom interfaces, for example, simplified or full-features interfaces and that individuals do not have to give up interfaces they are used to when replacing products.

With smartphones becoming more of a commodity worldwide, the use of smartphones as a platform for ubiquitous computing is promising. Due to Google's release of the Android Open Accessory Development Kit (ADK), a portal between the cyber world and the physical world made it possible to transform the ideas from EiA into the real world's working project. Having successfully implemented the soft controller in the virtual environment of Second Life [3, 5], our first prototype was to demonstrate how an idea tested in a virtual world can be made to work in the real life. Thus, a robot that can roam around to detect new smart objects and enable the user to immediately control these new objects mirrors its counterpart in the virtual world [6]. One and a half years after we had first successfully implemented the virtual prototype, technological advances and the ubiquity of smartphones caught up to provide the means to realize this idea in the real world.

We assume that in the near future, objects are associated with RFID tags, where each tag can uniquely identify the corresponding object. Using only this and a centralized database, we can obtain manufacturer's information about object such as object's XBee MAC address, a unique address assigned to each XBee, which will be needed for user-control. Within the proximity of the RFID reader, we can detect objects automatically, and through their unique MAC address, we can communicate with them wirelessly using only one controller, which in this case is the smartphone. Through the group of objects recognized by the RFID reader, we could infer about the user's environment, e.g. home, office, or schools, etc., and also the user's location with the phone's built-in GPS in order to provide better services or enable/disable certain capabilities of the objects for security purposes. This service is delivered to the user to satisfy his/her needs in response to the request originated from the real world or the virtual world in which this concept was first tested. As a result, the user has now achieved the goal of controlling the unknown objects of interests using a consistent flow. The virtual world was used for prototyping this flow first [3], and based on analogous technologies in the real world, we have shown how this flow can be realized in the real world [6] (Table 4.2).

A world where every object is a smart object which can be commanded, controlled and queried and where every state change can be recorded and replayed has many advantages. For instance, we can always ask questions about the past and recall specific answers. In heart catheter operations, we could ask how many heart operations involved three stents; whether there are correlations between patient age and surgery outcome; and whether some physicians performed better than others. If humans were instrumented with more monitors, then it is easier to monitor their health for wellness purposes, e.g. to reduce obesity or to watch over patients who might fall. Similarly, it is easier to remind patients to take their medications or prompt them in the next step in a recipe or in repairing their car. Therefore, there is considerable good that can come from a world in which computers can monitor and recognize human actions.

There is high likelihood that collecting this kind of data will create a permanent record of our life, all the way down to micro steps. An extreme case of this is a system that collects a record of all of one's actions. One of the authors has a complete email record back to 1995. That is a trace of one kind of communication and is helpful as a human memory augmentation. A record that keeps track of all traces of a person can effectively build an immortal avatar [89–91]. This kind of model aggregates many kinds of traces into a composite model, which can be viewed as a fully quantified self [92].

Given recent news stories on data aggregation, it should be clear that that there are security and privacy issues that must be solved if humans are to insure the ability to keep data secure and private.

Table 4.2 Virtual prototypes and real world implementations

	Virtual world (second life)	Real world
Active object (detector)	Prim controlled by avatar 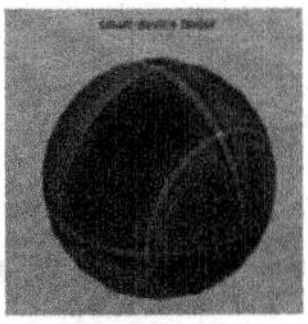	Robot with Arduino board 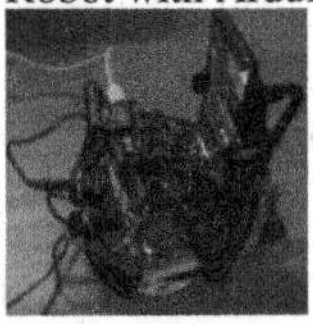
Owner object (controller)	Virtual controller in SL or on a web 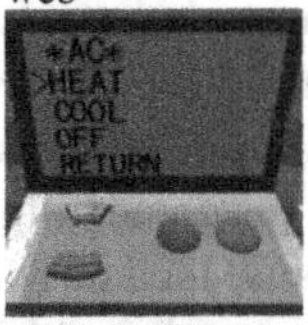	Application on Android phone (simulator) 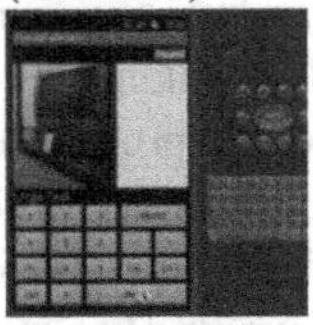
Passive object (controlled)	AC, bed, X-ray machine 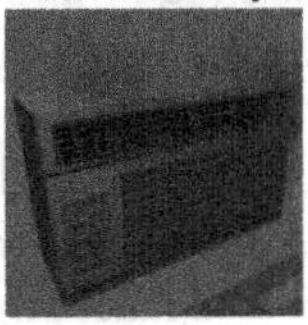	TV, LED 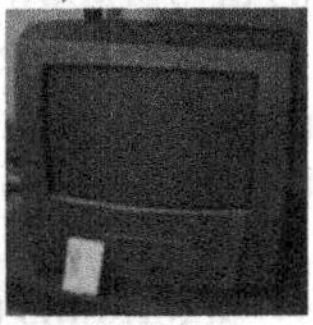
Identity	UUID of prim attached to object	RFID attached to object
Control	Linden Scripting Language	Google's ADK
Communication	Open channel (not secured)	XBee
API downloaded	Text base	Android program's plug-in

- In a world where everyone owns 5–10 networked smart objects, humans already spend considerable time installing security and other updates to their objects. What will happen when humans have 100s or 1000s of network objects? We cannot afford the time to spend on maintaining such worlds so we need better solutions.
- In that same world, we humans do not always have a clear understanding of what the updates do and whether they provide access to third parties. Once data leaks out into the open Internet or into another's system, what are the repercussions?
- In a world where third parties aggregate state that involves your personal data, and coupled with their ability to analyze patterns, how much control do individuals have over their own data.
- If third parties (insurance companies, criminals, the government, etc.) control data, to what extent is trust lost in transactions and in human dealings.

That is, like any other new technology, the ability to build a W2T world has great benefits if used wisely but can create many problems if abused. It is a manifest destiny that this world is coming; at the same time, it is our responsibility to understand this new world and design it to preserve our human digital rights.

4.2.7 From Human to Things: Recognition

Finally, the cycle restarts, and data collected during and after services are fed back into the W2T system [2]. Initially, we can teach the system to learn our personal preferences before it utilizes this knowledge to provide services to us. The question is how the systems can learn them from our behaviors. Image understanding is a more difficult problem than rendering a model with graphics because the model world can provide precise representations and can guarantee a well-defined family of ways to render a scene whereas images that come from the real world often contain artifacts that have no model correlate because the images are collected "in the wild". Therefore, if we want to map events in the real world into events inside computer representations of workflows, we have this extra layer of complexity.

We are in the early stages of using the Microsoft Kinect to recognize primitive objects and actions. As mentioned, Eguchi [8] and others have used Kinect libraries to train a computer to recognize a variety of objects but also Eguchi captured a sequence of frames of skeletal models from the Kinect and used support vector machine (SVN) algorithms to "recognize" and label primitive actions like walking, skipping, and running (see demo at [81]). Currently, we are working on the recipe scenario to first recognize the places and objects in an experimental kitchen (e.g., refrigerator, range, sink, etc.), kitchen equipment (e.g., pans and spoons), and ingredients (broccoli, potatoes). Then, the Kinect watches a human actor prepare a recipe and the participating objects and actions are labeled to create a very fine-grained workflow with primitive symbolically labeled steps like place the pan under the faucet, turn on the faucet, etc.). We repeat the recipe and labeling several times. This is research in progress. Our plan is to try to learn the individual actions and label them. Once labeled, we can view the primitive labelings as a string that can be recognized by a workflow grammar. The low level steps can be grouped similar to the way Orkin grouped steps to recognize higher level steps that make up typical recipes [82].

Even if this experiment is successful and we can recognize humans executing recipes, this work raises other questions. One interesting question is, if we can use the now-trained Kinect to recognize a step in a workflow, can we index all our recipe workflows so the Kinect can "guess" which workflows we might be executing from a larger set. For instance, if the Kinect sees you are boiling potatoes, this mid-level action might delimit which recipes are involved. A second question is, how can we rapidly learn by observing a much wider range or workflows that cover more of human experience. If you consider that humans can channel surf their TV and make a decision whether to go to the next channel or watch on, then, in that short time interval, they must be deciding that this is a reality show or a drama or a situation comedy and is or is not of interest.

Abstracting from this, we can consider that in our lives, until recently, computers have been situation unaware. They do not know what is happening around them and so cannot participate in our daily lives. There are already many special purpose exceptions: location-aware computing is a form of situation awareness where the GPS on our smartphone can identify our location which can be translated into augmented reality (e.g., labeling building nearby) or serving us location-sensitive ads. Similarly, cyber-physical systems can monitor our heart beat or blood sugar. Nevertheless, so far, these systems are special-purpose brittle one-offs that do not sense the situations and context of our lives. For participative computing to occur, in which computers understand the situation and can respond, they will need models and a way to recognize common activities, what we are calling human workflows.

4.3 Discussion

The world is getting smarter due to various rapidly developing technologies, so far being developed in semi-isolation. In such a world, surrounded by many artificial objects and services, it is important to figure out how those concepts are related together and how to use these new technologies to optimize our lives. The Everything is Alive project focuses on the problem. Our goal is to make everything alive to make our lives richer. Our work focuses on architectural frameworks and includes various aspects of pervasive computing such as smart world, smart objects, soft controllers, mobile computing, ontologies, psychology, virtual worlds, object recognition, human workflows, and mobile robot. In this chapter, we discussed four different perspectives of our project in terms of Ubiquitous Intelligence, Cyber-Individual, Brain Informatics, and Web Intelligence, and how those ideas interact. We also discussed how the EiA project fits into the endless cycle of Wisdom Web of Things by introducing future challenges as well.

As real world objects become smart, the boundary between the virtual and real world becomes blurred: we can use the same soft controller to control both virtual and real world objects. We can now have a 3D model of the real world which can be used to monitor and control objects nearby or at a distance. This implies that changes in the virtual world will be reflected in the real world, and vice versa.

In this virtual world, current technical difficulties can be temporarily suspended waiting for solutions in the future. An abstraction layer can be erected between the algorithms and the worlds so that the virtual world can be used as a test bed for real world implementations. The separation of platforms enabled us to make some assumptions not currently possible or still under development in the real world first; and then either we resolved them or tried to modify the logic to account for noise later. This demonstrates how technology will eventually catch up to concepts that were previously unreachable. We believe that now is the time for the Wisdom Web of Things and for Everything is Alive to flourish with the ubiquity of smartphones, advances in RFID and sensor research, Microsoft Kinect, Google Glass and other new technologies that connect computing to our everyday lives. So far, smartphones enable grand-scale data collection and analysis, and RFID identifies a physical object and serves as a link between the physical and virtual entities while the Microsoft Kinect resolves multiple issues in 3D modeling and provides a cheap but reliable platform on which to further develop ideas applicable to both worlds. However, in order to accomplish the goal, the adoption and inter-operability of smart objects will call for a more universal standard than our current approach to object communication, especially if we want to build smarter controllers, aka Web Intelligence.

With new technologies, we are increasingly provided tools and resources to share knowledge with others. Just as the invention of cars and airplanes provided us with greater mobility in our lives, and just as the invention of computers enabled us to share our experience with others more easily, the invention of smartphones has helped make it easier for us to share those information anywhere and anytime we want to. In other words, the world is becoming a much easier place for us humans to reach out to each other both physically and socially. With the knowledge pool getting larger by sharing, we are forming a centralized web of wisdom, which can be utilized to provide much and better services, those that can be provided by using smart devices and objects. In the world where everything is alive, we give clues as to how to make things around us coordinate in a harmonious way to achieve that goal.

References

1. C.W. Thompson, Everything is alive. IEEE Internet Comput. **8**, 83–86 (2004). doi:10.1109/MIC.2004.1260708
2. N. Zhong, J.H. Ma, R.H. Huang, J.M. Liu, Y.Y. Yao, Y.X. Zhang, J.H. Chen, Research challenges and perspectives on wisdom web of things (W2T). J. Supercomput. **64**, 862–882 (2013). doi:10.1007/s11227-010-0518-8
3. A. Eguchi, C.W. Thompson, Towards a semantic world: smart objects in a virtual world. Int. J. Comput. Inf. Syst. Indus. Manage. **3**, 905–911 (2011). http://www.mirlabs.org/ijcisim/regular_papers_2011/Paper102.pdf
4. J.D. Eno, C.W. Thompson, Virtual and real-world ontology services. IEEE Internet Comput. **15**, 46–52 (2011). doi:10.1109/MIC.2011.75
5. C.W. Thompson, Smart devices and soft controllers. IEEE Internet Comput. **9**, 82–85 (2005). doi:10.1109/MIC.2005.22
6. A. Eguchi, H. Nguyen, C.W. Thompson, Everything is alive: towards the future wisdom web of things. World Wide Web **16**, 357–378 (2013). doi:10.1007/s11280-012-0182-4
7. H. Nguyen, A. Eguchi, D. Hooten, In search of a cost effective way to develop autonomous floor mapping robots, in *2011 IEEE International Symposium on Robotic and Sensors Environments (ROSE)*, pp. 107–112 (2011). doi:10.1109/ROSE.2011.6058510
8. A. Eguchi, Object recognition based on shape and function: inspired by childrens word acquisition. Inquiry J. Undergrad. Res. Univ. Arkan **13** (2012). http://inquiry.uark.edu/issues/V13/2012a05.pdf
9. A. Eguchi, H. Nguyen, Minority game: the battle of adaptation, intelligence, cooperation and power, in *2011 Federated Conference on Computer Science and Information Systems (FedCSIS)*, pp. 631–634 (2011)
10. J. Robertson, C.W. Thompson, Everything is alive agent architecture. Int. Conf. Integr. Knowl. Intensive Multi-Agent Syst. **2005**, 21–25 (2005). doi:10.1109/KIMAS.2005.1427046
11. T. Gs, U. Kulkarni, SAP: self aware protocol for ubiquitous object communication. Int. J. Soft Comput. Eng. **1**, 7–12 (2011)

12. J. Eno, An intelligent crawler for a virtual world. thesis, University of Arkansas (2010–12). http://library.uark.edu:80/record=b2751498~S14. Thesis (Ph.D.)–University of Arkansas, Department of Computer Science and Computer Engineering (2010)
13. Y.Y. Yao, N. Zhong, J. Liu, S. Ohsuga, Web intelligence (WI), in *Proceedings of the First Asia-Pacific Conference on Web Intelligence: Research and Development*, WI'01 (Springer, 2001), pp. 1–17
14. J. Lertlakkhanakul, J. Choi, *Virtual Place Framework for User-centered Smart Home Applications* (Chap. 10, pp. 177–194. InTech, 2010-02-01). http://www.intechopen.com/books/smart-home-systems/
15. J. Wen, K. Ming, F. Wang, B. Huang, J. Ma, Cyber-i: vision of the individual's counterpart on cyberspace, in *Eighth IEEE International Conference on Dependable, Autonomic and Secure Computing*, 2009. DASC'09, pp. 295–302 (2009). doi:10.1109/DASC.2009.127
16. Acxiom. Consumer audience segmentation and visualization—personicx. http://www.acxiom.com/personicx/
17. Acxiom. Life stage segmentation system personicx (r) cluster perspectives (2010)
18. P. Martin, J. Haury, S. Yennisetty, D. Crist, M. Krishna, C.W. Thompson, *Mirror Worlds* (2010). http://csce.uark.edu/~cwt/DOCS/PAPERS/2003-2015/2010-04--X10
19. A. Hill, E. Barba, B. MacIntyre, M. Gandy, B. Davidson, Mirror worlds: Experimenting with heterogeneous AR, in *2011 International Symposium on Ubiquitous Virtual Reality (ISUVR)*, pp. 9–12 (2011). doi:10.1109/ISUVR.2011.28
20. N. Banerjee, S. Agarwal, P. Bahl, R. Ch, A. Wolman, M. Corner, Virtual compass: relative positioning to sense mobile social interactions, in *Pervasive'10 Proceedings of the 8th International Conference on Pervasive Computing* (2010)
21. K. Perkins. Virtual worlds as simulation platform, in *X10 Workshop on extensible virtual worlds* (2010). http://csce.uark.edu/~cwt/DOCS/WORKSHOPS/X10/ARCHITECTURE--Virtual-World-for-Simulation--Perkins.pdf
22. N. Zhong, J. Bradshaw, J. Liu, J. Taylor, Brain informatics. IEEE Intell. Syst. **26**, 16–21 (2011). doi:10.1109/MIS.2011.83
23. R. Desimone, Face-selective cells in the temporal cortex of monkeys. J. Cogn. Neurosci. **3**, 1–8 (1991). doi:10.1162/jocn.1991.3.1.1
24. D.D.I. Perrett, E.T. Rolls, W. Caan, Visual neurones responsive to faces in the monkey temporal cortex. Exp. Brain Res. **47**, 329–342 (1982). doi:10.1007/BF00239352
25. K. Tanaka, H. Saito, Y. Fukada, M. Moriya, Coding visual images of objects in the inferotemporal cortex of the macaque monkey. J. Neurophysiol. **66**, 170–189 (1991). PMID: 1919665
26. M. Stringer, G. Perry, T. Rolls, H. Proske, Learning invariant object recognition in the visual system with continuous transformations. Biol. Cybern. **94**, 128–142 (2006). doi:10.1007/s00422-005-0030-z
27. S.M. Stringer, E.T. Rolls, Learning transform invariant object recognition in the visual system with multiple stimuli present during training. Neural Networks Official J Int. Neural Netw. Soc. **21**, 888–903 (2008). doi:10.1016/j.neunet.2007.11.004. PMID: 18440774
28. I.V. Higgins, S.M. Stringer, The role of independent motion in object segmentation in the ventral visual stream: learning to recognise the separate parts of the body. Vis. Res. **51**, 553–562 (2011). doi:10.1016/j.visres.2011.01.016. PMID: 21320521
29. J.M. Tromans, M. Harris, S.M. Stringer, A computational model of the development of separate representations of facial identity and expression in the primate visual system. PLoS ONE **6**, e25,616 (2011). doi:10.1371/journal.pone.0025616
30. D. Roy, New horizons in the study of child language acquisition, in *Interspeech* (2009)
31. M. Meyer, P. DeCamp, B. Hard, D. Baldwin, D. Roy. Assessing behavioral and computational approaches to naturalistic action segmentation, in *Proceedings of the 32nd Annual Conference of the Cognitive Science Society*, pp. 2710–2715 (2010)
32. P. DeCamp, G. Shaw, R. Kubat, D. Roy, An immersive system for browsing and visualizing surveillance video, in *Proceedings of the international conference on Multimedia, MM'10*, pp. 371–380. ACM (2010). doi:10.1145/1873951.1874002

33. R.J. Dolan, T. Sharot, *Neuroscience of Preference and Choice: Cognitive and Neural Mechanisms*, 1st edn. (Academic Press, London; Waltham, MA, 2011)
34. P.A. Samuelson, A note on the pure theory of consumer's behaviour. Economica 61–71 (1938). http://www.jstor.org/stable/2548836
35. F. Gul, W. Pesendorfer, The case for mindless economics, in *The Foundations of Positive and Normative Economics*, pp. 3–42 (2008)
36. R. Elliott, J.L. Newman, O.A. Longe, J.F.W. Deakin, Differential response patterns in the striatum and orbitofrontal cortex to financial reward in humans: a parametric functional magnetic resonance imaging study. J. Neurosci. **23**(1), 303–307 (2003). http://www.jneurosci.org/content/23/1/303
37. L. Tremblay, W. Schultz, Relative reward preference in primate orbitofrontal cortex. Nature **398**(6729), 704–708 (1999). doi:10.1038/19525
38. C. Padoa-Schioppa, Range-adapting representation of economic value in the orbitofrontal cortex. J. Neurosci. **29**(44), 14004–14014 (2009). doi:10.1523/JNEUROSCI.3751-09.2009. http://www.jneurosci.org/content/29/44/14004
39. A. Eguchi, E. Bohannan, Who do you see in a mirror? cultural differences in identity perspectives, in *Advanced Research Poster Session* (University of Arkansas, 2011)
40. B. Landau, L.B. Smith, S.S. Jones, The importance of shape in early lexical learning. Cogn. Dev. **3**, 299–321 (1988). doi:10.1016/0885-2014(88)90014-7
41. D.G.K. Nelson, R. Russell, N. Duke, K. Jones, Two-year-olds will name artifacts by their functions. Child Development **71**, 1271–1288 (2000)
42. A. Eguchi, B. M. W. Mender, B. Evans, G. Humphreys, S. Stringer, Computational modelling of the neural representation of object shape in the primate ventral visual system. Front. Comput. Neurosci. **9**(100) (2015). doi:10.3389/fncom.2015.00100
43. A. Eguchi, S.A. Neymotin, S.M. Stringer, Color opponent receptive fields self-organize in a biophysical model of visual cortex via spike-timing dependent plasticity. Front Neural Circuits **8**, 16 (2014). doi:10.3389/fncir.2014.00016
44. A. Eguchi, S.M. Stringer, Computational modeling of the development of detailed facial representations along ventral pathway. BMC Neurosci. **15**(Suppl 1), P38 (2014). doi:10.1186/1471-2202-15-S1-P38
45. Y.Y. Yao, N. Zhong, J. Liu, S. Ohsuga, Web Intelligence (WI) Research Challenges and Trends in the New Information Age, pp. 1–17. No. 2198 in Lecture Notes in Computer Science. (Springer, Berlin Heidelberg, 2001)
46. N. Banerjee, S. Rollins, K. Moran, Automating energy management in green homes, in *Proceedings of the 2nd ACM SIGCOMM Workshop on Home Networks*, HomeNets'11, pp. 19–24. ACM (2011). doi:10.1145/2018567.2018572
47. T. Censullo, C.W. Thompson, Semantic world: ontologies for the real and virtual world, in *X10 Workshop on Extensible Virtual Worlds*, vol. 29 (2010). http://csce.uark.edu/~cwt/DOCS/WORKSHOPS/X10/CAPABILITIES--Ontologies-for-the-Real-and-Virtual-World--Censullo-Thompson.pdf
48. T. Berners-Lee, J. Hendler, O. Lassila, *The Semantic Web: Scientific american* (Scientific American, 2001)
49. G.A. Miller, WordNet: a lexical database for english. Commun ACM **38**, 39–41 (1995)
50. C.W. Thompson, D.R. Thompson, Identity management. IEEE Internet Comput. **11**, 82–85 (2007). doi:10.1109/MIC.2007.60
51. J. Hoag, C.W. Thompson, Architecting RFID middleware. IEEE Internet Comput **10**, 88–92 (2006). doi:10.1109/MIC.2006.94
52. S. McNulty, *The Amazon Fire Phone: Master your Amazon Smartphone Including Firefly, Mayday, Prime, and all the Top Apps* (Peachpit Press, 2014)
53. Logitech. Harmony Remotes—Choose Your Harmony Remote—Logitech. http://www.logitech.com/en-us/harmony-remotes
54. H. Cho, Y. Jung, H. Choi, H. Jang, S. Son, Y. Baek, Real time locating system for wireless networks using IEEE 802.15.4 radio, in *5th Annual IEEE Communications Society Conference on Sensor, Mesh and Ad Hoc Communications and Networks, 2008*. SECON'08, pp. 578–580 (2008). doi:10.1109/SAHCN.2008.75

55. C.W. Thompson, Virtual world architectures. IEEE Internet Comput. **15**, 11–14 (2011). doi:10.1109/MIC.2011.125
56. S. Williams, Virtual "university of arkansas" campus. thesis, University of Arkansas (2012). http://library.uark.edu:80/record=b3091177~S4. Thesis (BS)—University of Arkansas, Department of Computer Science and Computer Engineering (2012)
57. T.H. Kolbe, G. Groger, L. Plumer, CityGML: interoperable access to 3d city models, in P.D.P.v. Oosterom, D.S. Zlatanova, E.M. Fendel (eds.) *Geo-information for Disaster Management* (Springer Berlin Heidelberg, 2005), pp. 883–899
58. M. Philipose, K. Fishkin, M. Perkowitz, D. Patterson, D. Fox, H. Kautz, D. Hahnel, Inferring activities from interactions with objects. IEEE Pervasive Comput. **3**, 50–57 (2004). doi:10.1109/MPRV.2004.7
59. W. Deneke, W. N. Li, C. W. Thompson, Automatic composition of ETL workflows from business intents, in *Second International Conference on Big Data Science and Engineering (BDSE)* (2013–12)
60. C. Bizer, J. Lehmann, G. Kobilarov, S. Auer, C. Becker, R. Cyganiak, S. Hellmann, DBpedia—a crystallization point for the web of data. Web Semant. **7**, 154–165 (2009-09). doi:10.1016/j.websem.2009.07.002
61. S. Auer, C. Bizer, G. Kobilarov, J. Lehmann, R. Cyganiak, Z. Ives, DBpedia: a nucleus for a web of open data, in *The Semantic Web*, vol. 4825, Lecture Notes in Computer Science, ed. by K. Aberer, K.S. Choi, N. Noy, D. Allemang, K.I. Lee, L. Nixon, J. Golbeck, P. Mika, D. Maynard, R. Mizoguchi, G. Schreiber, P. Cudre-Mauroux (Springer, Berlin, Heidelberg, 2007), pp. 722–735
62. T. Sangameswaran, A deep search architecture for capturing product ontologies. thesis, University of Arkansas (2014). http://library.uark.edu:80/record=b3389396~S4. Thesis (Master)—University of Arkansas, Department of Computer Science and Computer Engineering (2014)
63. J. Pedro, P. Manzanares-Lopez, J. Malgosa-Sanahuj, Advantages and new applications of DHT-based discovery services in EPCglobal network, chap. 9. (InTech, 2011), pp. 131–156
64. D. Martin, M. Burstein, D. McDermott, S. McIlraith, M. Paolucci, K. Sycara, D. L. McGuinness, E. Sirin, N. Srinivasan. Bringing semantics to web services with OWL-S. World Wide Web **10**, 243–277 (2007). doi:10.1007/s11280-007-0033-x
65. D. Ferraiolo, J. Cugini, D.R. Kuhn, Role-based access control (RBAC): features and motivations, in *Proceedings of 11th annual computer security application conference*, pp. 241–248 (1995)
66. R.S. Sandhu, E.J. Coyne, H.L. Feinstein, C.E. Youman, Role-based access control models. Computer **29**(2), 38–47 (1996)
67. X. Wang, G. Lao, T. DeMartini, H. Reddy, M. Nguyen, E. Valenzuela. XrML eXtensible rights markup language, in *Proceedings of the 2002 ACM Workshop on XML Security, XMLSEC'02* (ACM, New York, NY, USA, 2002), pp. 71–79. doi:10.1145/764792.764803
68. B. Horling, V. Lesser, Using ODML to model multi-agent organizations, in *IEEE/WIC/ACM International Conference on Intelligent Agent Technology*, pp. 72–80 (2005). doi:10.1109/IAT.2005.139
69. E.D. Sacerdoti, Planning in a hierarchy of abstraction spaces. Artif. Intell. **5**, 115–135 (1974). doi:10.1016/0004-3702(74)90026-5
70. R.C. Schank, R.C. Schank, Scripts, plans, goals, and understanding: an inquiry into human knowledge structures. (L. Erlbaum Associates, distributed by the Halsted Press Division of Wiley, 1977)
71. D. Hollingsworth, U.K. Hampshire, Workflow management coalition the workflow reference model, in *Workflow Management Coalition*, vol. 68 (1993)
72. T. Andrews, F. Curbera, H. Dholakia, Y. Goland, J. Klein, F. Leymann, K. Liu, D. Roller, D. Smith, S. Thatte, et al., *Business Process Execution Language for Web Services* (2003). https://www.oasis-open.org/committees/download.php/2046/BPELV1-1May52003Final.pdf
73. P. Jiang, Q. Mair, J. Newman, Using UML to design distributed collaborative workflows: from UML to XPDL, in *Twelfth IEEE International Workshops on Enabling Technologies: Infrastructure for Collaborative Enterprises*, 2003. WET ICE 2003. Proceedings, pp. 71–76 (2003). doi:10.1109/ENABL.2003.1231385

74. O. Gilbert, S. Marsh, C.W. Thompson, Recognizing higher level activities from workflow traces, in *Freshman Engineering Honors Symposium* (2012)
75. D.C. Fallside, P. Walmsley, *XML Schema Part 0: Primer*. 2nd edn. (W3C recommendation, p. 16, 2004)
76. H. Katz, D.D. Chamberlin, *XQuery from the Experts: A Guide to the W3C XML Query Language*. (Addison-Wesley Professional, 2004)
77. M. Zeineldin, Defining, executing and visualizing representative workflows in a retail domain. Master's thesis, University of Arkansas. http://library.uark.edu:80/record=b2920438~S1
78. K. Perkins, Workflow simulation in a virtual world. Thesis, University of Arkansas (2011). http://library.uark.edu:80/record=b2812350~S14. Thesis (Master)—University of Arkansas, Department of Computer Science and Computer Engineering (2011)
79. K. Perkins, C.W. Thompson, Workflow in a virtual world, in *X10 Workshop on Extensible Virtual Worlds* (2010). http://csce.uark.edu/~cwt/DOCS/PAPERS/2003-2015/2010-04--X10WorkshoponExtensibleVirtualWorlds--WorkflowinaVirtualWorld--Perkins-Thompson.pdf
80. R. Ierusalimschy, *Programming in Lua*. (Lua, 2013)
81. C.W. Thompson, Everything is alive: demos. http://csce.uark.edu/~cwt/DOCS/VIDEOS/
82. J.D. Orkin, Collective artificial intelligence: simulated role-playing from crowdsourced data. Thesis, Massachusetts Institute of Technology (2013). Thesis (Ph.D.)—Massachusetts Institute of Technology, School of Architecture and Planning, Program in Media Arts and Sciences (2013). http://alumni.media.mit.edu/~jorkin/papers/orkin_phd_thesis_2013.pdf
83. E. Christensen, F. Curbera, G. Meredith, S. Weerawarana, et al., Web services description language (WSDL) 1.1. W3C (2001). http://www.w3.org/TR/2001/NOTE-wsdl-20010315
84. F. Curbera, M. Duftler, R. Khalaf, W. Nagy, N. Mukhi, S. Weerawarana, Unraveling the web services web: an introduction to SOAP, WSDL, and UDDI. IEEE Internet Comput. **6**(2), 86–93 (2002)
85. V. Chintaphally, K. Neumeier, J. McFarlane, J. Cothren, C.W. Thompson, Extending a natural language interface with geospatial queries. IEEE Internet Comput. **11**, 82–85 (2007). doi:10.1109/MIC.2007.124
86. H.R. Tennant, K.M. Ross, C.W. Thompson, Usable natural language interfaces through menu-based natural language understanding, in *Proceedings of the SIGCHI Conference on Human Factors in Computing Systems, CHI'83*, pp. 154–160. ACM (1983). doi:10.1145/800045.801601
87. C.W. Thompson, P. Pazandak, H. Tennant, Talk to your semantic web. IEEE Internet Comput. **9**, 75–78 (2005). doi:10.1109/MIC.2005.135
88. N. Farrer, Second Life Robot Command Language (2009). http://csce.uark.edu/~cwt/DOCS/STUDENTS/other/2009-02--SL-Robot-Command-Language-v0--Nicholas-Farrer.pdf
89. J. Gemmell, G. Bell, R. Lueder, S. Drucker, C. Wong, MyLifeBits: fulfilling the memex vision, in *Proceedings of the tenth ACM international conference on Multimedia, MULTIMEDIA'02*, pp. 235–238. ACM (2002). doi:10.1145/641007.641053
90. T. Kumar, C. W. Thompson, My immortal avatar, in *X10 Workshop on Extensible Virtual Worlds, 2010-04-29*. http://csce.uark.edu/~cwt/DOCS/WORKSHOPS/X10/APPLICATION--My-Immortal-Avatar--Kumar-Thompson.pdf
91. C.W. Thompson, P. Parkerson, DBMS[me] [life-time records]. IEEE Internet Comput. **8**, 85–89 (2004). doi:10.1109/MIC.2004.1297278
92. M. Swan, The quantified self: fundamental disruption in big data science and biological discovery. Big Data **1**(2), 85–99 (2013). doi:10.1089/big.2012.0002. http://online.liebertpub.com/doi/abs/10.1089/big.2012.0002
93. C.J. Spoerer, A. Eguchi, S.M. Stringer, A computational exploration of complementary learning mechanisms in the primate ventral visual pathway. Vis. Res. (2016) (in prep.)

Chapter 5
Context-Awareness in Autonomic Communication and in Accessing Web Information: Issues and Challenges

Francesco Chiti, Romano Fantacci, Gabriella Pasi and Francesco Tisato

Abstract In recent years, after the proposal of the Internet of Things and, later, of the Web of Things, context awareness is a central issue at various levels including devices, communications and applications. In this chapter we present an overview of the current state of research in autonomic communications by focusing on aspects of context awareness on which the emerging new paradigm of Context-Aware Autonomic Communication systems is based. As an example of application we also provide a synthetic analysis of the problem of contextual search and of the issues related to defining contextual search systems.

5.1 Introduction

Since the introduction of the expression *context-aware* by Schilit and Theimer with reference to distributed computing in the dynamic environment determined by the interaction of users with mobile and stationary computers [1], a big deal of research has addressed the problem of context awareness as a key issue in distributed and autonomous computing.

This research trend has recently culminated in the proposal of the Internet of Things (IoT) paradigm [2], which takes advantage of existing and evolving Internet and network developments; this paradigm can be considered as an advanced global network infrastructure with self-configuring capabilities. By means of suitable communication protocols, both physical and virtual devices, usually named things, are efficiently integrated into the information network so as to acquire an active role in business, information and social processes. In particular, they are enabled to autonomously interact and communicate among them, with the environment and even with applications in order to exchange data caught from the environment, and

F. Chiti · R. Fantacci
Università degli Studi di Firenze, Firenze, Italy

G. Pasi (✉) · F. Tisato
Università degli Studi di Milano Bicocca, Milan, Italy
e-mail: pasi@disco.unimib.it

N. Zhong et al. (eds.), *Wisdom Web of Things*, Web Information Systems Engineering and Internet Technologies Book Series,
DOI 10.1007/978-3-319-44198-6_5

to react to unpredictable events by running processes in an autonomic manner that triggers suitable actions.

On top of this new paradigm a shift from the Web of Data to the Web of Things (WoT) was proposed to leverage *"the existing and ubiquitous Web protocols as common ground where real objects could interact with each other"*; the aim was to define Web standards to make devices able to speak with other resources on the Web, *"therefore making it very easy to integrate physical devices with any content on the Web"* [3, 4].

In particular, tiny wireless sensors—which are widely available in almost all kinds of devices like Internet-capable-smart phones, cameras, cars, toys, medical instruments, home appliances, energy meters or traffic loops—promise to foster a significant expansion of the Internet. They are being adopted in several application domains, including intelligent agriculture, proactive health care, asset tracking, environmental monitoring, security surveillance, data center management and social networking. A large number of these applications require facilities for collecting, storing, searching, sharing and analyzing sensor data. The formerly introduced WoT paradigm involves assigning additional responsibilities to sensor nodes in addition to their usual sensing functionality, mainly security and quality of service (QoS) management, and network configuration.

In the above scenario, and strongly related to the Wisdom Web of Things as advocated in [5], the notion of context plays a prominent role; generally speaking, context can be related to any information that can be used to characterize the situation of an entity, including *location, identity, user preferences, activity* and *time*. In particular, it is a general, pervasive concept that may affect the definition of complex systems at various levels, from the physical device level to the communication level up to the characterization of both users and applications.

At the device level, context awareness has triggered the development of a new generation of smart communication devices having capabilities of detecting changes in the environment, as well as in the user or application needs, and adapt their functionalities accordingly.

At the communication level, novel research areas as Context-Aware Autonomic Communications have appeared, which can be considered as an up to date frontier of the well-known area of context-aware autonomic computing. In particular, by adopting basic principles of autonomic computing jointly with other principles related to mobile communications, new research challenges have been envisaged, thus broadening the interest in context-awareness and its use. Nowadays, the new developments in the field of context-aware autonomic communications related to IoT and WoT applications have attracted considerable interest from industries and from academia. By analogy to the autonomic human nervous system, which oversees vital functions based on context awareness without a direct conscious control, context-aware autonomic communications are able to handle the communications among devices by reducing or even by avoiding a direct human interaction.

At the application level, the applications must be able to adapt to the devices' locations and capabilities, and to react to any changes of them over the time by modifying *the quality/quantity of results*, or *the way in which computations are* performed. Moreover several applications could benefit of the knowledge of users preferences; as an example of applications that can benefit of context awareness, in this chapter we will focus on Information Retrieval.

Context awareness has at least two major facets when dealing with specific aspects of an ICT system (including both *computation* and *communication*). We can distinguish between *user-oriented* and *self-oriented* context awareness.

User-oriented context awareness means that an ICT system exposes context-aware services and applications to the users or, in general, to the surrounding environment. The context-aware aspect of Information Retrieval in distributed environments constitutes a notable example, which has focused on the development of techniques aimed at tailoring the search outcome to the users context, including her/his location and social relationships, so as to improve both the quality and the effectiveness of the search, and to overcome the "one size fits all" behavior of most current search engines. In this case the context includes information that is strongly related to the users' model.

On the opposite, *self-oriented* context awareness is a complex property in which the system exploits context information in order to enable and drive an autonomic behavior, i.e. to manage itself. For example, an autonomic system can maintain its performance within desired limits by dynamically *reconfiguring* itself using context information that may include the physical location of the computing nodes, their availability, the cost of the communication lines, the criticality of specific activities and so on.

Similar remarks apply to communication issues: a network may expose *user-oriented* context-aware communication services based on the location of mobile users even if the network itself has a static topology therefore it does not exploit *self-oriented* context awareness. On the opposite, a network based on mobile nodes may exploit context information (e.g., the location of the nodes) to autonomously reconfigure itself.

In this chapter we outline the current state of research in autonomic communications by focusing on both aspects of context awareness on which the emerging new paradigm of Context-Aware Autonomic Communication systems is based. As an example of application we also provide a synthetic analysis of the problem of contextual search and of the issues related to defining contextual search systems.

5.2 Context-Aware Autonomic Communications

According to the networking perspective, an autonomic communication system can be regarded as a collection of communication devices and entities that exhibit self-organizing, decentralized and adaptive communication behaviors [6]. They can dynamically modify their behavior based on information related to their contexts, such as location, battery level and available networking opportunities, as well as user preferences [7]. As a consequence, the communication protocol design has to evolve in order to supply connectivity demands of smart devices [8]. This has triggered novel communications paradigms, as those based on the cognitive radio technology, that use opportunistically the communication resources available at any given time, in order to guarantee a seamless connectivity and applications dependability. Specifically, autonomic communications imply a stronger interaction with context-aware approaches to improve networking properties. Smart network devices and software agents are used to collect context information related to the presence, the location, the identity, and the profile of users and services.

Nowadays, *wireless ad hoc networks* are the most widespread examples of context-aware autonomic communication systems [9]. According to this networking paradigm, the users devices dynamically self-organize into arbitrary and temporary network topologies, and they cooperatively provide the functionalities that are usually provided by the network infrastructure (i.e., routers in wired networks or access points in managed wireless networks). In particular, each node participates in the routing process by dynamically setting up temporary network paths, with intermediate nodes acting as routers forwarding data for other nodes over wireless links. Typically, the context-aware information is related to the traditional problems of wireless communications, as reliability lower than wired media, time-varying channels, interference, dynamic network topologies, energy-constrained operations, autonomous network management, and device heterogeneity [10]. All these problems may be overcome by leveraging the potentials of mobile ad hoc networking if networking functionalities make use of context information to adapt and optimize their operations. As a consequence, *cross-layering* approaches have to be adopted to allow the exchange of context information between different layers of the protocol stack [11]. To clarify the potential gains of context awareness in the design of ad hoc networks, in the following we specifically focus on routing and networking protocols as a specific use-case where context awareness provides important advantages.

5.2.1 Context-Aware Routing Strategies

Historically, context-awareness in mobile and wireless networking was mainly related to the physical context, namely to all those aspects that represent the devices status and the environments around the devices/users [12, 13]. The geographical location is a basic example of physical context. Therefore, within the past decade a growing interest has been dedicated to the design of *geographical routing protocols* that construct network paths using information about the location of the network nodes [14]. The simplest approach to the geographic routing is the *greedy* solution, in which each intermediate device relays messages to its neighbor geographically closest to the destination. While this solution ensures the minimization of routing complexity and overhead, it does not guarantee message delivery because, depending on the topology layout, it may be difficult to avoid loops or deadlocks. More sophisticated routing protocols based on the *location awareness* of nodes [15, 16] are able to guarantee delivery by taking advantage of graph planarization techniques that remove links between neighbors in such a way that loops are avoided. However, two major drawbacks affect the efficiency of geographic routing proposals. The first one is that each node must know exactly its position and the positions of other nodes in the network. This might be impractical in indoor environments or for battery-power tiny devices (e.g., sensors). Furthermore, location services for the dissemination of location-related information may consume excessive network resources, especially when high mobility causes rapid and unpredictable topology changes. One solution could be to assume that only a subset of nodes is aware of its locations (so-called *anchor nodes*), while all the others use local measurements and localization protocols to infer their location. However, dedicated hardware may be needed to measure distances between nodes. The second and most crucial drawback is that location aware routing schemes implicitly assume reliable links and nodes, which is not always true for wireless communications. Furthermore, there are several experimental studies that have demonstrated that physical proximity is not sufficient to guarantee high-quality links because of the complex and time-variable relationship between link distance and link throughput. Those considerations have motivated the investigation of routing protocols that construct the network topology without relying on the physical location of the nodes but taking advantage of other context information related to nodes and links between them. In this case the physical context is provided by a *routing metric*, which combines link-layer measurements to obtain a more accurate characterization of link properties. Therefore routing metrics are used to optimize the routing and forwarding the decision process.

The most intuitive and simple routing metric is the *hop count*. In this case, a path length is simply given by the number of links that a path has between the source node and the destination node. However, several cross-layer routing metrics have been developed to improve the performance of multi-hop routing by taking into account various categories of link and path properties. A first category consists of measures that describe the physical characteristics of each link in isolation, such as transmission rates or packet loss ratios. A second broader but more complex category of measures tries to quantify the interference between links of a same path or between links of nearby paths, especially in terms of bit and packet error rates. Finally, a third category of link metrics is concerned with the estimate of the effect of traffic load on link quality. A large number of routing metrics has been proposed by combining in different manners these physical measurements, and it is out of the scope of this chapter to review all of them. As a general observation we may notice that *load-aware routing metrics* help to provide load balancing between paths, and the use of less congested paths generally leads to better traffic performance. On the other hand, *interference-aware routing metrics* are best suited to estimate network-wide impact of traffic flows. Although there is already a large variety of ad hoc routing, there are still a few important areas that need further investigations. First of all, there is a lack of practical and scalable measurement frameworks that may provide accurate link measurements, especially as far as interference is concerned. As a matter of fact, most common measurements techniques rely on *active probing*, which is known to introduce an excessive overhead in the network, while losses of probe packets can easily result in underestimation of link qualities.

5.2.2 *Opportunistic Networks*

The previous discussion provided several examples for exploiting *physical context* information to design routing protocols for ad hoc networks. However, a more long-term direction for the design of context-aware autonomic communications will be the use of *user context*. The term user context generally refers to various aspects (dimensions) related to user, including location, preferences, and social relationships. From a formal point of view, *users' profiles* are defined as a representation of the considered users context. One of the most interesting evolutions of ad hoc networks, which may significantly benefit from user-context awareness are *opportunistic networks*. In opportunistic networks intermediate nodes store the messages when no forwarding opportunity exists (e.g. no other nodes are in the transmission range, or neighbors are not suitable for that communication), and they exploit direct contacts with other mobile devices to forward the data toward the destination. In this scenario, the social dimension of the users can be used to make more efficient routing decisions. For instance, people belonging to the same social community tend to spend significant time together. Then this information can be used to improve the performance of the content dissemination. One of the main drawbacks of user-centric networking is represented by the overhead introduced for collecting and managing the user-related information. For instance, statistics may be needed for each social community and for each data item to distribute. Thus, solutions that improve the scalability of this approach must be studied. Furthermore, suitable social-aware metrics are needed for selecting the most appropriate forwarder for each data item. Many existing solutions in this area use centrality metrics to measure the social importance of each node in the network. For instance, a centrality metric can be used to identify the best locations in the network to store content items.

5.2.3 *Machine-to-Machine Communications*

The spontaneous networking vision could be effectively supported by the recently introduced Machine-to-Machine (M2M) paradigm, which denotes the class of communications where two or more terminals discover each other and interact without any kind of human intervention [17]. An end-to-end communication is basically performed by a client entity that gathers information, by a network, that seamlessly supports the M2M communication, and by a server entity, that processes client requests and automatically takes decisions. M2M communications implicitly enable new service platforms fostering the development of self-organized networks, able to monitor certain events and automatically instruct actuation. This paves the way to the deployment of a vast number of services and applications based on M2M: as an example, environmental monitoring and civil protection can potentially take advantage of M2M communications for public safety purposes, while Smart Grid (SG) and Intelligent Transport System (ITS) represent novel solutions to optimize logistic and supply chain management systems. Further, M2M communications encourage the concept of *smart cities* that deals with the management and control of cities with the purpose of monitoring critical sites, handling traffic related problems or enhancing the overall energy efficiency.

In such a complex scenario, cellular networks, especially 4G systems, are extremely convenient due to the ubiquitous coverage and to the global connectivity provided by mobile operators. Although designed especially to meet the tight requirements of human-related applications, cellular systems are also able to allow M2M communications whose performance can be significantly improved by the context awareness exploitation.

Along with the Machine Type Communication (MTC) the ongoing 4G systems standardization provides the support to Device-to-Device (D2D) or *direct-mode* communications, enabling P2P transmission between devices in proximity. This functionality fosters a new generation of devices able to communicate with each other, without any kind of human intervention and without involving the cellular infrastructure for the user plane. On the other hand, D2D communications pose also several challenges. First of all, direct mode communications should be established without impairing traditional communications via base station, i.e. by avoiding possible *interferences* with other devices. Secondly, functionalities of peer and service discovery need to be introduced, since a device is typically not aware of other terminals in the proximity. A promising approach toward this integrated vision is represented by Multi-hop Cellular Networks (MCN), where D2D communications are accomplished by introducing more flexibility within a cellular network, due to the fact that direct links enable the communication among the terminals using multiple hops.

5.3 Context-Awareness and User Centric Information Management and Retrieval

The user-centric networking approaches and the M2M communication paradigm, which have been introduced in Sect. 5.2, pave the way for an efficient and effective development of user-centered and event-centered applications. Among the applications that can benefit of the above technologies an important one is that related to the task of accessing Web information that is relevant to specific needs and purposes.

Web search engines of first generation were based on a document centric approach, where the one size fits all paradigm was applied. Since its inception the Web is in constant and exponential growth, and it has offered users a view of interconnected (although somewhat complex) data and information items (documents), spread on the Internet. As outlined by Tim Berners-Lee, the realization of the Web was based on the following observation: *"It's not the computers (on the Internet) which are interesting, it's the documents!"* [18]. The WWW protocols (URI, HTTP, HTML) have then offered a means to send documents between Web servers and Web browsers, thus giving users an access to interconnected documents. We may say that the Web has instantiated a document-centric paradigm, where documents are stored and organized on machines connected to other machines, the contents of which the users aim at disclosing, to the main objective of fulfill their information needs.

However, as later outlined by Tim Berners-Lee, *"It isn't the documents which are actually interesting, it is the things they are about!"* [18]; this motivated the need for a semantic Web, where a semantic Web browser should be able to collect and to disclose to a user the information about a "thing" of interest, based on a search from many sources with a subsequent merge.

As outlined in the Introduction, the conception of the Internet of Things [2] has motivated the consequent proposal for an implementation of the Web of Things, as suggested by Guinard and Trifa, who have asserted [3]: *"we propose to leverage the existing and ubiquitous Web protocols as common ground where real objects could interact with each other. One of the advantages of using Web standards is that devices will be able to naturally speak the same language as other resources on the Internet, therefore making it very easy to integrate physical devices with any content on the Web."*

This poses the basis for a further shift from the document-centric view of data to a human-centric view of information, where "things" are owned by users who collect and organize information related to their lives.

Related to the task of Web Information Retrieval, this view has stimulated a shift from the document-centric perspective to a user-centric and context aware perspective.

As it has been outlined in the Introduction, context-awareness has two major facets: user-oriented and self-oriented. When thinking at an Information Retrieval Application the facet of user-oriented context-awareness has been deeply investigated in the literature and it has been referred to as personalization, which can be seen as an instantiation of contextualization, where the considered context is the user context. This contextualization is at the application level, and it does not imply a self-oriented context awareness, as discussed in Sect. 5.2. In fact a centralized Information Retrieval System may provide context-aware services without exposing a self-oriented autonomic behavior, if it is based on a server without self-management capabilities. On the opposite, a distributed information retrieval system may exhibit an autonomic context-aware behavior to ensure a high degree of availability and responsiveness, while the services it provides may be not context-aware (i.e. search may be independent on the user context).

Similar remarks apply to networking issues: a network may expose user-oriented context-aware communication services based on the location of mobile users even if the network itself has a static topology therefore it does not exploit self-oriented context-awareness. On the opposite, a network based on mobile nodes may exploit context information (i.e., the location of the nodes) to autonomously reconfigure itself, though it exposes end-to-end services based on classical static addresses.

Although this basic classification is inevitably coarse, it may help identifying what we are talking about when talking about context-awareness in a complex ICT system. In particular, it helps to understand that the general concept of context-awareness not only may involve different types of context information, but it can also be based on different technologies. For example, the context sensitive behavior of a recommender system for e-commerce can be based on context information stored in a large centralized database, while this solution may be hardly exploited for a distributed autonomic system that supports time and life critical applications.

In practice, the separation fades between user-oriented and self-oriented context-awareness, due to the fact that both aspects co-exist in an advanced ICT system. Therefore the ideal solution would be to devise a general set of concepts and mechanisms that can be exploited at different levels of abstraction, and at different system layers to support context-awareness. However, concrete solutions depend largely on both requirements and criticalities of specific application domains and of specific system layers, so that unification is a challenging issue.

5.3.1 Information Retrieval and User-Oriented Context Awareness

The notion of context has constituted an important issue in computer science, and it has been studied and formalized in several domains, such as artificial intelligence [19], distributed and mobile computing [1] and more recently in Information Retrieval [20, 21].

In Information Retrieval an important objective in contextualizing search is to define context-aware systems able to identify useful context information in a user unaware way, so as to overcome the "one size fits all" search paradigm, where a keyword-based query is considered as the only carrier of the users' information needs. Instead, a contextual Search Engine relies on a user-centric approach as it involves processes, techniques and algorithms that take advantage of contextual factors as much as possible in order to tailor the search results to the users context [22, 23].

A context-aware search system should produce answers to a specific query by also taking into account the contextual information formally expressed in a context model. The key notion of context has multiple interpretations in Information Retrieval [24]; it may be related to the characteristics and topical preferences of a specific user or group of users (in this case contextualization is referred to as personalization), or it may be related to spatio-temporal coordinates, it may refer to the information that qualifies the content of a given document/web page (for example its author, its creation date, its format etc.), or it may refer to a social or a socio- economic situation.

The development and increasing use of tools that either help users to express or to automatically learn their preferences, along with the availability of devices and technologies that can detect users location and monitor users actions, allow to capture elements of the users context.

To model new paradigms for contextual search in recent years a significant amount of research has addressed the two main issues of how to learn and to formally represent the context, and how to leverage the context model during the retrieval process. In particular, the above problems have been addressed based on the considered interpretation of context, leading to specific IR specializations such as personalized IR, mobile IR, social IR. The majority of the proposed approaches are related to personalization, i.e. to enhance the search outcome based on the availability of a user model, also called user profile.

An important and difficult problem to be addressed in personalized search is that often users switch from a search interest to another, and they alternate search related to long-term interests with search related to only temporary interests. In the case of a query that is not related to the users topical interest, the consideration of a user model is not useful, and may be even noisy and unproductive. Therefore a research challenge is to make search engines able to capture shifts in users interests.

In a contextual search the definition of the context model encompasses three main activities: acquisition of the basic information that characterizes the context, representation of the context information by means of a formal language (definition of the context model), and adoption of a strategy for updating the context model. To accomplish the first task two main techniques are employed: explicit and implicit [25–28]. The former requires an explicit user-system interaction, while the latter acquires information useful in defining the user profile without involving the user. By the explicit approach in fact the user is asked to be proactive and to directly communicate his/her personal data and preferences to the system. Concerning the implicit approach, several techniques have been proposed to automatically capture the user's interests, by monitoring the users actions, and by implicitly inferring from them the users preferences [28]. The proposed techniques range from click-through data analysis, query log analysis, analysis of desktop information, etc.

The formal representation of the information obtained by the context acquisition phase implies the selection of an appropriate formal language; to this aim in the literature several representations have been proposed, ranging from bag of words and vector representations, to graph-based representations [29], and, more recently, to ontology based representations [30–32].

The context model is employed to enhance search through specific algorithms, which make explicit use of the information in the context model to produce the search results related to a query. The three main classes of approaches proposed in the literature aim at: defining personalized retrieval models, reformulating the user query to enrich it with the context information, re-ranking search results based on the information represented in the context model [21–23, 27, 33].

5.4 Conclusions

The aim of this Chapter was to provide a general overview of a few key issues related to the notion of context in relation to the Internet of Things, the Web of Things and the Wisdom Web of Things. The proposed overview has tackled the two main layers of communication and applications, by specifically considering the applicative problem of accessing information on the Web through a contextual search approach.

While today some technologies represent a reality, and a considerable amount of research has been undertaken, much work has still to be done to implement an efficient and effective contextual approach to managing and accessing Web Information.

References

1. B.N. Schilit, M.M. Theimer, Disseminating active map information to mobile hosts. IEEE Netw. **8**(5), 22–32 (1994)
2. L. Atzori, A. Iera, G. Morabito, The internet of things: a survey. Comput. Netw. **54**(15), 2787–2805 (2010)
3. D. Guinard, V. Trifa, Towards the web of things: web mashups for embedded devices, in *Proceedings of the International World Wide Web Conferences*, Madrid, Spain (2009)
4. D. Guinard, V. Trifa, F. Mattern, E. Wilde, From the internet of things to the web of things: resource oriented architecture and best practices, in D. Uckelmann, M. Harrison, F. Michahelles (eds.), *Architecting the Internet of Things*, Springer, ISBN 978-3-642-19156-5, April 2011, pp. 97–129
5. N. Zhong, J.H. Ma, R.H. Huang, J.M. Liu, Y.Y. Yao, Y.X. Zhang, J.H. Chen, Research challenges and perspectives on Wisdom Web of Things (W2T). J. Supercomput. **1–21**, (Springer, 2010)
6. N. Ohta, A. Takahara, A. Jajszczyk, R. Saracco, Emerging technologies in communications. IEEE J. Sel. Areas Commun. **31**(9), 1–5 (2013)
7. Z. Movahedi, M. Ayari, R. Langar, G. Pujolle, A Survey of autonomic network architectures and evaluation criteria. Commun. Surv. Tutorials IEEE **14**(2), 464–490 (2012)
8. E. Gelenbe, R. Lent, A. Nunez, Self-aware networks and QoS. Proc. IEEE **92**(9), 1478–1489 (2004)
9. P. Makris, D. Skoutas, C. Skianis, A survey on context-aware mobile and wireless networking: on networking and computing environments integration. Commun. Surv. Tutorials IEEE **15**(1), 362–386 (2013)
10. O.G. Aliu, A. Imran, M.A. Imran, B. Evans, A survey of self organisation in future cellular networks. Commun. Surv. Tutorials IEEE **15**(1), 336–361 (2013)
11. A. Georgakopoulos, K. Tsagkaris, D. Karvounas, P. Vlacheas, P. Demestichas, Cognitive networks for future internet: status and emerging challenges. Veh. Technol. Mag. IEEE **7**(3), 48–56 (2012)
12. B.N. Schilit, D.M. Hilbert, J. Trevor, Context-aware communication. Wirel. Commun. IEEE **9**(5), 46–54 (2002)
13. J.J. Garcia-Luna-Aceves, M. Mosko, I. Solis, R. Braynard, R. Ghosh, Context-aware protocol engines for ad hoc networks. Commun. Mag. IEEE **47**(2), 142–149 (2009)
14. F. Cadger, K. Curran, J. Santos, S. Moffett, A survey of geographical routing in wireless ad-hoc networks. Commun. Surv. Tutorials IEEE **15**(2), 621–653 (2013)
15. T. Watteyne, A. Molinaro, M. Richichi, M. Dohler, From MANET to IETF ROLL standardization: a paradigm shift in WSN routing protocols. Commun. Surv. Tutorials IEEE **13**(4), 688–707 (2011)
16. V.C.M. Borges, M. Curado, E. Monteiro, Cross-layer routing metrics for mesh networks: current status and research directions. Comput. Commun. **34**(6), 681–703 (2011)
17. J. Kim, J. Lee, J. Kim, J. Yun, M2M service platforms: survey, issues, and enabling technologies. Commun. Surv. Tutorials IEEE pp. 99, 116 (2013)
18. T. Berners-Lee, *The Web of Things*. ERCIM News, number **72**, (January 2008)
19. J. McCarthy, Generality in artificial intelligence. Commun. ACM **30**(12), 1030–1035 (1987)
20. P. Ingwersen, K. Jrvelin, *The Turn: Integration of Information Seeking and Retrieval in Context* (Springer, Heidelberg, 2005)

21. G. Pasi, in *Contextual Search: Issues and Challenges, Information Quality in e-Health—7th Conference of the Workgroup Human-Computer Interaction and Usability Engineering of the Austrian Computer Society*, USAB 2011, Graz, Austria, November 25–26, Lecture Notes in Computer Science, 2011, vol. 7058. Information Quality in e-Health **23–30** (2011)
22. A. Micarelli, F. Gasparetti, F. Sciarrone, S. Gauch, S, Personalized search on the world wide web, in P. Brusilovsky, A. Kobsa, W. Nejdl (eds.), *Adaptive Web* 2007. LNCS, vol. 4321, pp. 195–230 (Springer, Heidelberg, 2007)
23. G. Pasi, Issues in personalizing information retrieval. IEEE Intell. Inf. Bull. (IIB) (December 2010)
24. L. Tamine-Lechani, M. Boughanem, M. Daoud, Evaluation of contextual Information retrieval effectiveness: overview of issues and research. Knowl. Inf. Syst. **24**, 134 (2010)
25. M. Claypool, D. Brown, P. Le, M. Waseda, Inferring user interest. IEEE Intern. Comput. **3239** (2001)
26. X. Shen, B. Tan, C.X. Zhai, Implicit user modeling for personalized search, in *International Conference on Information and Knowledge Management, CIKM 2005* (2005), pp. 824–831
27. J. Teevan, S. Dumais, E. Horvitz, Personalizing search via automated analysis of interests and activities, in *International ACM SIGIR Conference on Research and Development in Information Retrieval 2005* (2005), pp. 449–456
28. D. Kelly, J. Teevan, Implicit feedback for inferring user preference: a bibliography. SIGIR Forum **37**(2), 2003 (1828)
29. M. Daoud, L. Tamine-Lechani, M. Boughanem, Towards a graph-based user profile modeling for a session-based personalized search. Knowl. Inf. Syst. **21**(3), 365–398 (2009)
30. S. Calegari, G. Pasi, Personal ontologies: generation of user profiles based on the YAGO ontology. Inf. Process. Manage. **49**(3), 640–658 (2013)
31. A. Sieg, B. Mobasher, R. Burke, Web search personalization with ontological user profiles, in *International Conference on Information and Knowledge Management, CIKM 2007* (2007), pp. 525–534
32. M. Speretta, S. Gauch, Miology: a web application for organizing personal domain ontologies, in *International Conference on Information, Process and Knowledge Management, EKNOW 2009* (2009), pp. 159–161
33. G. Jeh, J. Widom, Scaling personalized web search, in *12th International World Wide Web Conference (WWW 2003)*, Budapest, Hungary (2003), pp. 271–279

Part II
Wisdom Web of Things and Humanity

Chapter 6
Ontology-Based Model for Mining User's Emotions on the Wisdom Web

Jing Chen, Bin Hu, Philip Moore and Xiaowei Zhang

Abstract The task of automatically detecting emotion on a web is challenging. This is due to the fact that a traditional web cannot directly interpret the meaning of semantic concepts or assess users emotions. We describe an ontology-based mining model for representation and integration of affect-related knowledge and apply it to detect user's emotions. This application is a typical use case of the broad-based Wisdom Web of Things (W2T) methodology. The model (named *BIO-EMOTION*) acts as an integrated framework for: (1) representation and interpretation of affect-related knowledge, including user profile, bio-signal data, situation and environment factors, and (2) supporting intelligent reasoning on users' emotions. To evaluate the effectiveness of the mining model, we conduct an experiment on a public dataset DEAP and capture a semantic knowledge base expressing both known and deduced knowledge. Evaluation shows that the model not only reaches higher accuracy than other emotion detection results from the same dataset but also achieves a comprehensive affect-related knowledge base which could represent things from both social world, physical world and cyber world in semantics. The ultimate goal of present research is to provide active, transparent, safe and reliable services to web users through their inner emotion. The model implements crucial sub-processes of W2T data cycle: from Things (acquisition of things in the hyper world) to Wisdom (performing intelligent reasoning on web users' emotion). A long-term goal is to achieve the whole W2T data cycle and to realize a holistic intelligent mining model used on the Wisdom Web.

J. Chen · B. Hu (✉) · P. Moore · X. Zhang
School of Information Science and Engineering,
Lanzhou University, Lanzhou 730000, China
e-mail: bh@lzu.edu.cn

J. Chen
e-mail: chenj12@lzu.edu.cn

P. Moore
e-mail: ptmbcu@gmail.com

X. Zhang
e-mail: zhangxw@lzu.edu.cn

N. Zhong et al. (eds.), *Wisdom Web of Things*, Web Information
Systems Engineering and Internet Technologies Book Series,
DOI 10.1007/978-3-319-44198-6_6

6.1 Introduction

In recent years with more people connected to the Internet, people are more likely to use the Web to find information pertinent to products and services. However, to make the Web capable of effectively interacting with users and improving user satisfaction requires users behaviors especially users cognitive behavior to be understood by the Web and some related resources to be captured. Often described as a vital part of human cognitive behaviors, one is expressing and understanding human emotions [83]. Emotional sensitivity in machines is believed to be a key element towards more human-like computer interaction. Therefore, one of the current issues in Artificial Intelligence and Web applications is to produce a wisdom web for efficient processing and understanding of users emotion and eventually for providing reliable services. Such a web could be very valuable as an intelligent platform providing active and transparent services to humans, which could be viewed as an application of Wisdom Web [99, 100]. In fact, many factors affect or reflect human emotions; specifically, sleep quality, age, gender and temperature could influence human emotions, and facial expression and physiological measures could reflect emotions. Here, it would be an issue how to gather and organize affect-related data, information and knowledge from humans, computers and physical world.

We have developed an ontology-based mining model, named *BIO-EMOTION* to address the above issue. The model can be a typical case of Wisdom Web of Things (W2T) [101] methodologies. The W2T is an extension of the Wisdom Web in the Internet of Things (IoT) [16, 93] age. The "Wisdom" means that each of things in the Web of Things (WoT) [27, 88] can be aware of both itself and others to provide the right service for the right object at the right time and context. Constructing the W2T for the harmonious symbiosis of humans, computers and things in the hyper world [52, 56] requires a highly effective W2T data cycle, namely from things to data, information, knowledge, wisdom, services, humans, and then back to things [101]. Multimodal affect-related data is gathered and represented in the model including demographic data, biological signals, environment information and other affect-related contexts. The information and knowledge extracted from the original data are represented in the model in semantics. The model provides an intelligent platform to competing emotion detection of a web user during his interaction with the Internet. The information from web users (in the social world), things (in the physical world) and computer systems (in the cyber world) are integrated into the model to realize their symbiosis, comprehensive knowledge representation and to provide input to intelligent reasoning on users emotions in accordance with an effective process of W2T data cycle. In this cycle, how to use multiple affect-related contexts for emotion detection would be one important task. Emotion exhibits certain sophisticated characteristics:

1. Emotion is hidden as a cognitive behavior, as though facial expression and gesture could merely sometimes portray it authentically;
2. The occurrences of emotion appear dynamically and in a very limited time;

3. Factors that influence emotional change are dispersed in highly imbalanced hyper world.

Towards measures of automatic emotion detection, numerous efforts have been deployed to the audiovisual channels such as facial expression or speeches. Using video to code gestures, body language, facial expressions and verbalizations, is a rich source of data; however, there is an enormous time commitment, which requires between 5 and 100 h of analysis for every hour of video [33]. Its analysis is generally event-based (user is smiling now), rather than continuous (degree of smile for every point in time) which is just important for exploring user emotions in web applications. The fact that humans easily and effortlessly perceive anger, or sadness, or fear in another persons face is not evidence that facial actions broadcast the internal state of the target person. Simply put, a face does not speak for itself. Several interesting findings indicate that certain affective states can be recognized by means of electroencephalogram (EEG). As an objective route, EEG signal always reflects the true emotional state of a person, while speech and facial appearance might be influenced by a person intentionally. Thus, EEG is an important indicator and knowledge of emotional experience in our model.

Since different theories on how emotions arise and are expressed exist, there is a variety of emotion models [74] which results in different interpretation of emotions across individuals even within the same culture [75]. Fortunately, thanks to the vast studies in psychology such as the proposal of six basic emotions by Ekman [31, 32] or the development of the International Affective Picture System (IAPS), this problem has been some extent alleviated by the employment of scientific categorization of emotions and the usage of standardized emotion elicitation facilities. IAPS provides a set of normative emotional description. In this system, emotions are regarded as points on the 2-D affective space, which is formed by the affective dimensions of valence and arousal. The affective space will be detailed in Sect. 6.3.1. Considering the above modeling characteristics, we propose an effective framework that synthesizes affect-related resources and incorporates several advanced data mining techniques. The main ideas, advantages and our contributions of this framework are as follows:

1. It is inspired by the theories of Affective Computing, Neuroscience and Wisdom Web of Things, providing a systematic solution by synthesizing domain knowledge, common sense knowledge, coming from humans, computers, and things in the physical world;
2. Brain is one of the most important organs of body and it has become a great source for the research of emotion assessment, thus EEG becomes important resource in the mining model. To fully explore powerful information hidden in EEG signals for emotion detection, multiple statistic features, time-frequency features and nonlinear dynamics features are extracted from raw EEG signals. Different from traditional human brain studies, the model emphasizes on a systematic approach for emotion assessment which involves multiple interrelated processes including EEG data collection, EEG data storage, data management, data description, data mining, information organization of EEG and knowledge utilization;

3. The affect-related knowledge is built in an ontology using description logics, where things in real world are defined as conceptual vocabularies, which provides a comprehensive and elegant knowledge base;
4. The model incorporates and integrates several data mining techniques, such as signal denoising, feature extraction and classification. C4.5 algorithm [77], one of Data Mining technique, is used to produce reasoning rules. Construction of decision tree (DT) using the tuples leads to generation a set of compact rules by traversing each path from root toward leaf nodes. The model drives an inference engine to perform decision-making on the rule base. The deduced knowledge is then described in the *BIO-EMOTION* to complete comprehensive knowledge expression and storage;
5. Massive experiments in a public dataset DEAP show that our model, on the one hand, could deduce user emotions with a higher accuracy and a lower false positive rate than most emotion-related models, outperforming the existing rule-based system. On the other hand, our model performs well in knowledge representation of both known knowledge and deduced knowledge, and in completing a sound W2T data cycle. Experimental results show that the models underlying reasoning on 2-D affective space (valence dimension and arousal dimension respectively) reaches average accuracy of 75.19 and 81.74 %.

The remainder of this work is organized as follows. Section 6.2 gives an overview of related research. Section 6.3 presents the *BIO-EMOTION* model, in which comprehensive representation of affect-related knowledge is supported by an intelligent reasoning approach. The application of the ontology-based mining model on the DEAP dataset [49] is described in Sect. 6.4. Section 6.5 discusses experimental results and presents future work aimed at solving drawbacks of the model. Finally, Sect. 6.6 gives a conclusion.

6.2 Related Work

Emotion is a complex phenomenon for which no definition that is generally accepted has been given. These affect-related phenomena have traditionally been studied in depth by disciplines such as philosophy or psychology. Emotional sensitivity in machines is believed to be a key element towards more human-like computer interaction and the past decades have shown an increasing interest in interdisciplinary methods that automatically recognize emotions. In order for web users to benefit from web services, knowledge mining techniques have been proposed to represent and organize affect-related knowledge from the hyper world.

This section explores the state of the art in two domains the present research is closely related to: approaches to emotion detection and techniques of building knowledge mining model.

6.2.1 Previous Studies on Emotion Detection

The research literature related to emotion detection has been surveyed previously. These surveys have very different foci, as is expected in a highly interdisciplinary field that spans psychology, computer science, engineering, neuroscience, education, and many others.

The psychological literature related to emotion detection is probably the most extensive. Journals such as Emotion, Emotion Review, and Cognition and Emotion provide an outlet for reviews, and are good sources for researchers with an interest in emotion. Recent reviews of emotion theories include the integrated review of several existing theories (and the presentation of his core affect theory) by Russell [79], a review of facial and vocal communication of emotion also by Russell [79], a critical review on the theory of basic emotions and a review on the experience of emotion by Barrett [7, 8], and a review of affective neuroscience by Dalgleish et al. [23]. The Handbook of Cognition and Emotion [24], the Handbook of Emotions [54], and the Handbook of Affective Sciences [26] provide broad coverage on affective phenomena.

In recent studies in computer science and engineering, D'Mello and Graesser [21] considered a combination of facial features, gross body language, and conversational cues for detecting some of the learning-centered affective states. Classification results supported a channel judgment type interaction, where the face was the most diagnostic channel for spontaneous affect judgments (i.e., at any time in the tutorial session), while conversational cues were superior for fixed judgments (i.e., every 20 s in the session). Pantic and Rothkrantz [70] and Sebe et al. [84] provided reviews of multimodal approaches (mainly face and speech) with brief discussions of data fusion strategies. Zeng et al. [97] reviewed the literature on audiovisual detection approaches focusing on spontaneous expressions, while others [20, 70] focused on reviewing work on posed (e.g., by actors) emotions. A set of text-based approaches to analyzing emotion was reviewed [20]. Ko et al. [48] employed EEG relative power values and Bayesian network for recognizing 5 types of basic emotions. Murugappan et al. [63] used statistical features from discrete wavelet transform feature extraction and fuzzy c-means clustering for distinguishing four basic emotions, namely happy, surprise, fear and disgust. Results indicated that reduced number of EEG channels reduces computational complexity and yields better results. In a study about cerebral asymmetry, Davidson et al. found that disgust caused less alpha power in the right frontal region than happiness, while happiness caused less alpha power in the left frontal region [25]. Moreover, Kostyunina and Kulikov found that alpha peak frequency differs among emotions. For joy and anger they observed an increase in alpha peak frequency while sorrow and fear caused a decrease compared to the baseline condition [51]. Aftanas et al. [2] reported significant changes in EEG synchronization and desynchronization for certain frequency bands in connection with different emotional states. An user-dependent system for arousal classification based on frequency band characteristics was developed [15]. With this system, classification rates around 45 % on three arousal categories could be achieved. The effectiveness of the different marketing strategies may be evaluated by monitoring brain activity resulting from consumers observing different advertisements and products [3, 67]. This is mainly driven by the fact that people cannot (or do not want to) fully explain their preferences when explicitly asked; as human behavior can be (and is) driven by processes operating below the level of conscious awareness [12]. The change in the human brain signal, denoted as EEG, is observed to examine consumers' cognitive or affective processes in response to prefabricated marketing stimuli [4, 9, 46, 68]. The importance of the left frontal region is also indicated in an experiment relating the smelling of favorite and dislikeable odors to EEG power change suggesting an association between theta wave and alpha wave from the frontal regions and preferences [95].

6.2.2 Building Knowledge Model Techniques

A set of concept maps and associated resources about a particular domain of knowledge is referred to as a Knowledge Model [11]. Arthur Anderson Business Consulting [5] proposed a schematic representation of the relationships among data, information, knowledge, and wisdom, and stated that data, information, and knowledge are necessary for dealing with regular affairs, whereas wisdom is necessary for dealing with irregular affairs and adopting appropriate actions when faced with a changing environment. According to their view, knowledge modeling not only manages knowledge, but also encourages individuals to utilize knowledge effectively while working. Based on adaptive network-based fuzzy inference system (ANFIS) modeling, a derived fuzzy knowledge model is proposed for quantitatively estimating the depth of anesthesia (DOA) [98]. By using ANFIS, fuzzy if-then rules are obtained to express the complex relationship between the three derived parameters and anesthesia states. These rules are then used to construct a derived fuzzy knowledge model for providing a single variable to represent the DOA.

Since traditional web usage only records requested URLs but not the semantics of contents requested by the users, it is difficult to use such record for tracking the users actual web access behaviors, emotions, and interests. Ontology can be defined as the formal specification of knowledge in a specific domain. In traditional knowledge engineering and in emerging Semantic Web research, ontologies play an important role in defining the semantics of data. The use of ontology in computer science can be traced to Artificial Intelligence (AI) research in the 1960s [81]. Ontology techniques which are used in our research are first introduced followed by related studies in this domain.

Ontology defines a set of representational terms that associate the names of entities (e.g., classes, relations, functions or other objects) in an area of interest (universe of discourse) in a human-readable formalism describing meaning and formal axioms that constrain the interpretation with well-formed use of the terms. In computer science and information systems, an ontology is a representation of a knowledge model with semantic detail and structure. Formally, ontology is built on logical theory to represent objects and supports inference and reasoning thereby providing the basis upon which a degree of computational intelligence can be realized. An important concept that underpins ontological models is semantics and semantic relationships between objects and entities. Ontologies based on Description Logics paradigm include definitions of concepts (OWL classes), roles (OWL properties) and individuals. The most common language to formalize Semantic Web ontologies is OWL (Ontology Web Language) [60], a proposal of the W3C. The goal of this standard is to formalize the semantics that was created ad hoc in old frame systems and semantic networks.

OWL has three increasingly expressive sub-languages: OWL Lite, OWL DL, and OWL Full. OWL Lite is the simplest subset of OWL, specially designed to provide a quick migration path for other taxonomical structures. OWL DL is the subset of OWL designed for applications that need the maximum expressiveness without losing computational completeness and decidability. It is based on Description Logics, a particular fragment of first-order logic, in which concepts, roles, individuals, and axioms that relate them (using universal and existential restrictions, negation, etc.) are defined. These entailments may be based on a single document or multiple distributed documents that we combine using the import OWL mechanisms. The OWL DL reasoning capabilities rely on the good computational properties of DLs. OWL DL has support for poly hierarchical automatic classification.

Java is probably the most important general-purpose language for developing Semantic Web applications, and it is also the language in which the original voice synthesizer was made, so the choice was obvious. However, there are at least two very promising Java frameworks available. One of them is Sesame [1], an open source RDF framework with support for RDF Schema inferencing and querying. The other one is Jena [43], another open source framework with a programmatic environment for RDF, RDFS, OWL, SPARQL, and its own rule-based inference engine. Sesame has a local and remote access API, several query languages (included SPARQL) and it is more oriented to offer flexible and fast connections with storage systems. Jena has also RDF and OWL APIs, tools to deal with RDF/XML, N3 and N-Triples formats, an SPARQL query engine and also some persistent storage functionality. It is important to consider that Jena is a useful tool for exploring the strong relation between SPARQL queries and OWL-DL ontologies [44].

For our purposes, both ontology-based knowledge representation performance and inference support for Description Logics are taken into consideration. The architecture of Sesame is probably easier to extend than the architecture of Jena, but from the point of view of the client building a wrapper for the functionality of the underlying framework, Jena is the most intuitive and usable API.

Ontologies are built in a machine readable formalism [37] for Web services to enable reasoning and inference over various data as input and return as output (which have the characters of W2T proposed in Zhong et al. [101]) based on entailment and subsumption. Once Web services are described semantically it allows for large parts of the Web service usage process to be automated. Apparently, a potential issue lies in the failure on some system designers who had attempted to bring more meaning to web resources but without a solid formal underpinning. However, suitable rules can be defined to transform the separated ontological knowledge into a relational network. In response, diverse valid research initiatives in distinct application fields (e.g. Mathieu [59]; Francisco et al. [34]; Lpez et al. [53]) have been proposed. Additionally, there is a W3C Emotion Markup Language Incubator Group, working on the definition of valid representations of those aspects of emotional states that appear to be relevant for a number of use cases in emotion scenarios. Mathieu [59] presented a semantic lexicon in the field of feelings and emotions. This lexicon is described with an ontology. Words in the lexicon are emotionally labeled as positive, negative and neutral. With the support of ontology technologies, users can retrieve information in a semantic manner [18]. Focusing on speech, Galunov et al. [36] presented an ontology for speech signal recognition and synthesis where emotion is taken into account. On the other hand, focusing on the context, Benta et al. [6] presented an ontology-based representation of the affective states for context aware applications which allows expressing the complex relations between affective states and context elements. Although these kinds of approaches have relevance in their respective fields, they lack properly expression of the multimodal nature of human emotions (Lpez et al. [53]). In this sense, Cearreta et al. [14] modeled user context by dividing it into several parts and focusing on emotion-related aspects in each part. Dai and Mobasher [22] used domain ontology to enhance web usage mining for traditional web usage logs, but the mapping from requested URLs to ontological entities lacks reliability, especially for dynamic websites. Oberle et al. [66] proposed another framework for semantic enrichment of web usage logs by mapping each requested URL to one or more concepts from the ontology of the underlying website. It clusters groups of sessions with specific user interests from the semantically enhanced weblogs, and applies association rule mining to the semantically enhanced weblogs. Eirinaki et al. [29] obtained concept-logs (C-logs) by enriching each webserver log record with keywords from a taxonomy representing the semantics of the requested URLs. C-logs were analyzed in [62] with MINE RULE (a query language for association rule mining) for discovering access patterns. Also, Fraternali et al. [35] created conceptual logs by combining the server log data with the conceptual schema of the web application. Most semantic web usage mining techniques focus only on discovering simple usage statistics and common access patterns of user groups. Further, the discovered knowledge should be represented as ontology to enable Semantic Web applications.

6.2.3 Discussion

The combination of knowledge modeling and Emotion Recognition is an interesting approach toward providing the right service for the right object at a right time and time. Brain signals seem to reflect the "inner" and real emotions, but there is limited EEG-based research in the ontological modeling area, even though a variety of statistical techniques are emerging for analysis of spatiotemporal patterns in EEG research [28]. According to Dou et al. [28], they introduced a framework for mining ERP (event-related potentials) ontologies based on clustering, classification and association rule mining. Their goal is to address basic scientific questions in ERP research using ontology-based classification. On the one hand, we classify and label brain signal patterns which can lead to refinement of these concepts and association rules. On the other hand, we map low-level EEG signals to high-level human emotions in semantics. Specifically, we extract and label EEG features for each user, identify important metrics for emotion recognition and define the reasoning rules showing corresponding relationships between EEG patterns and user emotions. Given the above, a DL ontology-based model BIO-EMOTION for mining web users emotion is proposed.

6.3 Building the *BIO-EMOTION* Model

An affect-related knowledge model, named *BIO-EMOTION*, is proposed for automatic reasoning and recognition of web users emotions to eventually support the Wisdom Web. The model uses ontology techniques to construct comprehensive knowledge including knowledge related to Affective Computing and common sense knowledge. The *BIO-EMOTION* provides an upper ontological model expressing abstract concepts (OWL Classes), properties (Datatype Properties and Object Properties), and instances (Individuals) of each abstract class. All elements of the ontology identify and specify concrete things in the hyper world. For instance, if one type of things in the real-world such as brain regions, electrodes or EEG features extracted from raw EEG signals could be represented as a set which contains many instances, such a set will be described as a Class in the ontology; whereas if it refers to a concrete object, it will be described as an Individual. The model also provides inference mechanism incorporating C4.5 algorithm upon the ontological knowledge base to explore new knowledge. The model first expresses facts or known knowledge in the ontological knowledge base, and then performs reasoning to explore new knowledge under the help of C4.5 algorithm. The whole process of the model construction exactly achieves sub-processes of W2T from "Things to Data to Information to Knowledge to Wisdom", in which intelligent reasoning makes the model reach the wisdom level. We know that constructing the W2T for the harmonious symbiosis of humans, computers and things in the hyper world also requires completing sub-processes from Wisdom to Services to Humans to Things. Indeed, once the model is used in a specific application such as telemedicine for monitoring users emotional experiences, the model would easily complete these services-related subprocesses for there is a very specific target of how to provide specific services.

6.3.1 Building Conceptual Knowledge Base in the BIO-EMOTION

Ontology "transforms" things from real world into "data" world. Depending on the expressivity of Web Ontology Language (OWL), ontological representations range from simple taxonomies defining term hierarchies to sophisticated concept networks with complex restrictions in the relations. We know that enormous facts exist and they could be directly represented in the ontological model without mining. These facts form the foundational knowledge base. Building these knowledge or facts completes sub-processes of W2T data cycle: (1) "Things to Data": various data of things are collected into an ontology-based conceptual knowledge base; these data include high time-resolution data of things coming from EEG sensors, the Web accessible historic data of things stored on the Web, and the data of Web produced on the Web; (2) "Data to Information": information related to both sensor data and Web data are extracted and reorganized to generate multi-aspect and multi-granularity data information after data integration, and storage. The obtained information is also described and stored in our ontology-based knowledge base; (3) "Information to Knowledge": the valuable affect-related knowledge is explored and extracted from data information, which are also represented in the knowledge base; (4) "Knowledge to Wisdom": based on the obtained knowledge, we focus on affect-related reasoning to detect user emotions and to support Wisdom Web. However, ontological knowledge base cannot perform reasoning itself; to make our model at its wisdom level, we incorporate a Data Mining method, C4.5 algorithm, into the model (detailed in Sect. 6.3.2). One challenge, at this stage of knowledge representation, is to develop and test a framework for separating, expressing and classifying complex patterns that are superposed in measured EEG data. The model *BIO-EMOTION* describes things by different dimensions and includes various specifications on different levels of conversion mechanism.

The first and indispensable level is to conceptualize facts or known knowledge in the hyper world. This level primarily involves data collection, information extraction and knowledge expression of things coming from hyper world. A DL ontology is developed depending on the following elements: Classes, which represent the basic ideas of the domain; instances or *Individuals*, which are concrete occurrences of objects; relations, roles, or *Properties*, which represent binary connections between individuals or individuals and typed values. Complex concept and relation expressions can be derived inductively from atomic primitives by applying the constructors defined by the logic. First-order logic (or DL) is implemented in the ontology-based model for its powerful functions of knowledge expressing and supporting reasoning. The ontology-based knowledge base consists of 84 *Classes* and 38 *Property* definitions. Figure 6.1 shows a representation of some key elements (represented as *Classes*, *Individuals* and *Properties*) defined in the ontology of the *BIO-EMOTION* model. The key top-level elements of the ontology-based model consist of Classes and Properties like *#Emotion, #Biosignals, #EEG_Features, #User*, and *#Situation (Classes)* with *<extractedFrom>*, *<hasEEGFeature>*, and *<hasEmotion> Properties*. Descriptions of the principal elements and their functions are as follows:

- ***#Emotion***: This *Class* defines users' emotional states. Two main opposite representing approaches are categorical and dimensional:

1. The categorical approach is used when searching for specific emotional states. There exist a small number of emotions that are basic, hard-wired in our brain, and

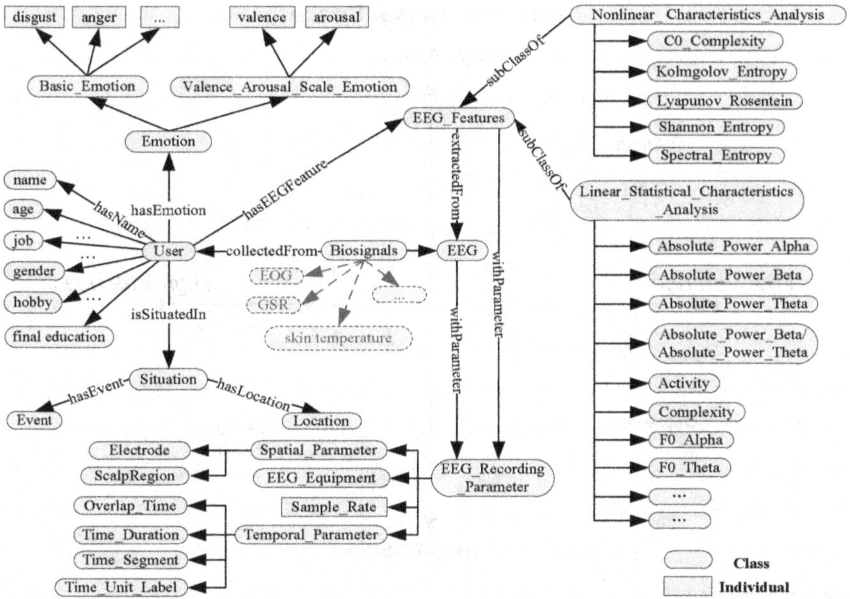

Fig. 6.1 Overview of the ontology-based model *BIO-EMOTION*

recognized universally. Ekman conducted various experiments and concluded that six basic emotions can be recognized universally, namely, happiness, sadness, surprise, fear, anger, and disgust [30].

2. According to the dimensional approach, affective states are not independent from one another; indeed, they are related to one another in a systematic manner. In this approach, the majority of affect variability is covered by two dimensions: valence and arousal [61, 80]. The valence dimension (V) refers to how positive or negative the emotion is, and ranges from unpleasant feelings to pleasant feelings of happiness. The arousal dimension (A) refers to how excited or apathetic the emotion is, and ranges from sleepiness or boredom to frantic excitement. Psychological evidence suggests that these two dimensions are intercorrelate [55, 69]. More specifically, there exist repeating configurations and interdependencies within the values that describe each dimension. The combination of these two dimensions forms four emotional categories (HVHA, HVLA, LVLA, and LVHA) which incorporate several categorical emotions as shown in Fig. 6.2.

The model represents emotions from the above two approaches: categorical approach through *#Basic_Emotion* and dimensional approach through *#Valence_Arousal_Scale_Emotion*. The Class *#Basic_Emotion* describes discrete emotional states, such as anger, disgust or fear. The Class *#Valence_Arousal_Scale_Emotion* focus on two dimensions: valence and arousal. To be specific, *#Basic_Emotion* and *#Valence_Arousal_Scale_Emotion* are expressed as two sub-classes of the super-class *#Emotion*, and the *Individuals* like *#calm, #anger, #arousal*, and

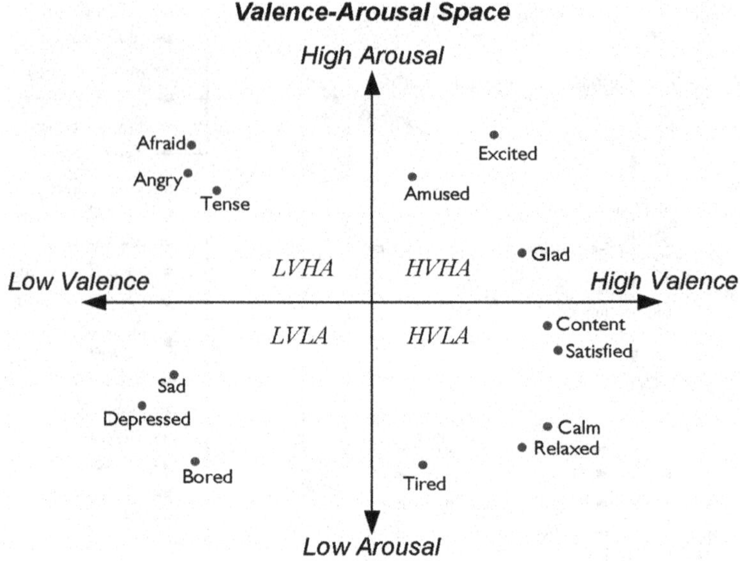

Fig. 6.2 Valence-Arousal space

#valence are represented as instances of *#Basic_Emotion* and *#Valence_Arousal_Scale_Emotion* respectively.

In the categorical approach, each affective display is classified into a single category, thus complex affective state or blended emotions may be too difficult to handle [96]. Instead, in the dimensional approach, emotion transitions can be easily captured, and observers can indicate their impression of moderate (less intense) and authentic emotional expressions on several continuous scales. Moreover, it derives from theory that valence and arousal are two orthogonal, independent dimensions of the emotional stimulus. This leads to an assumption that any emotion-related bio-signals may initially get differentiated according to one of the aforementioned dimensions (e.g., their valence dimension), and then, the other (e.g., their arousal dimension), leading to clear and theory-supported pathway for subsequent signal discrimination/classification [64]. Hence, dimensional approach has proven to be more useful in several domains (e.g., affective content analysis [94]) compared with the categorical approach. Considering viability of dimensional approach, we emphasize this approach in the present research.

- ***#Biosignals*** and ***#EEG_Features***: As we know, an interruption in human-computer interaction with the purpose to explicitly ask a web user about his current feeling could modify his true feeling. Such interruption should be avoided by suitable approaches, i.e., continuous monitoring other objects which could reflect users' emotions. Bio-signals are known to include emotion information that can be used for emotion assessment. They comprise the signals originating from the central nervous system and autonomic nervous system. It has been shown that emotional markers are stored in EEG signals. As brain signals can be hardly deceived by voluntary control and are available all the time, *BIO-EMOTION* is embedded

EEG signals and multiple features extracted from EEG signals as primary context information to deduce user emotions. EEG signal acts as decisive contextual information which is represented as subclass of *#Biosignals*. The multi-aspect EEG signal analysis is implemented for understanding complex brain information in depth, and for uncovering the emotion reactivity of thinking centric cognitive functions. Here, multiple EEG features, which are actually extracted from raw EEG signal using linear and nonlinear dynamics approaches, are expressed as subclasses of *#EEG_Features*. These features include spectral energy from different frequency bands, C_0 Complexity and Shannon Entropy, etc. (see Sect. 6.4.1 for details of the extracted features and their calculation). The model drives underlying data processing modules to obtain concrete values of these. *#EEG_Features* is connected to *#User* via a *Property <hasEEGFeature>* and to *#EEG* via another *Property <extractedFrom>*. In OWL subclass means necessary implication. In other words, if *#Activity* is a subclass of *#EEG_Features* then all instances of *#Activity* are instances of *#EEG_Features*, without exception—if something is an instance of *#Activity* then this implies that it is also an instance of *#EEG_Features*. And if *#Activity* is a subclass of *#EEG_Features* and *#EEG_Features* has a relation of *<hasEEGFeature>* with *#User* then *#Activity* also has the same relation with *#User*. To specify the representation of Classes and Individuals in the ontology, the description of one sub-class of EEG features *#Max_Power_Beta* and one of its instances are detailed in Figs. 6.3 and 6.4. Since several physiological signals (electrooculogram (EOG), skin temperature, Galvanic Skin Response (GSR),

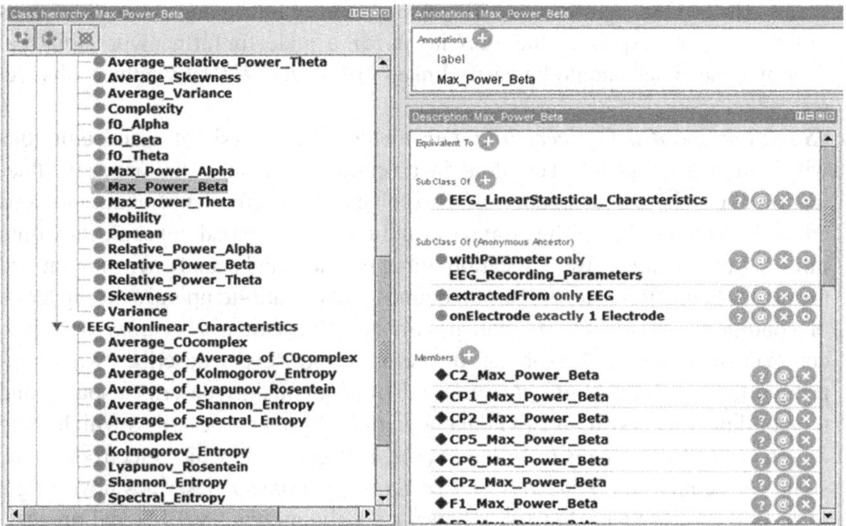

Fig. 6.3 Description of the Class *#Max_Power_Beta*. *#Max_Power_Beta* is a sub-class of *#EEG_LinearStatistical_Characteristics*; this kind of feature (instances of *#Max_Power_Beta*) can be extracted only from EEG signals and each feature sequence is extracted only and exactly from one EEG channel

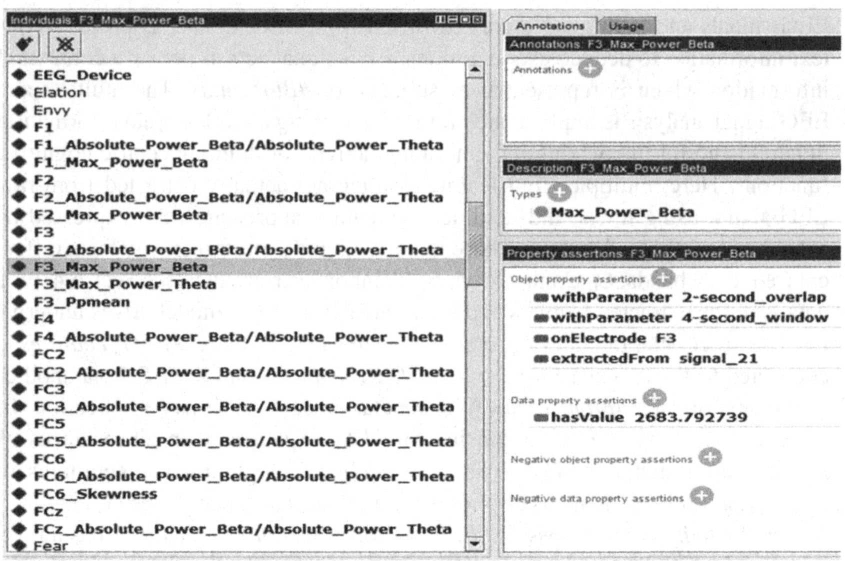

Fig. 6.4 Description of the instance of *#Max_Power_Beta*. The feature (instance) is extracted from an EEG channel named 'signal_21' on electrode F3 and its calculation has some restrictions: each value is calculated by sliding 4-s windows with a 2-s overlap

respiration amplitude, electrocardiogram (ECG), blood volume, and electromyograms (EMG)) are also sensitive to and may convey information about emotions [39, 45], we have expressed them as Classes in the model for further work, thus real data of these signals could be easily linked to *BIO-EMOTION* via these abstract sets.

- ***#Situation*** and ***#EEG_Recording_Parameter***: The analysis of users' emotions will be more accurate when combined with contexts as contexts influence the fluctuation of psychological signals and also enhance the performance of autonomous emotion detection [87]. The context in the model is a broad concept, including information about the user's location, time, physical and social environment and the device being used, etc. *#Situation* defines users' spatio-temporal states in terms of conditions, circumstances, and proximate information. *#Location* describes contexts such as the whereabouts of the user, and *#Event* describes what happens to the user, etc. *#EEG_Recording_Parameter* mainly describes spatial and temporal parameters about EEG data. *#Spatial_Parameter* describes which scalp region each EEG signal is recorded in (*#ScalpRegion*) and which electrode(s) the signal is recorded on (*#Electrode*). *#Temporal_Parameter* describes how long a recording lasts (*#Time_Duration*), how long a sliding window of signal processing is (*#Time_Segment*) and how long EEG signals could be overlapped when processed (*#Overlap_Time*). Besides, *#Sample_Rate* is represented as an instance of *#EEG_Recording_Parameter*, which details the sampling rate of a recording.

- ***#User***: Emotion is highly dependent on specific users, and we cannot give a precise detection of the specific underlying emotion even if external environment as an impact factor is seriously considered. It is vital that a model captures users' demographic characteristics ranging from the very basic features such as: *gender, age*, or *native language* to more complex socio-cultural parameters including the *level of formal education* and *family income*. These demographic characteristics are represented as *Classes* which are linked to *#User* through *Object Properties*. The *#User* is incorporated into the model to hold the demographic parameters with their related *Literal Values*, and it is the central element which links *#Situation, #Biosingals*, and *#EEG_Features* to *#Emotion*.

6.3.2 Intelligent Reasoning

Upon the conceptual knowledge representation, the second level is intelligent reasoning level. The model *BIO-EMOTION* describes things from the hyper world as different conceptual entities and superclass-subclass relationships. After numerous facts are represented in the ontology, the model drives an inference engine to deduce affect-related new knowledge just depending on these enormous built conceptual data and heterogeneous information.

With the changing of user preference and the contexts in the hyper world, Wisdom Web should provide active, transparent, safe, and reliable services based on users current requirement. In our model, recognition of web users emotion has historically two approaches: (1) direct user interviews, or (2) rule-based reasoning approach. Many reasoning techniques can provide more sensitive and objective metrics for emotion recognition when compared with users verbal responses in interviews [92]. Rule-based approach is often a classic AI reasoning technique used in smart web with predicate logic. It has been recognized that advanced reasoning capabilities require integrating some human-level capabilities such as robustness, autonomous interaction with their environment, communication with natural language, planning, learning, discovery and creativity. Our model is built just for being used on the Wisdom Web, so we should integrate automatic reasoning rather than human intervention in our model. The model performs the rule-based reasoning upon the ontology-based conceptual knowledge introduced in Sect. 6.3.1.

EEG data and multiple features extracted from the data are huge, thus feature selection is also a crucial step of building reasoning rules. Too large feature vectors used in reasoning process will highly affect its efficiency, which should be tackled especially in such Wisdom Web application. But when and how does the model drive a feature selection process? We use the users historical data to calculate the relevance of a feature to each affective state in terms of its F-score value, and mark those features, which have relatively higher score, in the model. Naturally, the historical data should not be too old because human EEG patterns change along years. The features with higher discrimination would be the basis of generating reasoning rules. C4.5 is a widely used classification algorithm the reasoning rules in this model are generated based on. Construction of DT using the tuples leads to generation a set of compact rules by traversing each path from root toward leaf nodes. The generated rules are inserted in the rule base to be employed in the next analysis phase. During this process, a great deal of semantic information generated is stored in the ontology-based knowledge base. When a new recognition task comes, the model will query these features with higher discrimination in the ontology and use this relatively small number of features to perform reasoning. In such an environment, we perform semantic queries on the already built knowledge in the ontology to obtain antecedent information of reasoning rules and use an inference engine to produce new information by automatic querying the rule set.

Reasoning involves two elements: rules and facts. Rules are in the form of *IF* → *Then*, where "*IF*" represents a matched condition or conditions, and "= *Then* =" means the triggered operation(s) when the condition(s) is matched. Facts express the current context of the hyper world, and are applied to matching the condition parts of rules. The rules are written based on Description Logic. When facing the massive and distributed knowledge in W2T, a C4.5 algorithm is proposed as the reasoning algorithm. A simplified example of a tree-like structure generated by C4.5 is depicted in Fig. 6.5. An inference rule described in first-order logical language corresponding to Fig. 6.5. is depicted as follows:

```
  String rule =
''[Rule1:(?EEG_feature1 rdf:type base: Kolmogorov_Entropy)
(?EEG_feature1 base:hasValue ?value1)
lessThanOrEqual(?value1, 2.3718)
(?EEG_feature1 base:onElectrode ?electrode1)
(?electrode1 rdfs:label ''CP4'')
(?variable1 rdf:type base:Gender)
(?variable1 base:hasValue ?value2)
equal(?value2, ''Male'')
(?EEG_feature2 rdf:type base:Max_Power_Alpha)
(?EEG_feature2 base:hasValue ?value2)
lessThanOrEqual(?value2, 1.74329)
(?EEG_feature2 base:onElectrode ?electrode2)
(?electrode2 rdfs:label ''O2'')
(?emotion rdf:type base:Emotion)
(?emotion base:hasSymbol ''1'') →
(?user base:hasEmotion ?emotion)]''.
```

Variables (prefixed by "?") in a reasoning rule represent things in the hyper world (a specific value of users' EEG features, the name of an EEG feature and an electrode that some features are extracted from, etc.). These variables in reasoning rules could be linked to the knowledge in the ontology using SPARQL queries, and the model performs reasoning using Jena API. As the descriptions of the ontology and the reasoning rule set are serialized in XML/RDF, we could use namespaces to specify particular properties of some resources. The namespace identified by the URI-Reference

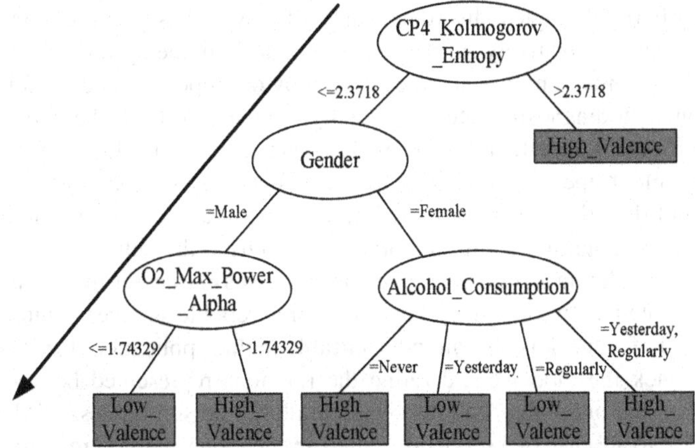

Fig. 6.5 A simplified rule-based decision on valence in the *BIO-EMOTION*. '*CP4_Kolmogorov_Entropy*' refers to the feature *Kolmogorov Entropy* calculated on electrode CP4. '*O2_Max_Power_Alpha*' refers to the feature of maximum alpha band power calculated on electrode O2

http://www.w3.org/2000/01/rdf-schema# is associated with the prefix 'rdfs'. We also use the prefix 'rdf' to refer to the RDF namespace *http://www.w3.org/1999/02/22-rdf-syntax-ns#* [10]. The vocabulary '*base*' is defined as the namespace of *BIO-EMOTION* itself. Each component (a statement in a pair of parentheses) of a rule is described in the form of *subject-predicate-object* expressions. These expressions are known as *triples* in RDF terminology [47]. The *subject* denotes the conceptual knowledge, and the *predicate* denotes traits or aspects of the knowledge and expresses a relationship between the subject and the object. For example, a *subject* denotes a variable named "EEG_feature1" in the first row of the shown rule, a *predicate* denoting "has the type of", and an *object* denoting a variable named "Kolmogorov_Entropy".

When completing this intelligent reasoning, or the "Knowledge to Wisdom" sub-process, the model could offer affect-related knowledge reasoning. For a given emotion analysis task, the model initially drives data processing methods to clean user data and extract EEG features to produce tuples, then drives an inference engine on reasoning rule set for exploring new knowledge, and then adds these new knowledge to the *BIO-EMOTION model*.

6.3.3 Service Construction

The service level involves service construction and service integration. Having completed the sub-processes of "Things to Wisdom", the model could supply services according to specific applications. For instance, frequent mood changes may be indicators of early psychological disorders, since affective states of depression, anxiety, and chronic anger negatively influence the human immune system [83]. Efficient monitoring of human emotional states may provide important and useful medical information with diagnostic value, especially for the elderly or the chronically ill people. Here, the object the model provides services to is the elderly or the chronically ill people. Depending on which affective states users are in, the model could provide relief directly to web users, or link the user to a doctor online and pass the data of the users cognitive status and other symptoms to the online doctor.

The above modeling techniques depict the processes of transforming data of things into an integrated knowledge model and providing reliable services to humans. Particularly, users feedback is also an indispensable in this application. Upon receiving user's feedback the model could refine the relations represented between different entities in the ontology. This step just completes the sub-process of "Human to Things". Due to absence of a service-oriented application in current research, service construction cannot be detailed.

The whole affect-related knowledge modeling implements a W2T data cycle: from things to conceptual knowledge, services, humans, and then back to things. Owing to ontology-based knowledge representation and organization abilities, a tremendous amount of affect-related knowledge and relations could be integrated into a comprehensive model *BIO-EMOTION* for mining web users' emotions. Owing to the rule-based reasoning approach C4.5 algorithm, the model achieves mining new knowledge and relations.

6.4 Model Instantiation

In this section, we illustrate the instantiation of the model BIO-EMOTION with a user-case. A Database for Emotion Analysis Using Physiological Signals (DEAP) [17] containing multimodal physiological signals is used in this model to explain the performance of the model. The physiological signals in this database are GSR, EEG, respiration amplitude, skin temperature, ECG, blood volume by plethysmograph, EMG of Zygomaticus and Trapezius muscles, and EOG. Among these variable bio-informatics, brain information can be seen as the origin of human emotions. It has been shown that emotional markers are present in EEG signals. Most cognitive processes take place within a few hundred milliseconds, so fine-grained representation of the time course of brain activity is extremely important. In addition, with the advent of dense-array methodologies, modern EEG methods are now characterized by high spatial (scalp topographic), as well as high temporal dimensionality. Consequently, we mainly evaluate EEG signals and express a substantial amount of information about EEG signals in the model *BIO-EMOTION*.

We first processed the raw EEG signals from the dataset and extracted various statistical, linear and nonlinear features from a 4-s sliding window of signals. Since the amount of features extracted is extremely large (the *curse of dimensionality problem*) we performed *dimensionality reduction* using F-score, which is crucial for

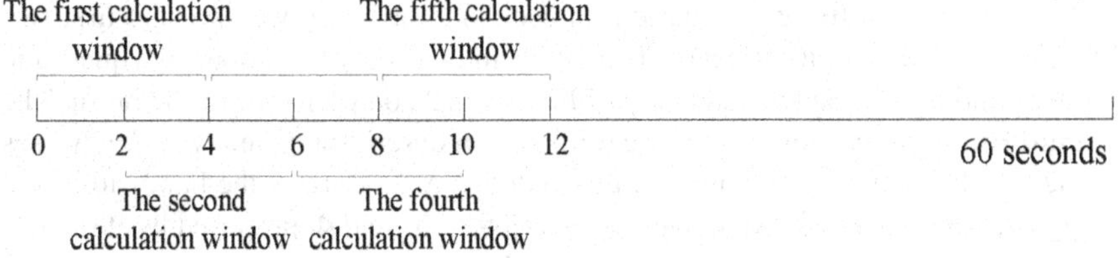

Fig. 6.6 Extracting features from sliding windows

remaining reasoning efficiency. Finally, a small amount of feature tuples were used to generate the reasoning rule set with emotional states as consequent parameters of these rules. These rules were built depending on calculation of information gain ratio in C4.5 algorithm [77]. When a new task of emotion analysis comes, the model applies reasoning rules from a rule set to deduce web users' emotions upon conceptual knowledge from the ontology.

6.4.1 Data Collection and Pre-processing

EEG and peripheral physiological signals coming from 32 healthy participants were recorded using a Biosemi ActiveTwo system[1] on a dedicated recording PC (Pentium 4, 3.2 GHz). EEG was recorded at a sampling rate of 512 Hz using 32 active AgCl electrodes (placed according to the international 10–20 system) [49]. Forty videos were presented in 40 trials; each trail consists of 1-min display of the music video and self-assessment for arousal and valence. The arousal and valence scales are from 1 to 9. Two different binary recognition problems were posed: the detection of low/high arousal and low/high valence. To this end, the users ratings during the experiment are used as the ground truth. The ratings for each of these scales are divided into two categories (low and high). On the 9-point rating scales, the threshold was placed in the middle as Koelstra et al. [49] did in their research.

Brain data represents a mixture of "signal" (functional brain patterns) and "noise". Data cleaning methods can help separate signal from noise and disentangle overlapping patterns. A *Band-pass* filter was used to smooth the signals and eliminate EEG signal *drifting* and EMG *disturbances* [72], and a self-adaptive wavelet algorithm eliminating EOG disturbances [71]. The raw signals were trimmed to a fixed time length of 60 s. Features were extracted by sliding 4-s windows with a 2-s overlap (Fig. 6.6). EEG features were extracted from different approaches:

1. Features from time and frequency domains including absolute spectral energy from different frequency bands (alpha, beta and theta bands), relative spectral energy, maximum spectral energy, center frequency of each band, Hjorth parameters (*activity, mobility*, and *complexity*) and hemispheric asymmetry, etc.

[1] http://www.biosemi.com.

To compare non-linear correlation on each side of brain, we used the first two Hjorth descriptors [40, 41] namely activity and mobility to compute the quadratic mean and the dominant frequency of EEG signals on each side of the brain. The third Hjorth descriptor was to The third Hjorth descriptor called *complexity* uses the fourth-order spectral moment m4 to define a measure of the bandwidth of a signal, which uses the multichannel descriptors $\sum$ and Φ proposed by [90, 91]. Let us consider the spectral moment of order zero and two

$$m_0 = \int_{-\pi}^{\pi} S(\omega)d\omega = \frac{1}{T}\int_{t-T}^{t} f^2(t)dt \tag{6.1}$$

$$m_2 = \int_{-\pi}^{\pi} \omega^2 S(\omega)d\omega = \frac{1}{T}\int_{t-T}^{t} (\frac{df}{dt})^2 dt \tag{6.2}$$

where $S(\omega)$ is the power density spectrum and $f(t)$ the EEG signal within an epoch of duration T ($T = 4s$). Three Hjorth parameters are given by

$$\text{Activity: } h_0 = m_0 \tag{6.3}$$

$$\text{Mobility: } h_1 = \sqrt{\frac{m_2}{m_0}} \tag{6.4}$$

$$\text{Complexity: } h_2 = \sqrt{\frac{m_4}{m_2} - \frac{m_2}{m_0}} \tag{6.5}$$

h_0 represents the square of the quadratic mean and h1 reflects the dominant frequency. The discrete forms of these quantities, $h_0(k)$ and $h_1(k)$ at sampled time k, are computed within a sliding window of 4 s length. More specifically, activity describes the rhythmic *activity* that either increases or decreases in amplitude-frequency; *mobility* describes the curve shape by measuring the relative average slope, and *complexity* measures the frequency domain irregularity.
An EEG hemispheric asymmetry index was derived [76], which reflects the log alpha power density difference in corresponding regions of the two hemispheres (i.e., alpha power). Thus, higher asymmetry scores represent lower amounts of alpha activity and relatively greater activity in the left hemisphere for a particular region. The asymmetry score has been shown to have acceptable psychometric properties [89]. In *BIO-EMOTION*, asymmetries of spectral power density from three bands are all calculated and expressed.

2. Statistics including mean value, standard deviation, skewness, kurtosis, peak-to-peak amplitude.
   Skewness is a measure of symmetry or the lack of symmetry in an epoch of EEG data. A distribution of EEG data in an epoch is symmetric if the waveform looks the same to the left and right of the center point.
   Kurtosis is a measure of whether one-epoch EEG data are peaked or flat relative to a normal distribution. That is, one-epoch EEG recordings with high kurtosis

tend to have a distinct peak near the mean, decline rather rapidly, and have heavy tails. One-epoch EEG recordings with low kurtosis tend to have a flat top near the mean rather than a sharp peak. A uniform distribution in an epoch would be the extreme case.

Peak-to-peak amplitude is defined as the difference in voltage between maximum and minimum voltage of a wave [65]. The feature is calculated to characterize the distribution of values in a 4-s epoch.

3. Features from nonlinear dynamics domains, including Shannon Entropy, Spectral Entropy, C_0 Complexity, the largest Lyapunov exponent, Kolmogorov Entropy.

   Shannon Entropy [86] may be interpreted as the measure of impurity in a signal. Shannon Entropy (ShEn) denoted by H_{Sh} characterizes probability density function of a signal and is defined as

$$H_{Sh} = -\sum_{i} P_i \log P_i \tag{6.6}$$

   where i ranges over all amplitudes of the signal, P_i indicates the probability of the signal having amplitude a_i. Generally, probability density function of the practical signal is not readily known and should be estimated over the discrete values of a_i. There are several methods for estimating probability density function [86] and when the discrete values of amplitude of the signal are available at sufficient number of time intervals, the use of histogram is a convenient technique. For the number of available signal samples N, the amplitude range of signal is linearly divided into k bins such that the ratio k/N remains constant. Usually, the normalized value of H_{Sh} is used

$$ShEn = \frac{H_{Sh}}{\log k} \tag{6.7}$$

   In this work, the constant ration k/N is taken as 0.01.

   Spectral Entropy (SpEn) is based on the power spectrum of EEG waves and describes the irregularity of the signal spectrum. The entropy of the power spectrum denoted by H_{sp} is defined as

$$H_{sp} = -\sum_{i=f_l}^{f_h} P_i \log P_i \tag{6.8}$$

   where P is the power density over a defined frequency band of the signal, f_l and f_h are the lower and upper frequency and power is normalized such that $\sum P_n = 1$ [42]. H_{sp} is also used in the normalized form as

$$SpEn = \frac{H_{sp}}{\log N_f} \tag{6.9}$$

where N_f is the number of frequencies within the defined band $[f_i, f_h]$. In this work the frequency band is specified as [3, 45] Hz.
C_0 Complexity was introduced to quantify time dynamics of order/disorder states of the EEG signals and activated/deactivated states of cerebral cortex, for its moderate coarse graining procedure. C_0 Complexity is a nonlinear measure of time series proposed by Gus group [17]. For a time series, complexity can be obtained as follows:
For a time series with size described as $\{f(k), k = 0, 1, 2, \ldots, N-1\}$, discrete Fourier transformation is

$$F_N(n) = \frac{1}{N}\sum\sum_{k=0}^{N-1} f(k)W_N^{-nk}, \; n = 0, 1, 2, \ldots, N-1 \tag{6.10}$$

here,

$$W_N = \exp(\frac{2\pi i}{N}), \; i = \sqrt{-1} \tag{6.11}$$

The mean squared value of $\{F_N(n), n = 0, 1, 2, \ldots, N-1\}$ is

$$G_N = \frac{1}{N}\sum_{n=0}^{N-1} |F_N(n)|^2 \tag{6.12}$$

Defined $Y(n)$ as follows:

$$Y(n) = \begin{cases} F_N(n) \; if |F_N(n)|^2 > rG_N \\ 0 \qquad\; if |F_N(n)|^2 \le rG_N \end{cases} \tag{6.13}$$

r is a positive real number. Here, we take r to be 1. The inverse discrete Fourier transformation of $\{Y(n), n = 1, 2, \ldots, N-1\}$ is

$$y(k) = \sum_{n=0}^{N-1} Y(n)W_N^{nk}, \; k = 0, 1, 2, \ldots, N-1 \tag{6.14}$$

C_0 Complexity could be defined as follows:

$$C_0 = \frac{\sum_{k=0}^{N-1} |f(k) - y(k)|^2}{\sum_{k=0}^{N-1} |f(k)|^2} \tag{6.15}$$

For a random time series with zero mean, its C_0 Complexity approaches to 1 with increasing length, for a periodic time series, its C_0 Complexity approaches to 0 with increasing length and for any time series, its complexity is a real number between 0 and 1. Thus, C_0 Complexity can be regarded as a "randomness finding" complexity measurement of time series [13]. The more random signal has the higher C_0 Complexity.

The Lyapunov exponent (λ) is used to discriminate between chaotic dynamics and periodic signals. It is a measure of the rate at which the trajectories separate from one another. Thus, λ provides a qualitative and quantitative characterization of dynamical behavior, and are related to the exponentially fast divergence or convergence of nearby orbits in phase space. Lyapunov exponents quantify the mean rate of divergence of neighbored trajectories along various directions in phase space. If a system has one or more positive Lyapunov exponents, then the future state of the system with an uncertain initial condition cannot be predicted. This type of system is known as chaotic. A positive Lyapunov exponent effectively represents a loss of system information [19]. For converging trajectories, the corresponding Lyapunov exponents are negative. A zero exponent means the orbits maintain their relative positions and they are on stable attractors. Finally, a positive exponent implies the orbits are on a chaotic attractor. The algorithm of Rosenstein is used to extract largest Lyapunov Exponent from EEG data [78].
Let X_0 and $X_0 + \Delta x_0$ be the two EEG data points in a space. Let us assume that, each of them will generate an orbit in that space and the separation between the two orbits is Δx. This separation has the form $\Delta x(X_0, t)$ and will behave erratically. The mean exponential rate of divergence of two initially close orbits is given by

$$\lambda = \lim_{t\to\infty} \frac{1}{t} \ln \frac{|\Delta(X_0, t)|}{|\Delta X_0|} \tag{6.16}$$

The maximum value of λ is called the largest Lyapunov exponent and is useful for distinguishing among the various types of orbits.
Kolmogorov Entropy measures the average rate of information loss in phase space, and quantifies the dynamic properties of trajectories in the reconstructed phase space of single channel EEG [50]. Kolmogorov Entropy estimation is based on phase space reconstruction. Kolmogorov Entropy refers to the order-2 Kolmogorov entropy, K_2, proposed by Grassberger and Procaccia [38]. Consider the time series $\{\overset{\omega}{X}_i\}_{i=1}^N$, where $\overset{\omega}{X}_i = \overset{\omega}{X}(t = i\tau)$. We could reconstruct the trajectory from d measurements of any single coordinate. The correlation integrals can be defined as follows:

$$C_d(\varepsilon) = \lim_{N\to\infty} \frac{1}{N^2} [number\ of\ pairs(n, m)\ with(\sum_{i=1}^{d} |X_{n+i} - X_{m+i}|^2)^{1/2} < \varepsilon] \tag{6.17}$$

The K_2 entropy can easily be calculated from the equation with the correlation integrals [38]:

$$K_2 = \lim_{\varepsilon\to 0} \lim_{d\to\infty} \frac{1}{\tau} \ln[\frac{C_d(\varepsilon)}{C_{d+1}(\varepsilon)}] \tag{6.18}$$

If all EEG features from 32 electrodes are analyzed in each reasoning process, it will generate an enormous amount of computing, thus the features described above were extracted merely on 11 remarkable channels according to [49, 73, 82]. We normalized each feature sequence by subtracting its minimum value and dividing the difference by the range of the attribute and then multiplying by 10. Then F-score, a feature selection filter method, was used to measure the discrimination of different categories. Given a feature vector x_k, $k = 1, 2, \ldots, m$, if the number of high valence and low valence are $n_{highvalence}$ and $n_{lowvalence}$ ($n_{highvalence} + n_{lowvalence} = m$) respectively, then the F-score of the ith feature on valence dimension is defined as:

$$F(i) \equiv \frac{(\overline{x}_i^{(highvalence)} - \overline{x}_i)^2 + (\overline{x}_i^{(lowvealence)} - \overline{x}_i)^2}{\frac{1}{n_{highvalence}-1}\sum_{k=1}^{n_{highvalence}}(x_{k,i}^{(highvalence)} - \overline{x}_i^{highvalence})^2 + \frac{1}{n_{lowvalence}-1}\sum_{k=1}^{n_{lowvalence}}(x_{k,i}^{(lowvalence)} - \overline{x}_i^{(lowvalence)})^2} \tag{6.19}$$

where $\overline{x}_i$, $\overline{x}_i^{(highvalence)}$, and $\overline{x}_i^{(lowvalence)}$ are the average value of ith feature sequence, the average value of ith feature sequence categorized as high valence and the average value of the ith feature sequence categorized as low valence, respectively; $x_{k,i}^{(highvalence)}$ is the kth high valence instance of the ith feature sequence, and $x_{k,i}^{(lowvalence)}$ is the kth low valence instance if the ith feature sequence. The numerator indicates the discrimination between the different emotion sets, and the denominator indicates the discrimination within each of the two sets. The larger the F-score value, the more likely the feature is discriminative. Features regarded as irrelevant to user emotions will not be marked in the ontology and not be selected for reasoning task. The arousal F-score of the ith feature sequence is the same as valence one, which is defined as:

$$F(i) \equiv \frac{(\overline{x}_i^{(higharousal)} - \overline{x}_i) + (\overline{x}^{(lowarousal)_i - \overline{x}_i})^2}{\frac{1}{n_{higharousal}-1}\sum_{k=1}^{n_{higharousal}}(x_{k,i}^{(higharousal)} - \overline{x}_i^{higharousal})^2 + \frac{1}{n_{lowarousal}-1}\sum_{k=1}^{n_{lowarousal}}(x_{k,i}^{(lowarousal)} - \overline{x}_i^{(lowarousal)})^2} \tag{6.20}$$

Therefore, we used this score as a feature selection criterion. In our experiment, the threshold value was set at 3.30 on both valence and arousal dimensions. For the purpose of getting higher emotion recognition, we used a discretization method *PKIDiscretize* in the Waikato Environment for Knowledge Analysis (WEKA) to discretize numeric attributes using equal frequency binning after F-score feature selection. The next step is constructing the inference rules based on C4.5 algorithm, which is detailed in the next subsection.

6.4.2 Rule-Based Inference

A core of the model *BIO-EMOTION* mentioned above is ontology techniques including information integration and knowledge expression since we should "translate" all affect-related things from the hyper world as ontological resources. The ontology relies on well-defined knowledge to reach the logical consistency. Another core, mentioned in this section, is ontology-based inference involved with concept extraction, relation discovery (non-taxonomic relation discovery [57, 58] and axiom acquisition [85]). An ontology itself cannot reach intelligent reasoning level for it is separated from inference engine, so a method of data mining or reasoning is deployed for discovering affect-related knowledge. Since the model applies DL to express things in the hyper world into the ontology and the deduced knowledge should have consistent representing way of the knowledge as the ontology, the model constructs logical inference rules to complete intelligent reasoning. After inference rule sets have been built based on users' historical data, when the inference engine receives a users new EEG signals and his other contextual factors, reasoning would be run on the rules to generate results.

Inference rules in this case are built depending on a small number of EEG features and other contexts in the ontology. A rule set generated from a decision tree is a set of *IF* → *THEN* statements. In current research, a result is deduced when the user's EEG features and other contexts are routed down the tree according to the values of each attribute in successive nodes. When a leaf is reached a rule will be generated with a specific emotional state assigned to this leaf. The C4.5 algorithm is used in our research to generate these rules. The principal motivating factors for use of the C4.5 algorithm include:

- DT C4.5 algorithm generates is an effective representation tool of decisions;
- DT provides good interpretability of knowledge;
- It breaks down a complex decision-making process into a collection of simpler decisions;
- The algorithm selects features which are most relevant to differentiate each affective state;
- The algorithm is a rule-based method and its expression could be transformed to *IF* → *THEN* statement seamlessly.

Using 'rich' ontology-based knowledge, the model uses the C4.5 algorithm to construct inference rule set. We have identified the most significant EEG features by pre-processing methods mentioned above to avoid redundant rules. The EEG features of each individual are used for generating personalized inference rules by the J48 classifier (a Java implementation of C4.5 Classifier) in WEKA. The confidence factor used for pruning is set at C=0.25, whereas the minimum number of instances per leaf is set at M=2. Containing EEG-related information (electrodes, feature names and the values, etc.), user profile (age, vision and level of alertness, etc.) and other contexts (EEG device, experimental time, etc.), each rule is generally extremely long. A simplified example of a tree generated by C4.5 is depicted in Fig. 6.5. The example has omitted a large number of EEG-related information, but it holds the same structure as a real rule in the model and can give a clear understanding of the inference rules. The reasoning reaches an average detection rate of 75.19 % on valence and 81.74 % on arousal based on a ninefold cross validation.

Particularly, when a user's new EEG signals and other contexts are entered into the *BIO-EMOTION* model, data processing methods will be driven to clean (EEG) data and store data in semantics; feature extraction methods are triggered to calculate EEG features which will be then stored in the ontology; finally an inference engine is driven to deduce the users emotions by acquiring needed knowledge (or information) from the ontology and finding paths from the root of trees to leaves (or from inference rules). The inference engine would match the needed information acquired from the ontology to the resources in the inference rules. Figure 6.5 shows routing down a decision tree along the arrow, and when a leaf is reached the category of a users one emotional dimension, *Valence*, is obtained which is assigned as the *Low_Valence* to the leaf. Due to the massive information in the ontology and in the rule set in real situations, we here suppose a scenario to explain the process of reasoning (or routing down a tree). In such a scenario, when an elderly user is watching a documentary in the bedroom, his EEG signals are detected directly from sensors. Obviously, high-level emotional states cannot be directly acquired from sensors which should deduced from the low-level EEG signals, personal profile and environmental information. The *BIO-EMOTION* characterizes intelligent technologies of W2T. The model is powerful for knowledge representation and reasoning through inference rules; both knowledge and inference rules are expressed using DL. Here, when the elderly user is watching a violent scene in that film, the values of EEG features are: "*CP4_Kolmogorov_Entropy* = 2.247, *Cz_Mobility* = 0.8032, *O2_F0_Beta* = 3.987, *O2_Max_Power_Alpha* = 1.534", and some other contexts are: "*Gender* = *1*, *Alcohol_Consumption* = 2 and *Tobacco_Consumption* = *1*." (Here, '1' in 'Gender' indicates that he is a man; '2' in 'Alcohol_Consumption' indicates that the user consumed alcohol yesterday, and '1' in 'Tobacco_Consumption' indicates that the user never consumes tobacco.) This tuple could be classified into the *Low_Valence* by hypothetically checking in a rule set which includes the rule shown in Fig. 6.5. It is noted that several information like "*O2_F0_Beta*" and "*Alcohol_Consumption*" are not appeared in the decision tree (Fig. 6.5), that is because there is a process of feature selection before building rules. Thus during the reasoning process, unselected information in that tuple would not be queried and extracted from the ontology. Finally, the deduced emotion result is added back to the ontology model as a new axiom or assertion.

6.5 Performance Evaluation and Future Work

In our research, we have proposed an innovative ontology-based model for mining web users emotion using brain informatics. We succeeded in expressing emotion-related knowledge by ontology techniques and applying inference rules for reasoning. We also realized a combination of both emotion recognition from EEG signals and semantic representation of affect-related knowledge in an ontology-based model. The whole running mechanism of the *BIO-EMOTION* model is graphically illustrated in Fig. 6.7. The *Ontology-based Conceptual Knowledge Base* and *Inference Rule Set* are two core elements: the first one contains all affect-related knowledge and the other consists of inference rules used for producing new knowledge. The running process of the model is shown in the graph at the top. The whole process needs to interact with

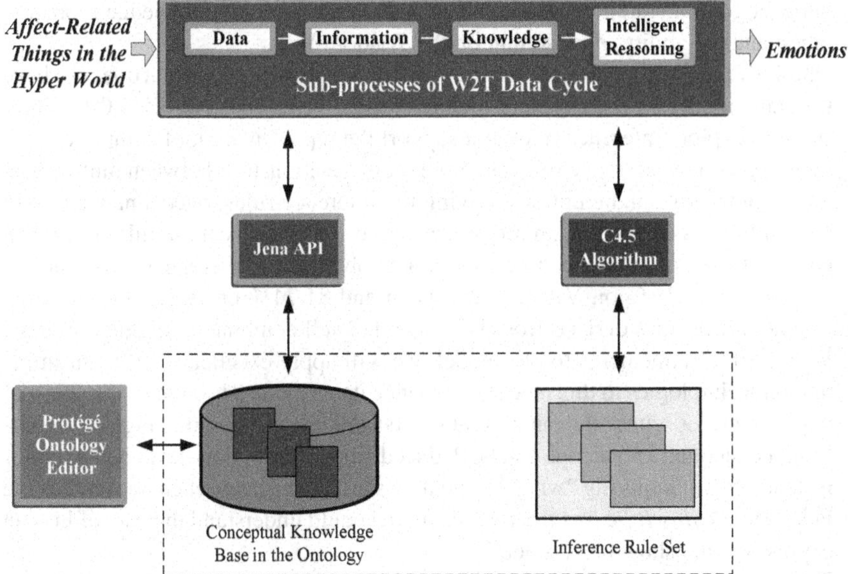

Fig. 6.7 Running mechanism of the model *BIO-EMOTION*

the ontology (including storing information in the ontology or querying information from the ontology). The model drives C4.5 algorithm to generate inference rules after abundant affect-related knowledge have been represented in the ontology. These inference rules are stored in a rule set.

Here, we give a discussion on both the highlights and drawbacks of the model *BIO-EMOTION*.

- The *BIO-EMOTION* model addresses a core issue of how to ensure the harmonious symbiosis of heterogeneous things in nature. An ontology-based model for mining web users emotion on the Wisdom Web is proposed, which contains and represents multiple affect-related contexts. Under this framework, emotion becomes a measurable and analyzable entity. The model realizes a systematic mapping from low-level brain information to human emotions and realizes sub-processes of W2T data cycle from "Things to Wisdom". *BIO-EMOTION* model has achieved the essential part in the whole cycle from *Things*, like low-level EEG signals from real world, to *Wisdom* which refers to deducing human emotions based on multiple affect-related contexts. The small sub-processes from "Wisdom to Things" have not been achieved in this work for the absence of a specific application. We will, at the next step, make this model to implement the whole data cycle oriented toward a specific application, for instance, telemedicine or online consumers.
- This model is highly informative for representing abundant semantic resources which correspond to things in the social world, the physical world and the cyber world. Figure 6.1 gives a proper and semantic representation of conceptual

knowledge in hierarchies which enhances both the logic of knowledge representation and the ability of reasoning on the Wisdom Web.

- Ontology is a great tool for semantic knowledge representation, but it does not have the same ability as Data Mining methodologies have. Thus, we used C4.5 algorithm to explore inference rules and support the representation of comprehensive knowledge. The inference rules specify precise relationships between multimodal affect-knowledge and emotions. Giving the inference rules, once a new emotion recognition task comes in, an inference engine would query these rules to find an answer. Based on inference rules, the model obtained an average accurate detection rate of 75.19 % on Valence dimension and 81.74 % on Arousal dimension. The inference rules derived from DT could be well combined with the ontology. With further refinements to our model, we will apply excellent intelligent information technologies to this model to enhance its wisdom. Through the creation of reasoning rules within the entailment of first-order logic, a wide range of higher-level, conceptual knowledge can be deduced from relevant low-level contexts; for instance, when inquiring "what are the user's affective states when he watches the video called *May It Be by En-ya?*", the model could understand the way of human expression and show the answers.
- The consequent parameter of all inference rules is assigned as an emotional state but not related be other affect-related information, which is really a limitation of the model. The next phase of the *BIO-EMOTION* model building is focused on multi-aspect knowledge reasoning. On the other hand, we would explore more excellent data cleaning and mining methods which could reduce information redundancy and improve inference ability.

6.6 Conclusion

We have introduced an ontology-based mining model, in which the ontology is built for the interaction of web information and knowledge sharing and inference rules generated from C4.5 algorithm are used for exploring the possible relations between multiple information and emotions. The aim of building this model is to support intelligent applications on the Wisdom Web and realize the organic amalgamation and harmonious symbiosis among humans, computers and things in the hyper world. The model achieves the main sub-processes of the W2T data cycle: from *Things* (e.g., EEG signals from real world) to *Wisdom* (e.g., intelligent reasoning). Emotion becomes a measurable and analyzable entity in the model. A realistic use case illustrates how the *BIO-EMOTION* model could be performed on the Wisdom Web. This shows the usefulness of the proposed ontology-based mining model. Our research contribution is, on the one hand, constructing a semantic ontology representing affect-related knowledge which would be linked to things from hyper world and on the other hand, generating logical inference rules to exploit potential information. Indeed, ontology techniques have already enabled major scientific progress in biomedical research and they are also a rapidly growing area in bioinformatics and neuro-informatics research. We expect that the *BIO-EMOTION* model could be extended to other neuroscience-, Affective Computing- and Wisdom Web-related research and to support other biomedical ontology-based knowledge sharing and representation efforts.

Acknowledgments This work was supported by the National Basic Research Program of China (973 Program) (No.2014CB744600), the National Natural Science Foundation of China (No.60973138 and No.61003240), the International Cooperation Project of Ministry of Science and Technology (No.2013DFA11140), the National Basic Research Program of China (973 Program) (No.2011CB711000), and Gansu Provincial Science & Technology Department (No. 1208RJYA015). The authors would like to acknowledge European Community's Seventh Framework Program (FP7/2007–2011) for their public DEAP database.

References

1. Aduna. Sesame (2012). http://www.openrdf.org
2. L. Aftanas, N. Reva, A. Varlamov, S. Pavlov, V. Makhnev, Analysis of evoked EEG synchronization and desynchronization in conditions of emotional activation in humans: temporal and topographic characteristics. Neurosci. Behav. Physiol. **34**(8), 859–867 (2004)
3. D. Ariely, G.S. Berns, Neuromarketing: the hope and hype of neuroimaging in business. Nat. Rev. Neurosci. **11**(4), 284–292 (2010)
4. G.M.M Aurup. *User Preference Extraction from Bio-signals: An Experimental Study* (Concordia University, 2011)
5. Author Anderson Business Consultation, *Zukai knowledge management* (Toyo Keizai, Tokyo, 1999)
6. K.-I. Benta, A. Raru, M. Cremene, Ontology based affective context representation, in *Proceedings of the 2007 Euro American Conference on Telematics and Information Systems* (ACM, 2007), p. 46
7. L.F. Barrett, Are emotions natural kinds? Perspect. Psychol. Sci. **1**(1), 28–58 (2006)
8. L.F. Barrett, B. Mesquita, K.N. Ochsner, J.J. Gross, The experience of emotion. Ann. Rev. Psychol. **58**, 373 (2007)
9. N. Bourdaud, R. Chavarriaga, F. Galn, J. del R. Millan, Characterizing the EEG correlates of exploratory behavior. IEEE Trans. Neural Syst. Rehabil. Eng. **16**(6), 549–556 (2008)
10. D. Brickley, R.V. Guha, *RDF Vocabulary Description Language 1.0: RDF Schema* (2004). http://www.w3.org/TR/rdf-schema/
11. A.J. Caas, G. Hill, J. Lott, *Support for Constructing Knowledge Models in CmapTools*. Technical Report No. IHMC CmapTools 2003-02) (Institute for Human and Machine Cognition, Pensacola, FL, 2003)
12. G.A. Calvert, M.J. Brammer, Predicting consumer behavior: using novel mind-reading approaches. IEEE Pulse **3**(3), 38–41 (2012)
13. Y. Cao, Z. Cai, E. Shen, W. Shen, X. Chen, G. Gu, T. Shou, Quantitative analysis of brain optical images with 2D C0 complexity measure. J. Neurosci. Methods **159**(1), 181–186 (2007)
14. I. Cearreta, J.M. Lpez, N. Garay-Vitoria, Modelling multimodal context-aware affective interaction, in *Proceedings of the Doctoral Consortium of the Second international Conference on ACII* (2007), pp. 57–64
15. G. Chanel, J. Kronegg, D. Grandjean, T. Pun, Emotion assessment: arousal evaluation using EEGs and peripheral physiological signals, in *Multimedia Content Representation, Classification and Security* (Springer, 2006), pp. 530–537
16. H. Chaouchi, *The Internet of Things: Connecting Objects* (Wiley, 2013)

17. F. Chen, J. Xu, F. Gu, X. Yu, X. Meng, Z. Qiu, Dynamic process of information transmission complexity in human brains. Biol. Cybernet. **83**(4), 355–366 (2000)
18. Y.-L. Chi, S.-Y. Peng, C.-C. Yang, Creating Kansei engineering-based ontology for annotating and archiving photos database, in *Human-Computer Interaction. Interaction Design and Usability* (Springer, 2007), pp. 701–710
19. S. Claesen, R. Kitney, Estimation of the largest Lyapunov exponent of an RR interval and its use as an indicator of decreased autonomic heart rate control, in *Computers in Cardiology 1994* (IEEE, 1994), pp. 133–136
20. R. Cowie, E. Douglas-Cowie, N. Tsapatsoulis, G. Votsis, S. Kollias, W. Fellenz, J.G. Taylor, Emotion recognition in human-computer interaction. IEEE Sign. Process. Mag. **18**(1), 32–80 (2001)
21. S.K. D'Mello, A. Graesser, Multimodal semi-automated affect detection from conversational cues, gross body language, and facial features. User Model User-Adap. Inter. **20**(2), 147–187 (2010)
22. H.K. Dai, B. Mobasher, Using ontologies to discover domain-level web usage profiles. Semant. Web Min. **35** (2002)
23. T. Dalgleish, B.D. Dunn, D. Mobbs, Affective neuroscience: past, present, and future. Emot. Rev. **1**(4), 355–368 (2009)
24. T. Dalgleish, M.J. Power, J. Wiley, *Handbook of Cognition and Emotion* (Wiley Online Library, 1999)
25. R.J. Davidson, P. Ekman, C.D. Saron, J.A. Senulis, W.V. Friesen, Approach-withdrawal and cerebral asymmetry: Emotional expression and brain physiology: I. J. Pers. Soc. Psychol. **58**(2), 330 (1990)
26. R.J. Davidson, K.R. Scherer, H. Goldsmith, *Handbook of Affective Sciences* (Oxford University Press, 2003)
27. T.S. Dillon, A. Talevski, V. Potdar, E. Chang, Web of things as a framework for ubiquitous intelligence and computing, in *Ubiquitous Intelligence and Computing* (Springer, 2009), pp. 2–13
28. D. Dou, G. Frishkoff, J. Rong, R. Frank, A. Malony, D. Tucker, Development of NeuroElectroMagnetic ontologies (NEMO): a framework for mining brainwave ontologies, in *Proceedings of the 13th ACM SIGKDD International Conference on Knowledge Discovery and Data Mining, 2007* (ACM, 2007), pp. 270–279
29. M. Eirinaki, M. Vazirgiannis, I. Varlamis, SEWeP: using site semantics and a taxonomy to enhance the Web personalization process, in *Proceedings of the Ninth ACM SIGKDD International Conference on Knowledge Discovery and Data Mining, 2003* (ACM, 2003), pp. 99–108
30. P. Ekman, *Emotions in the Human Faces*, 2nd edn. (Cambridge University, Press, 1982)
31. P. Ekman, *Are there Basic Emotions?* (1992a)
32. P. Ekman, An argument for basic emotions. Cogni. Emot. **6**(3–4), 169–200 (1992b)
33. C. Fisher, P. Sanderson, Exploratory sequential data analysis: exploring continuous observational data. Interactions **3**(2), 25–34 (1996)
34. V. Francisco, P. Gervs, F. Peinado, Ontological reasoning to configure emotional voice synthesis, in *Web Reasoning and Rule Systems* (Springer, 2007), pp. 88–102
35. P. Fraternali, M. Matera, A. Maurino, Conceptual-level log analysis for the evaluation of web application quality, in *Web Congress, 2003. Proceedings. First Latin American, 2003* (IEEE, 2003), pp. 46–57
36. V. Galunov, B. Lobanov, N. Zagoruiko, Ontology of the subject domain, in *Speech Signals Recognition and Synthesis SPECOM* (2004)
37. N. Gibbins, S. Harris, N. Shadbolt, Agent-based semantic web services. Web Semant. Sci. Serv. Agents World Wide Web **1**(2), 141–154 (2004)
38. P. Grassberger, I. Procaccia, Estimation of the Kolmogorov entropy from a chaotic signal. Phys. Rev. A **28**(4), 2591–2593 (1983)
39. F. Hnig, A. Batliner, E. Nth, Real-time recognition of the affective user state with physiological signals, in *Proceedings of the Doctoral Consortium, Affective Computing and Intelligent Interaction* (2007)

40. B. Hjorth, EEG analysis based on time domain properties. Electroencephalogr. Clin. Neurophysiol. **29**(3), 306–310 (1970)
41. B. Hjorth, The physical significance of time domain descriptors in EEG analysis. Electroencephalogr. Clin. Neurophysiol. **34**(3), 321–325 (1973)
42. T. Inouye, K. Shinosaki, H. Sakamoto, S. Toi, S. Ukai, A. Iyama, Y. Katsuda, M. Hirano, Quantification of EEG irregularity by use of the entropy of the power spectrum. Electroencephalogr. Clin. Neurophysiol. **79**(3), 204–210 (1991)
43. Jena. Apache Jena. *HP Labs Semantic Web Toolkit* (2011). http://jena.sourceforge.net/
44. Y. Jing, D. Jeong, D.-K. Baik, SPARQL graph pattern rewriting for OWL-DL inference queries. Knowl. Inf. Syst. **20**(2), 243–262 (2009)
45. C.M. Jones, T. Troen, Biometric valence and arousal recognition, in *Proceedings of the 19th Australasian Conference on Computer-Human Interaction: Entertaining User Interfaces, 2007* (ACM, 2007), pp. 191–194
46. M. Kawasaki, Y. Yamaguchi, Effects of subjective preference of colors on attention-related occipital theta oscillations. Neuroimage **59**(1), 808–814 (2012)
47. G. Klyne, J.J. Carroll, *Resource Description Framework (RDF): Concepts and Abstract Syntax* (2004). http://www.w3.org/TR/rdf-concepts/
48. K.-E. Ko, H.-C. Yang, K.-B. Sim, Emotion recognition using EEG signals with relative power values and Bayesian network. Int. J. Control Autom. Syst. **7**(5), 865–870 (2009)
49. S. Koelstra, C. Muhl, M. Soleymani, J.-S. Lee, A. Yazdani, T. Ebrahimi, T. Pun, A. Nijholt, I. Patras, Deap: a database for emotion analysis using physiological signals. IEEE Trans Affect. Comput. **3**(1), 18–31 (2012)
50. Kolmogorov. An entropy per unit time as a metric invariant of automorphisms, in *Dokl. Akad. Nauk SSSR* (1959), pp. 754–755
51. M. Kostyunina, M. Kulikov, Frequency characteristics of EEG spectra in the emotions. Neurosci. Behav. Physiol. **26**(4), 340–343 (1996)
52. T. Kunii, J. Ma, R. Huang, Hyperworld modeling, in *Proceedings of International Conference Visual Information Systems (VIS 96)* (1996), pp. 1–8
53. J.M. Lpez, R. Gil, R. Garca, I. Cearreta, N. Garay, Towards an ontology for describing emotions, in *Emerging Technologies and Information Systems for the Knowledge Society* (Springer, 2008), pp. 96–104
54. M.D. Lewis, J.M. Haviland-Jones, L.F. Barrett, *Handbook of Emotions* (Guilford Press, 2010)
55. P. Lewis, H. Critchley, P. Rotshtein, R. Dolan, Neural correlates of processing valence and arousal in affective words. Cerebral Cortex **17**(3), 742–748 (2007)
56. J. Ma, R. Huang. Improving human interaction with a hyperworld, in *Proceedings of the Pacific Workshop on Distributed Multimedia Systems (DMS'96)* (1996), pp. 46–50
57. A. Maedche, S. Staab, Discovering conceptual relations from text, in *Ecai*, vol. 325 (2000), p. 27
58. A. Maedche, S. Staab, *Ontology Learning* (Springer, 2004)
59. Y.Y. Mathieu, Annotation of emotions and feelings in texts, in *Affective Computing and Intelligent Interaction* (Springer, 2005), pp. 350–357
60. D.L. McGuinness, F. Van Harmelen, *OWL Web Ontology Language Overview* (W3C Recommendation, 2004)
61. A. Mehrabian, J.A. Russell, *An Approach to Environmental Psychology* (The MIT Press, 1974)
62. R. Meo, P.L. Lanzi, M. Matera, R. Esposito, Integrating web conceptual modeling and web usage mining, in *Advances in Web Mining and Web Usage Analysis* (Springer, 2006), pp. 135–148
63. M. Murugappan, M. Rizon, R. Nagarajan, S. Yaacob, D. Hazry, I. Zunaidi, Time-frequency analysis of EEG signals for human emotion detection, in *4th Kuala Lumpur International Conference on Biomedical Engineering 2008* (Springer, 2008), pp. 262–265
64. M.A. Nicolaou, H. Gunes, M. Pantic, Continuous prediction of spontaneous affect from multiple cues and modalities in valence-arousal space. IEEE Trans Affect. Comput. **2**(2), 92–105 (2011)

65. E. Niedermeyer, The normal EEG of the waking adult, in *Electroencephalography: Basic Principles, Clinical Applications, and Related Fields*, vol. 167 (2005)
66. D. Oberle, B. Berendt, A. Hotho, J. Gonzalez, Conceptual user tracking, in *Advances in Web Intelligence* (Springer, 2003), pp. 155–164
67. R. Ohme, D. Reykowska, D. Wiener, A. Choromanska, Analysis of neurophysiological reactions to advertising stimuli by means of EEG and galvanic skin response measures. J. Neurosci. Psychol. Econ. **2**(1), 21 (2009)
68. R. Ohme, D. Reykowska, D. Wiener, A. Choromanska, Application of frontal EEG asymmetry to advertising research. J. Econ. Psychol. **31**(5), 785–793 (2010)
69. A.M. Oliveira, M.P. Teixeira, I.B. Fonseca, M. Oliveira, Joint model-parameter validation of self-estimates of valence and arousal: Probing a differential-weighting model of affective intensity, in *Proceedings of the 22nd Annual Meeting of the International Society for Psychophysics* (2006), pp. 245–250
70. M. Pantic, L.J. Rothkrantz, Toward an affect-sensitive multimodal human-computer interaction. Proc. IEEE **91**(9), 1370–1390 (2003)
71. H. Peng, B. Hu, Q. Liu, Q. Dong, Q. Zhao, P. Moore, User-centered depression prevention: an EEG approach to pervasive healthcare, in *2011 IEEE 5th International Conference on Pervasive Computing Technologies for Healthcare (PervasiveHealth)* (2011a), pp. 325–330
72. H. Peng, B. Hu, Y. Qi, Q. Zhao, M. Ratcliffe, An improved EEG de-noising approach in electroencephalogram (EEG) for home care, in *2011 IEEE 5th International Conference on Pervasive Computing Technologies for Healthcare (PervasiveHealth)* (2011b), pp. 469–474
73. P.C. Petrantonakis, L.J. Hadjileontiadis, Adaptive extraction of emotion-related EEG segments using multidimensional directed information in time-frequency domain, in *Engineering in Medicine and Biology Society (EMBC), 2010 Annual International Conference of the IEEE* (IEEE, 2010), pp. 1–4
74. R.W. Picard, Affective computing: challenges. Int. J. Hum.-Comput. Stud. **59**(1), 55–64 (2003)
75. R.W. Picard, E. Vyzas, J. Healey, Toward machine emotional intelligence: analysis of affective physiological state. IEEE Trans Pattern Anal. Mach. Intell. **23**(10), 1175–1191 (2001)
76. R. Pivik, R. Broughton, R. Coppola, R. Davidson, N. Fox, M. Nuwer, Guidelines for the recording and quantitative analysis of electroencephalographic activity in research contexts. Psychophysiology **30**(6), 547–558 (1993)
77. J.R. Quinlan, *C4. 5: Programs for Machine Learning*, vol. 1 (Morgan kaufmann, 1993)
78. M.T. Rosenstein, J.J. Collins, C.J. De Luca, A practical method for calculating largest Lyapunov exponents from small data sets. Physica D: Nonlin. Phenomena **65**(1), 117–134 (1993)
79. J.A. Russell, Core affect and the psychological construction of emotion. Psychol. Rev. **110**(1), 145 (2003)
80. J.A. Russell, M. Lewicka, T. Niit, A cross-cultural study of a circumplex model of affect. J. Pers. Soc. Psychol. **57**(5), 848 (1989)
81. S.J. Russell, P. Norvig, J.F. Canny, J.M. Malik, D.D. Edwards, *Artificial Intelligence: A Modern Approach*, vol. 74 (Prentice hall Englewood Cliffs, 1995)
82. M. Sabeti, R. Boostani, S. Katebi, G. Price, Selection of relevant features for EEG signal classification of schizophrenic patients. Biomed. Sign. Process. Control **2**(2), 122–134 (2007)
83. P. Salovey, J.D. Mayer, Emotional intelligence. Imagination Cogn. Pers. **9**(3), 185–211 (1989)
84. N. Sebe, I. Cohen, T.S. Huang, Multimodal emotion recognition. Handb. Pattern Recogn. Comput. Vis. **4**, 387–419 (2005)
85. M. Shamsfard, A.A. Barforoush, Learning ontologies from natural language texts. Int. J. Hum.-Comput. Stud. **60**(1), 17–63 (2004)
86. C.E. Shannon, A mathematical theory of communication. ACM SIGMOBILE Mobile Comput. Commun. Rev. **5**(1), 3–55 (2001)
87. C. Stickel, M. Ebner, S. Steinbach-Nordmann, G. Searle, A. Holzinger, Emotion detection: application of the valence arousal space for rapid biological usability testing to enhance universal access, in *Universal Access in Human-Computer Interaction. Addressing Diversity* (Springer, 2009), pp. 615–624

88. V. Stirbu, Towards a restful plug and play experience in the web of things, in *2008 IEEE International Conference on Semantic Computing* (IEEE, 2008), pp. 512–517
89. A.J. Tomarken, R.J. Davidson, R.E. Wheeler, L. Kinney, Psychometric properties of resting anterior EEG asymmetry: temporal stability and internal consistency. Psychophysiology **29**(5), 576–592 (1992)
90. J. Wackermann, Towards a quantitative characterisation of functional states of the brain: from the non-linear methodology to the global linear description. Int. J. Psychophysiol. **34**(1), 65–80 (1999)
91. J. Wackermann, C. Allefeld, On the meaning and interpretation of global descriptors of brain electrical activity. Including a reply to X. Pei, et al. Int. J. Psychophysiol. **64**(2), 199–210 (2007)
92. T. Wehrle, K.R. Scherer, *Towards computational modeling of appraisal theories*, in *Appraisal Processes in Emotion: Theory, Methods, Research* (Oxford University Press, New York, 2001)
93. E. Welbourne, L. Battle, G. Cole, K. Gould, K. Rector, S. Raymer, M. Balazinska, G. Borriello, Building the internet of things using RFID: the RFID ecosystem experience. IEEE Internet Comput. **13**(3), 48–55 (2009)
94. Y-H. Yang, Y-C. Lin, Y-F, Su, H.H. Chen, Music emotion classification: a regression approach, in *2007 IEEE International Conference on Multimedia and Expo* (IEEE, 2007), pp. 208–211
95. E.Yokomatsu, S-i. Ito, Y. Mitsukura, J. Cao, M.A. Fukumi, Design of the preference acquisition detection system, in *SICE, 2007 Annual Conference* (IEEE, 2007), pp. 2804–2807
96. C. Yu, P.M. Aoki, A. Woodruff, *Detecting User Engagement in Everyday Conversations.* arXiv preprint cs/0410027 (2004)
97. Z. Zeng, M. Pantic, G.I. Roisman, T.S. Huang, A survey of affect recognition methods: audio, visual, and spontaneous expressions. IEEE Trans. Pattern Anal. Mach. Intell. **31**(1), 39–58 (2009)
98. X.-S. Zhang, R.J. Roy, Derived fuzzy knowledge model for estimating the depth of anesthesia. IEEE Trans. Biomed. Eng. **48**(3), 312–323 (2001)
99. N. Zhong, J. Liu, Y. Yao, In search of the wisdom web. IEEE Comput. **35**(11), 27–31 (2002)
100. N. Zhong, J. Liu, Y. Yao. Web intelligence (WI): a new paradigm for developing the Wisdom Web and social network intelligence, in *Web Intelligence* (Springer, 2003), pp. 1–16
101. N. Zhong, J.H. Ma, R.H. Huang, J.M. Liu, Y.Y. Yao, Y.X. Zhang, J.H. Chen, Research challenges and perspectives on Wisdom Web of Things (W2T). J. Supercomput. 1–21 (2013)

Chapter 7
Multi-level Big Data Content Services for Mental Health Care

Jianhui Chen, Jian Han, Yue Deng, Han Zhong, Ningning Wang, Youjun Li, Zhijiang Wan, Taihei Kotake, Dongsheng Wang, Xiaohui Tao and Ning Zhong

Abstract Systematic brain informatics studies on mental health care produce various health big data of mental disorders and bring new requirements on the data acquisition and computing, from the data level to the information, knowledge and wisdom levels. Aiming at these challenges, this chapter proposes a brain and health big data center. A global content integrating mechanism and a content-oriented cloud service architecture are developed. The illustrative example demonstrates significance and usefulness of the proposed approach.

J. Chen · J. Han · H. Zhong · N. Wang · Y. Li · Z. Wan · D. Wang
The International WIC Institute, Beijing University of Technology, Beijing, China

J. Chen
e-mail: chenjianhui@bjut.edu.cn; chenjhnh@mail.tsinghua.edu.cn

J. Han
e-mail: hanjian0204@emails.bjut.edu.cn

H. Zhong
e-mail: z.h0912@emails.bjut.edu.cn

N. Wang
e-mail: wangningning@emails.bjut.edu.cn

Y. Li
e-mail: lyj@ncut.edu.cn

Z. Wan
e-mail: wandndn@gmail.com

N. Zhong et al. (eds.), *Wisdom Web of Things*, Web Information Systems Engineering and Internet Technologies Book Series,
DOI 10.1007/978-3-319-44198-6_7

7.1 Introduction

E-health care has become a hot issue and drawn great attentions from both research and industry. Its goal is to improve the quality and reduce the cost of medical services by modern information and computing technologies. The increasing ability to obtain digital information in health care has led to health big data. At present, e-health care systems have not limited to recording and managing of medical process information, such as digital medical records and hospital information systems. Enhancing the acquisition and computing of health big data to provide intelligent medical services has been an important trend in e-health care. Because of the powerful capabilities of data storage and computing, cloud computing [1, 14] has played an important role on e-health care. It can be used to develop the web-based epilepsy analytic system for supporting data mining of clinical examinations [29]. It can also be integrated with wearable body sensor components to develop intelligent health care services for diagnosis of chronic illness [19].

Mental health care is a focus of e-health care. Comparing with other disorders, mental disorders have distinct characteristics, such as the high incidence rate, long treatment cycle, high recurrence rate, complex pathogeny, etc., and bring new requirements of e-health care, especially the acquisition and computing of mental health big data. In order to understand pathology of mental disorders in depth and develop new clinical diagnosis technologies, brain informatics (BI) [42, 43] adopts a systematic methodology to study mental disorders from macro, meso and micro points of view. Systematic studies product multi-level and multi-aspect mental health big data and bring new requirements of systematic brain data management. It is necessary to

Y. Deng
The Industry Innovation Center for Web Intelligence, Suzhou, China
e-mail: nos2013@163.com

Z. Wan · N. Zhong · T. Kotake
The Department of Life Science and Informatics, Maebashi Institute of Technology, Maebashi-city 371-0816, Japan

T. Kotake
e-mail: kotake@maebashi-it.org

D. Wang
Institute of Intelligent Transport System, School of Computer Science and Engineering, Jiangsu University of Science of Technology, Zhenjiang, China
e-mail: dswang@bjut.edu.cn

X. Tao
Faculty of Health, Engineering and Sciences,
The University of Southern Queensland, Toowoomba, Australia
e-mail: xtao@usq.edu.au

N. Zhong (✉)
Beijing Advanced Innovation Center for Future Internet Technology, The International WIC Institute, Beijing University of Technology, Beijing, China
e-mail: zhong@maebashi-it.ac.jp; zhongn@bjut.edu.cn

effectively integrate multi-level mental health big data and provide multi-level and content-oriented data services for different types of users by an open and extendable mode. In our previous studies [45], the Data-Brain-based brain data center has been constructed to realize systematic brain data management. However, it mainly focuses on data sharing and reuse of neuroimaging data among research groups, and cannot meet those new requirements.

This chapter analyzes new requirements of systematic brain data management brought by systematic BI studies on mental health care, and proposes a brain and health big data center. Wisdom as a service, a content-oriented cloud service architecture for mental health care is developed as the core technology of the big data center to effectively organize, manage and utilize health big data of mental disorders based on the storage and computing capabilities of "cloud". The remainder of this chapter is organized as follows. Section 7.2 discusses background and related work. Section 7.3 analyzes new requirements brought by systematic BI studies on mental health care and proposes a brain and health big data center. Section 7.4 designs a content integrating mechanism of health big data. Based on the preparations, Sect. 7.5 presents the content-oriented cloud service architecture and Sect. 7.6 provides an illustrative example. Finally, Sect. 7.7 gives concluding remarks.

7.2 Background and Related Work

7.2.1 From Cloud Computing to Wisdom as a Service

The Internet, the mobile Internet, the Internet of Things [4, 37], and the Web of Things [11, 33] connect humans, computers, and other devices to form an immense network and result in a hyper-world consisting of the social, cyber, and physical worlds. How to make each "things" in the network "wisdom", i.e., developing the Wisdom Web of Things (W2T) [46], becomes a core issue for realizing the harmonious symbiosis of humans, computers, and things in the hyper-world, where the "wisdom" means that each "thing" is aware of itself and others to provide the right service for the right object at the right time and context. This is a new goal of Web intelligence (WI) [38, 41] in the hyper-world age and its core is a W2T cycle, namely, "from things to data, information, knowledge, wisdom, services, humans, and then back to things".

Constructing such a W2T cycle relies on large-scale converging of intelligent IT applications, which needs an open and scalable architecture to meet seven factors of intelligent IT applications—that is, the infrastructure, platform, software (developing and scheduling abilities), data, information, knowledge, and wisdom. They can be divided into two types: system resources and contents. Cloud computing provides an open and service-oriented architecture for system resources of IT applications, including the infrastructure, platform and software, by Infrastructure as a Service (IaaS), Platform as a Service (PaaS) and Software as a Service (SaaS), respectively.

Furthermore, it is necessary to develop an open and interoperable intelligence service architecture for contents of IT applications, including data, information, knowledge and wisdom.

Wisdom as a service (WaaS) [8] was proposed for the above requirement. It includes four service layers, namely, data as a service (DaaS), information as a service (InaaS), knowledge as a service (KaaS), and wisdom as a service (Waas). Its realization needs a WaaS standard and service platform, with four components according to the four service layers. Each component includes a software platform and a standard system for realizing all services in the corresponding service layer.

WaaS is an open intelligent IT architecture and oriented to the contents of IT applications, i.e., big data. It is independent of cloud computing and focuses on the DIKW (the data, information, knowledge, and wisdom) organization and transformation to realize wisdom from big data. It is also based on cloud computing and obtains the needed computing, storage, and communication resources, as well as developing and scheduling abilities, by IaaS, PaaS and SaaS services. Binding WaaS with cloud computing, both system and content-level demands of intelligent IT applications can be met in a unified, pay-as-you-go manner for supporting the developing of intelligent IT applications. A large number of intelligent IT applications will appear and converge into an open and sharing network to realize the W2T cycle.

7.2.2 Brain Information for Mental Health Care

Brain informatics (BI) [42, 43] is a new interdisciplinary field to study human information processing mechanism systematically from both macro and micro points of view by cooperatively using experimental and computational cognitive neuroscience and WI centric advanced information technologies [38, 41]. It focuses on human thinking centric cognitive functions and clinical diagnosis and pathology of human brain, mind and mental related diseases. A systematic methodology is adopted and includes four core issues, namely, systematic investigation of complex brain science problems, systematic design of cognitive experiments, systematic human brain data management, and systematic human brain data analysis and simulation [44].

Mental health care is also a core issue of BI. Guided by the systematic methodology, BI is studying brain and mental disorders, such as depression, from macro (i.e., behavior and symptomatology), meso (i.e., brain function and structure) and micro (i.e., molecule, neuron and gene) points of view. Some preliminary fruits have been achieved [21, 22]. At present, the application of wearable health devices is an important characteristic of BI studies on mental health care. Various wearable health devices, such as the wearable EEG belt, are used as new physical examination devices to obtain macro and meso levels of brain and mental data. These wearable health data are integrated with clinical physical examination data, as well as various medical information and knowledge sources, including medical records, experimental reports, LOD (Linked Open Data) medical data sets [10], SNOMED CT [12], PubMed [28], and DrugBank [20].

Such a systematic study needs a powerful brain data center. Our previous studies have developed a Data-Brain and a Data-Brain-based brain data center [6, 45]. The Data-Brain is a domain-driven conceptual modeling of brain data for modeling a whole process of systematic BI studies. It is used as a multi-dimension framework to integrate data, information and knowledge coming from the whole BI research process. However, the existing Data-Brain-based brain data center is oriented to BI studies on human thinking-centric cognitive functions and mainly focuses on data sharing and reuse of neuroimaging data among research groups. It cannot effectively support systematic BI studies on mental health care, which are involved with multi-level contents and services of mental health big data. It is necessary to extend the Data-Brain-based brain data center for developing a brain and health big data center.

7.3 Developing a Brain and Health Big Data Center

7.3.1 New Requirements Brought by Systematic Brain Informatics Studies on Mental Health Care

Systematic BI studies on mental health care bring new requirements on the acquisition and computing of mental health big data, from the data level to the information, knowledge and wisdom levels. They can be described as follows:

- comprehensive data collection and targeted data management: Systematic BI studies on mental health care are involved with multi-level health data, from behavior and symptomatology data to molecule, neuron and gene data. All of data need to be collection in the round. However, these data cannot be managed by using a unified mode. Because of the differences of data formats, data sources, acquisition environments and mining tools, it is necessary to adopt different data collection, storage and management methods for these heterogeneous data.
- broad information integration: Complex pathogeny is an important characteristic of mental disorders. Their diagnosis and evaluation are often based on an index system rather than a or several indexes. Hence, identifying multi-aspect and multi-level indexes and their relationships to form a unified index system becomes a core objective during systematic BI studies on mental health care. In order to realize this objective, it is necessary to broadly integrate multi-aspect health information, including features found in experimental data, content information of medical records, personal information, etc., into a unified health information sources for the finding of mental disorder-related indexes and their relationships.
- domain-driven knowledge integration: Studies on mental health care are interdisciplinary and involved with multi-aspect domain knowledge. It is also a kind of important mental health big data and should be formally collected or described to support various knowledge-driven applications, including resource exchange, resource integration, experiment data mining, etc. Furthermore, all domain knowledge should be integrated into a global knowledge framework by a domain-driven

approach. The core issue is to develop a global conceptual model of mental health big data based on system BI methodology.

- multi-level wisdom service: BI mental health care studies focus on not only pathology studies but also clinical diagnosis. Potential users are more diversified than traditional study-oriented brain databases, including patients, patients' family members, doctors, nurses, researchers, developers, etc. They bring various service requirements about mental health big data. A data mining experts often needs raw clinic or experimental data for algorithm experiments; a doctor often needs mining results and corresponding patients' information, and a patient just needs a diagnosis results and evidences. It is necessary to provide different levels of mental health big data for different users. Service should also be "wisdom". The right service is provided for the right object at the right time and context.

Generally speaking, in systematic BI mental health care studies, mental health big data include not only multi-level physiological data but also various health information and knowledge. Effectively integrating multi-level mental health big data and providing multi-level and content-oriented data services for different types of users by an open and extendable mode become new requirements of developing the brain big data center.

7.3.2 *The System Framework of Brain and Health Big Data Center*

A brain and health big data center needs to be constructed for the above requirements. As shown in Fig. 7.1, it mainly includes two components: the brain and health database and the wisdom service platform.

The brain and health database is a multi-level database which is used to store health big data obtained from system BI studies on brain and mental disorders. It consists of a group of health databases, an integrated information base, and an integrated knowledge base.

Health databases are the basis of the brain and health database, and involved with three types of databases: clinical examinations databases which are used to store and manage multi-level brain and mental data obtained from diversified clinical examinations, wearable databases which are used to store and manage raw data obtained from diversified wearable health devices, and medical information databases which are used to store and manage patient-related medical information obtained from diversified medical information systems, such as digital medical record systems.

There are an integrated information base and an integrated knowledge base on these health databases. The integrated information base includes semantic medical information and brain informatics provenances [7, 47], index databases and case databases. Semantic medical information is obtained by importing outer semantic medical information sources or transforming patient-related medical information of medical information databases. Brain informatics provenances are semantic

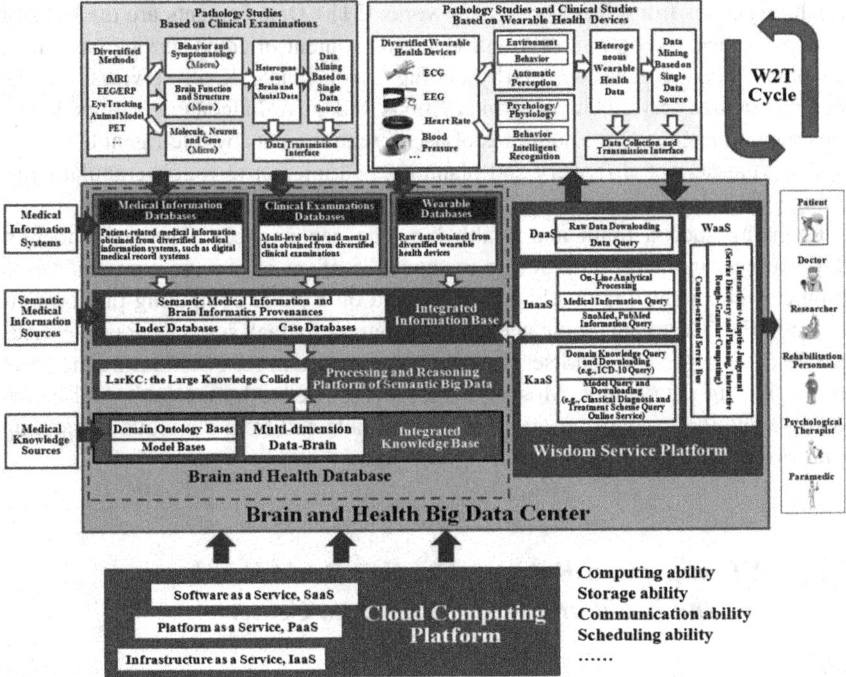

Fig. 7.1 The System Framework of Brain and Health Big Data Center

metadata of brain and mental data which are stored in clinical examinations databases or wearable databases. The integrated knowledge base includes various domain ontology bases and model bases, in which all of domain ontologies are integrated based on a multi-dimension Data-Brain.

The wisdom service platform is the service portal of brain and health big data center. Guided by the WaaS architecture, it is divided into four service layers: DaaS, InaaS, KaaS and WaaS. The DaaS, InaaS and KaaS layers include various data content services based on multi-level mental health big data stored in the brain and health database. For examples, classical diagnosis and treatment scheme can be constructed as medical models to provide model query services.

The WaaS layer includes two components: the content-oriented service bus and the "Interactions+Adaptive Judgement" component. It is constructed based on a meta-equation:

$$Wisdom = Interactions + Adaptive\ Judgement \\ + Data\ Contents,$$

which originates from Skowron et al.'s works [31].[1] Data contents are the basis of wisdom. Hence, the bottom of WaaS layer is a content-oriented service bus which can obtain needed data contents by calling DaaS, InaaS, KaaS services. On the content-oriented service bus, the "Interactions+Adaptive Judgement" component is constructed to generate the solutions of users' requirements by intelligent technologies, such as service discovery and planning, and interactive rough-granular computing [18, 31].

Realizing such a brain and health big data center needs a large number of IT resources, including computing resources, storage resources, communication resources, etc. Hence, it should be constructed on a cloud computing platform, as shown in Fig. 7.1, to obtain the needed IT resources by IaaS services, PaaS services and SaaS services. The PaaS services are most important for constructing the brain and health big data center. Most of IT resources needed by the brain and health database and the wisdom service platform are obtained from the cloud computing platform by calling corresponding PaaS services.

7.3.3 A Comparison Between Existing Brain Databases and the Brain and Health Big Data Center

Brain science is a data-driven study in which brain databases play an important role. Tradition Web-based brain databases focus on storing and sharing multi-level experiment data, from the gene level [26], the cell level [25] to the system level [36]. In recent years, the long-term community-oriented databasing of brain data [15] and data curation [16] become new trends in brain database studies. Developing a brain research portal to furthest improve the availability and value of brain data by data description, data organization and data preprocessing for effectively supporting brain science studies, especially systematic studies which integrate multiple groups of experiments, become an important issue. Many important brain research portals have been constructed. Different from tradition Web-based brain databases [9, 17], which are oriented to storing and sharing of experiment data, existing brain research portals focus on research sharing. They can provide not only experiment data but also data-related information, such as experimental paradigm and analytical results, and various domain knowledge, including ontologies and models. Furthermore, research resources belonging to different experiments are often integrated to provide a systematic and global study. For examples, NIF (Neuroscience Information Framework) [24] integrates various neuroinformatics resources by domain ontologies to provide the resource query based on semantics; BrainMap [3] stores a large number of analytical results obtained by neuroimaging studies, i.e., brain activations, to support the meta-analysis [35].

[1] Skowron et al. proposed "Wisdom = Interactions + Adaptive Judgement + Knowledge". In the WaaS architecture, all of big data, from data to information and knowledge, are data resources for bringing "Wisdom". Hence, we change "Knowledge" to "Data Contents" in this study.

From Web-based databases to research portals, experiment data are no longer the only core contents of brain databases. Both provenances [30] and domain ontologies become important brain data resources in brain databases. However, existing brain databases still only focus on a specific type of brain data resources, such as experiment data and analytical results, and provide services related to this type of brain data resources. The brain and health big data center is oriented to those four levels of requirements of health big data stated in Sect. 3.1. Compared with existing brain databases, it has the following two characteristics and innovations:

- a global content integrating mechanism of mental health big data: Different from existing brain databases, which focus on a specific type of brain data resources, the brain and health big data center includes three levels of mental health big data, from diversified experiment data to various experiment data-related information and domain knowledge. All of them are regarded as core contents of mental health big data for storing and utilizing respectively. A global content integrating mechanism is designed to integrate multi-level mental health big data. By using this content integrating mechanism, multi-level contents of mental health big data can be represented and organized uniformly to construct a brain data and knowledge base for meeting multi-level and multi-aspect service requirements about mental health big data.
- a content-oriented cloud service architecture of mental health big data: Different from existing brain databases, which provide services based on a specific type of brain data resources, the brain and health big data center provides multiple levels of big data services, from raw data downloading to on-line analytical processing and domain knowledge query, based on the integrated multi-level mental health big data. A content-oriented cloud service architecture is developed to realize multi-level services of mental health big data. By using this content-oriented service architecture, multi-level big data services can be developed and deployed with a unified and open mode for meeting various service requirements brought by systematic BI studies on mental health care.

Owing to the above two characteristics, the brain and health big data center is no longer a traditional Web-based brain database or research portal oriented to a or several specific functions, such as experiment data sharing, resource query, meta-analysis, parallel analysis, etc. It is an open and extendable platform, on which anyone focusing on any aspect of studies, clinical practices and industries of mental health care can publish, share and trade his or her achievements and productions, for supporting the large-scale research cooperation, achievement promotion and industrialization. These two characteristics also become core research issues of the brain and health big data center. They will be discussed in the following sections.

7.4 A Global Content Integrating Mechanism of Mental Health Big Data

The global content integrating mechanism of mental health big data is an important characteristics and core research issue of the brain and health big data center. As stated in Sect. 3.1, the brain and health big data center should realize the information and knowledge levels of integrations though heterogeneous raw data and patient-related medical information need to be stored and managed, independently. Hence, this global content integrating mechanism includes two levels: the knowledge integration and the information integration.

7.4.1 A Top-Down Integration Approach

Studies on brain databases focus on information and knowledge-level integration by using ontologies and provenances because most of brain data are unstructured. They often adopt a bottom-up integration approach. Aiming at a specific system function, ontologies and provenances are constructed to describe a specific level of brain big data, such as raw data, mining results and information resources. They are only function components rather than a part of brain big data. Their structures and contents are decided by the system function. Hence, most of ontologies in traditional brain databases are term ontologies which mainly provide domain term sets for supporting the semantic query. Related provenances mainly focus on describing single data set or analysis workflow.

Different from traditional brain databases oriented to a or several specific functions, the brain and health big data center is an open and extendable platform for supporting the large-scale research cooperation, achievement promotion and industrialization. All levels of mental health big data, including ontologies and provenances, should be regarded as data resources and integrated together to describe the whole systematic BI studies rather than a specific system function. Hence, a top-down approach is necessary to realize information and knowledge-level integration. It will be introduced in the following subsections.

7.4.2 The Data-Brain Based Knowledge Integration

The Data-Brain is used to realize the knowledge level of integration in mental health big data. It is a domain-driven conceptual model of brain data, which represents multi-aspect relationships among multiple human brain data sources, with respect to all major aspects and capabilities of human information processing systems, for systematic investigation and understanding of human intelligence [5, 6]. Previous studies have constructed a thinking-oriented Data-Brain, which includes four dimensions corresponding to the four core issues of BI methodology for integrating all domain knowledge during the whole process of thinking-centric BI studies.

Similarly, the Data-Brain oriented to mental disorders can also be constructed to integrate all domain knowledge during systematic BI studies of mental health care. It also includes the following four dimensions:

- The *function dimension*, denoted by FD, is a set of concepts, relationships and axioms, and used to model the systematic investigation during BI studies of mental health care. It is a set of concepts, relationships and axioms, and includes two types of concepts: cognitive functions and mental disorders.
- The *experiment dimension*, denoted by ED, is a set of concepts, relationships and axioms, and used to model the systematic experimental design during BI studies of mental health care. It mainly includes three types of concepts: experimental tasks, measuring instruments and subjects.
- The *data dimension*, denoted by DD, is a set of concepts, relationships and axioms, and used to model the systematic brain data management during BI studies of mental health care. It includes three types of concepts: data concepts, information concepts and knowledge concepts corresponding to multi-level mental health big data.
- The *analysis dimension*, denoted by AD, is a set of concepts, relationships and axioms, and used to model the systematic data computing, including analysis, simulation and intelligent applications during BI studies of mental health care. It mainly includes two types of concepts: computing tasks and analytic tools.

By using the domain-driven conceptual modeling process [45], the multi-dimension Data-Brain can be constructed and its each dimension is an upper ontology to integrate multi-aspect domain ontologies during each core issue of systematic studies. For example, a segment of the function dimension is shown in Fig. 7.2. The Data-Brain and integrated domain ontologies form a global conceptual model to model the whole systematic BI studies on mental health care.

7.4.3 The Brain Informatics Provenances Based Information Integration

BI Provenances is used to realize the integration level of integration in mental health big data. They are the metadata describing the origin and subsequent processing of various human brain data in systematic BI studies [7, 47], including data provenances and analysis provenances:

- Data provenances are metadata that describes the BI data origin by integrating multi-aspect experiment information, including subjects information, how experimental data of subjects were collected, what instrument was used, etc. By using data provenances, description information of raw data in clinical examinations databases and wearable databases and contents information in medical information

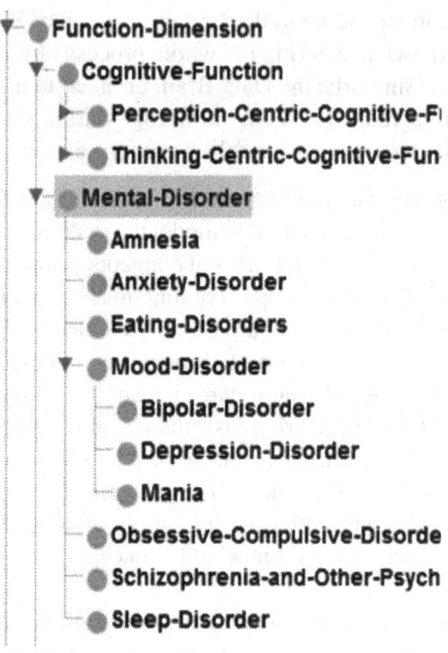

Fig. 7.2 A segment of the function dimension

databases, such as medical records, can be integrated into a unified information sources.

- Analysis provenances are metadata that describes what processing in a brain dataset has been carried out, including what analytic tasks were performed, what experimental data were used, what data features were extracted, and so on. By using analysis provenances, features found in raw data, outer medical information sources, such as LOD medical data sets, can be integrated into a unified information sources.

By recording the whole life cycle of raw data, BI provenances can integrate multi-aspect health information, which are obtained from information systems, digital records, literatures and outer information sources, into a unified health information sources for supporting the discovery of mental disorder-related indexes and their relationships.

Constructing BI provenances can adopt a domain-driven approach. The four ontological dimensions of the Data-Brain and their own domain ontologies form a knowledge-base which includes multi-aspect domain knowledge about heterogeneous brain and mental data, not only data themselves, but also data productions and data processing. By adding relationships among these dimensions, holistic conceptual schemata can be obtained for guiding the development of BI provenances.

For example, to provide a general conceptual schema for BI data provenances, the function, experiment and data dimensions are connected by the following two relations:

- has-experimental-purpose. It is between experimental task concepts in an experiment dimension and the corresponding mental disorders concepts in a function dimension, which describes an experimental purpose.
- has-result-data. It is between experiment concepts in an experiment dimension and the corresponding raw data concepts in a data dimension, which describes results of an experiment.

By using the above two relations, mental disorder related concepts and experiment design related concepts are connected to the corresponding original data concepts. They form a general conceptual schema for describing the BI data origin, as shown in Fig. 7.3. Based on this schema, BI data provenances can be constructed by collecting related information and creating instances of concepts and relations.

By using BI provenances as a bridge, the knowledge level of mental health big data, namely, the Data-Brain and its own domain knowledge, can be integrated with the data level of mental health big data, namely, brain and mental data obtained by clinical examination devices and wearable health devices, and patient-related medical information. Multi-level contents of mental health big data can become a whole for developing the content-oriented cloud service architecture.

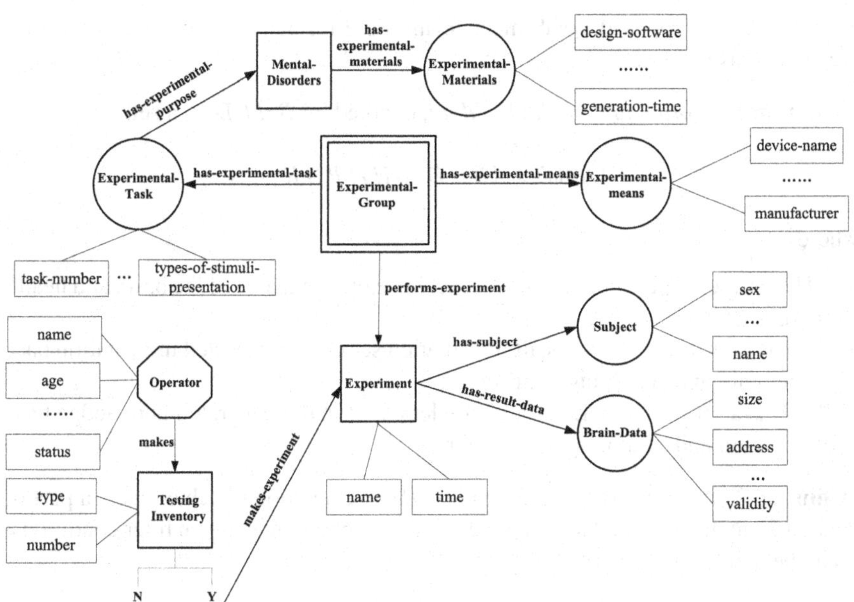

Fig. 7.3 An example of data provenances schema

7.5 Wisdom as a Service: A Content-Oriented Cloud Service Architecture For Mental Health Care

The content-oriented cloud service architecture for mental health care is another important characteristics and core research issue of the brain and health big data center. Based on the WaaS architecture [8], various content-oriented cloud services can be divided into four layers, namely, the DaaS, InaaS, KaaS and WaaS. Realizing such a content-oriented cloud service architecture is involved with multi-aspect work, including service definition, service encapsulation, service registering, etc. Exiting Web service technologies and semantic Web service technologies [23, 27] provide effective methods for service encapsulation, service registering, service publishing, service call, and service communication. Hence, our study focuses on service definition, description, discovery and planning. The detail will be discussed in this section.

7.5.1 Service Definition and Description

To describe the proposed WaaS mechanism more formally, some basic definitions are defined as follows.

Definition 1 A *brain and health big data*, denoted by $BHBD$, is a set:

$$BHBD = \{BHD, BHI, BHK\},$$

where,

- BHD is a set which includes all data set in health databases of the brain and health big data center;
- BHI is a set which includes all information set in the integrated information base of the brain and health big data center;
- BHK is a set which includes all knowledge set in the integrated knowledge base of the brain and health big data center.

Definition 2 A *data service*, denoted by DS, is a function which extracts a part of data set from the brain and health big data center according to given filter conditions. It can be defined as:

$$DS(BHD, \sigma(attr, \upsilon)) = BHD' = \{BHD_i | BHD_i \in BHD, \\ \forall attr_j \in attr \wedge \sigma_j(BHD_i.attr_j, \upsilon_j) = true\}.$$

where,

- $attr = (attr_1, attr_2, ..., attr_m)$ is an attribute list in which each $attr_i$ is an attribute of the data set BHD_i or BI provenances of BHD_i;

- $\sigma(attr, \upsilon) = (\sigma_1(attr_1, \upsilon_1), ..., \sigma_m(attr_m, \upsilon_m))$ is a filter condition list and each $\sigma_j(attr_j, \upsilon_j)$ is a filter condition on the attribute $attr_j$, where σ_j is an operator to define a kind of relationships among attribute values of $attr_j$, such as "=", and υ_i is an attribute value of $attr_j$.

Similarly, an *information service* can be defined as $IS(BHI, \sigma(attr, \upsilon)) = BHI' = \{BHI_i | BHI_i \in BHI, \forall attr_j \in attr \wedge \sigma_j(BHI_i.attr_j, \upsilon_j) = true\}$, where each $attr_j$ is an attribute of the information set BHI_i, and a *knowledge service* can be defined as $KS(BHK, \sigma(attr, \upsilon)) = BHK' = \{BHK_i | BHK_i \in BHK, \forall attr_j \in attr \wedge \sigma_j(BHK_i.attr_j, \upsilon_j) = true\}$, where each $attr_j$ is an attribute of metadata of the knowledge set BHK_i.

All data, information and knowledge services can be constructed by semantic Web service technologies, whose core idea is to annotate the descriptions of services by formal ontologies. By using the Data-Brain and domain ontologies integrated into the Data-Brain, service descriptions can be defined as follows.

Definition 3 A *data service description*, denoted by DSD, is a three-tuple:

$$DSD = (Name, Type, Attr),$$

where,

- $Name$ is the identifier of the data service;
- $Type$ represents the data type provided by the data service and is a concept in the data dimension of the Data-Brain;
- $Attr$ is a sub-set of attribute set of $Type$ and used to construct filter conditions.

Similarly, an *information service description* can be defined as $ISD = (Name, Type, Attr)$, where $Type$ represents the information contents provided by the information service and is a or a group of concepts and their relationships in the Data-Brain, and an *knowledge service description* can be defined as $KSD = (Name, Type, Attr)$, where $Type$ represents the knowledge contents provided by the knowledge service and is a model concept or a top concept of domain ontology in the Data-Brain.

Data, information and knowledge services are to obtain existing big data contents from the brain and health database. These data contents are constructed by offline computing before receiving service requests. Based on these offline computing services, context and user-related big data content services, namely wisdom services, can be developed by online computing technologies, such as user interest-based literature recommendation and user-centric query refinement [40]. The wisdom service and its description can be defined as follows.

Definition 4 A *wisdom service*, denoted by WS, is a function which transforms existing big data contents to new big data contents by online computing. It can be defined as:

$$WS(bhbd) = \{bhbd'\},$$

where $bhbd$ and $bhbd' \subset BHBD$.

Definition 5 A *wisdom service description*, denoted by WSD, is a three-tuple:

$$WSD = (Name, WInput, WOutput),$$

where,

- $Name$ is the identifier of the wisdom service;
- $WInput = \{WInput_1, ..., WInput_n\}$ represents initial big data contents, namely, the input of the wisdom service, and each $WInput_i$ is a concept in the set which consists of all $DSD.Type$, $ISD.Type$ and $KSD.Type$.
- $WOutput$ represents obtained big data contents, namely, the output of the wisdom service, and is a concept in the data dimension of the Data-Brain.

Data services, information services, knowledge services and wisdom services form a multi-level and content-oriented cloud service architecture.

7.5.2 Service Discovery and Planning

The Data-Brain based service descriptions make it possible to automatically discover and planning content-oriented cloud services according to users' service requests. By using the semantic based service planning technologies [7, 23, 27], the whole process can be described as follows.

Firstly, service requests should be described based on the Data-Brain and domain ontologies integrated in the Data-Brain.

Definition 6 A *service request*, denoted by SR, is a two-tuple:

$$SR = (RInput, Results),$$

where,

- $RInput$ is a set of concepts or attributes in the Data-Brain and represents the input conditions of service request. They can be information submitted by users, such as query conditions. They can also be information submitted by systems, such as context information, user information;
- $Results$ is a concept in the set which consists of all $DSD.Type$, $ISD.Type$, $KSD.Type$ and $WSD.WOutput$.

Secondly, regarding $SR.RInput$ as the initial space, $SR.Results$ as the objective space and data, information, knowledge and wisdom services as atomic operations, content-oriented cloud services can be found and organized to build a topology graph by typical problem-solving methods. The pseudo codes of the algorithm are shown in Algorithm 1. The $CanMatch(SRTS, input)$ is to check if each element of $input$

can find a "matching" element of $SRTS$. Because all elements in $SRTS$ and $input$ are concepts or attributes in the Data-Brain, the "matching" doesn't mean that the same concept or attribute. The sub-class, sub-attribute and including relationship can also be regarded as the "matching". The "add" is an incremental addition, namely, only adding new nodes and edges. Relevant edges are the edges from node cs_i to those nodes whose $Type$ or $WOutput$ are matching elements of $SRTS$ during performing the function $CanMatch(SRTS, input)$.

Algorithm 1 Services Discovery and Planning

```
Input: a service request SR
Output: a topology graph TG.
Initialize an empty Topology Graph TG;
Initialize an empty service request type set SRTS;
For each rinput_i in SR.RInput do
  add rinput_i into SRTS;
End For
While (SRTS <> empty) do
  Initialize New-SRTS = empty;
  For each available content-oriented service cs_i do
    If cs_i is a wisdom service then
      input = cs_i.WInput;
      output = cs_i.WOutput
    else
      input = cs_i.Attr;
      output = cs_i.Type
    End If
    If CanMatch(SRTS, input) == true then
      add cs_i as a node and relevant directed edges into TG;
      add output into New-SRTS;
    End If
  End For
  Add elements of SRTS which have not been matched into New-SRTS;
  Initialize SRTS = New-SRTS;
  For each nss_i in New-SRTS do
    If CanMatch(nss_i, SR.Results) == true
      make cs_i corresponding to nss_i as the target node;
      make SRTS == empty;
      break;
    End If
  End For
End While
```

Thirdly, the obtained topology graph includes many redundant nodes which cannot find a path to the target node. They can be removed by finding all simple paths from start nodes to the target node and deleting nodes and edges out of simple paths in the topology graph. The new topology graph is just the service workflow to realize the service request.

7.6 The Illustrative Example

Medical literatures are important information sources for clinical and pathology studies of mental disorders. Aiming at a mass amount of literatures, a literature recommendation system is useful to doctors, researchers and developers which focus on studies of mental disorders. In this section, an illustrative example will be used to describe how to realize a user interest-based literature recommendation on the WaaS architecture.

The user interest-based literature recommendation mainly includes the following seven steps:

- transforming literature information in PubMed to semantic information sources,
- constructing BI provenances,
- querying user's BI provenances,
- querying literatures which meet a or several given conditions,
- constructing the user model by using BI provenances,
- computing literature weight vectors,
- computing literature recommendation values (i.e., similarity degrees).

These seven steps can be divided into two stages: offline computing and online computing. In this illustrative example, the goal of the literature recommendation is set as "recommending literatures on PubMed for Professor Wang who is a psychiatrist".

Offline computing: The first two steps, namely, transforming literature information and constructing BI provenances, should be completed before submitting service requests. Because semantic data set of PubMed literature information can be downloaded from the web site of PubMed, constructing BI provenances become the only work during the offline computing stage.

As stated in Sect. 4.2, constructing data provenances is just to collect related information and create instances of concepts and relations guided by Fig. 7.3. In this case study, user's publications are regarded as information sources. Some rule-based templates have developed to realize information extraction from literatures.

Online computing: The last five steps should be completed after submitting service requests. These online computing operations can be realized based the WaaS architecture. The corresponding content-oriented cloud service workflow is shown in Fig. 7.4. As shown in this figure, the five steps are realized by two information services and three wisdom services:

(1) The information service $IS{:}PQ(BIP, PQ_{Filter})$: the $IS{:}PQ$ is a BI provenance query service which can provide BI provenances according to the query condition PQ_{Filter}. In this case study, $PQ_{Filter} = (=(author, ''Gang\ Wang''), in(publication\ date,$ [2012, 2014])) means to choose BI provenances which were constructed by extracting study-related information from Professor Wang's publications in 2012, 2013 and 2014 years. The number of involved literatures is 13. The BIP represents BI provenances in the brain and health big data center.

(2) The wisdom service $WS{:}UM(BIP)$: the $WS{:}UM$ is an interest-based user modeling service which can provide the interest-based user model by computing

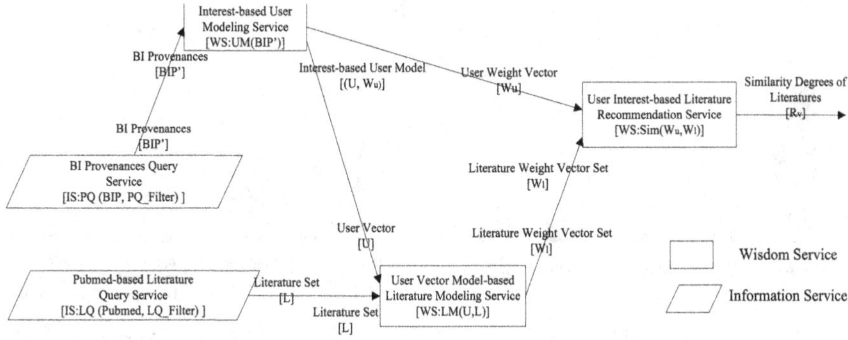

Fig. 7.4 The content-oriented service workflow for realizing user interest-based literature recommendation

users' interests on BI provenances BIP. An interest-based user model is a two-tuple:

$$IUM = (U, W_u),$$

where $U = (e_1, e_2, e_3, ...)$ is a user vector to represent users' interests, in which each e_k represents the users' interest on the element E_k of BI provenances; $W_u = (w_{e1}, w_{e2}, w_{e3}, ...)$ is a user weight vector to quantificationally represent users' interests, in which each w_{ek} represents the retained interest value of the users' interest e_k. In this case study, four elements of BI provenances $E_1 = Mental\_Disorder$, $E_2 = Research\_Means$, $E_3 = Experimental\_Material$, and $E_4 = Subject$ are defined based on domain experts' suggestions. This means that user research interests are described from four aspects including mental disorder types, experimental means, experimental tasks, and subject types. The retained interest value w_{ek} is computed by using the retained interest formula RI [13]:

$$RI(e_k(i), n) = \sum_{j=1}^{n} y_{e_k(i)}, j \times AT_{e_k(i)}^{-b}$$

where $e_k(i)$ is a possible value of E_k and represents a candidate user interest on E_k; n is the number of time periods; $T_{e_k(i)}$ is the number of time periods since appearance and represents the duration of influence of $e_k(i)$; $y_{e_k(i)}, j$ is the appearance frequency of the candidate interest $e_k(i)$ in the time period j; A is used to control the difference of retained interest with current interest, and makes them have the minimum difference; b is used to control the decaying speed on lost interests.

In this case study, three time periods were defined, namely, 2012, 2013 and 2014 years. The value of A is 0.855 and the value of b is 1.295 according to previous studies [39, 40]. By computing on BI provenances BIP, all candidate user interests and their retained interest values on four elements of BI prove-

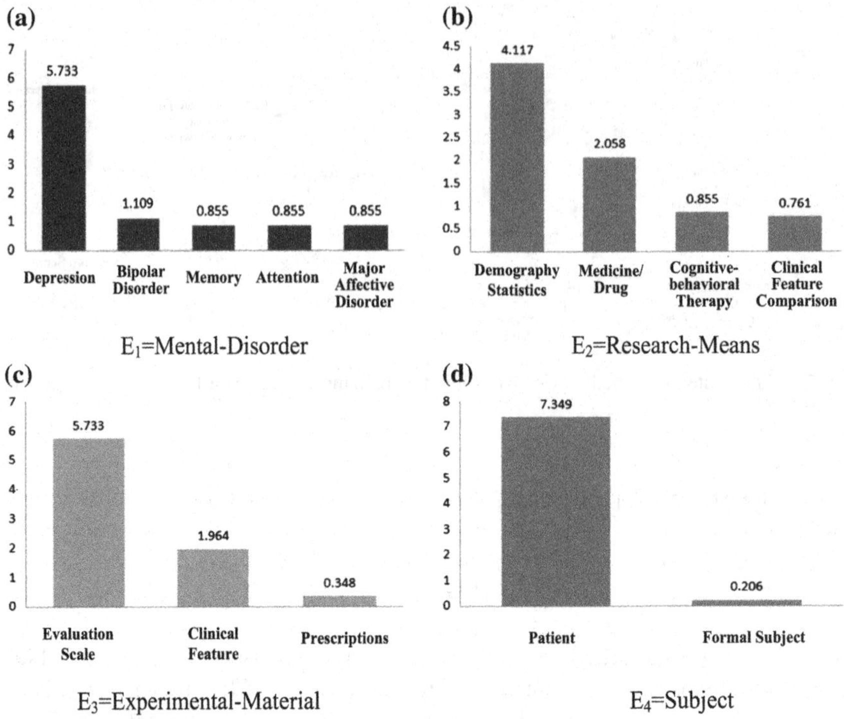

Fig. 7.5 All candidate user interests and their retained interest values

nances are shown in Fig. 7.5. By choosing use interests with the max retained interest values, Professor Wang's interest-based user model $IUM_{wang}(U, W_u) = ((Depression, Demography\ Statistics, Evaluation\ Scale, Patient), (5.733, 4.117, 5.733, 7.349))$ can be obtained.

(3) The information service $IS{:}LQ(PubMed, LQ_{Filter})$: the $IS{:}LQ$ is a PubMed-based literature query service which can provide semantic literature information in PubMed according to the query condition LQ_{Filter}. Considering the huge literature number in PubMed, this case study chose 1000 literatures which include the word "Depression", namely, the highest user interest on this kind of *Mental Disorder*, in the title, the abstract or keywords, to reduce redundant calculating works, i.e., $LQ_{Filter} = (including(title, "Depression"), including(abstract, "De\text{-}pression"), including(keywords, "Depression"), in(publi\text{-}cation\ date, [2012, 2014]))$.

(4) The wisdom service $WS{:}LM(U, W_l)$: the $WS{:}LM$ is a user vector model-based literature modeling service which can provide the literature weight vectors of objective literatures based on a given user vector. A literature weight vector, denoted by W_l, can be defined as follows:

$$W_l = (w_{l1}, w_{l2}, w_{l3}, \ldots)$$

where w_{li} is the literature weight value corresponding to the element e_i of the given user vector $U = (e_1, e_2, ...e_i)$. It is computed by using the following formula:

$$w_{li} = \alpha * w_{ti} + \beta * w_{ki} + \gamma * w_{abi},$$

where w_{ti} is the number of e_i in the title of the literature; w_{ki} is the number of e_i in keywords of the literature; w_{abi} is the number of e_i in the abstract of the literature.

The α, β and γ are weight coefficients when the element e_i appears in the title, key words and the abstract, respectively. In our study, their values are set as "0.5", "0.333" and "0.167" based on repeated experiments and domain experts' result assessments.

(5) The wisdom service $WS{:}Sim(W_u, W_l)$: the $WS{:}Sim$ is a user interest-based literature recommendation service which can provide similarity degrees of literatures based on a user weight vector and a group of literature weight vectors. The similarity degree of literatures is computed by using the following cosine similarity formula:

$$Sim(U, L) = (\sum_{i=1}^{n} w_{ui} * w_{li})/(\sqrt{\sum_{i=1}^{n} w_{ui}^2} * \sqrt{\sum_{i=1}^{n} w_{li}^2})$$

Based on definitions stated in Sect. 5.1, information services and wisdom services can be described based on the Data-Brain:

The information service $IS{:}PQ$ can be described as $(IS{:}PQ, "BI\_Provenances", ("author", "publication\ date", ...))$ where "BI Provenances" is an information concept in the Data-Brain and represents the type of information sources provided by this service; "author" and "publication date" are attributes of the concept "BI Provenances" and are used to define filter conditions. Similarly, the information service $IS{:}LQ$ can be described as $(IS{:}LQ, "Semantic\_Literature\_Information", ("title", "abstract", "keywords"))$.

The wisdom service $WS{:}UM$ can be described as $(WS{:}UM, "BI\_Provenances", "Interest\_based\_User\_Model")$ where "BI Provenances" is an information concept in the Data-Brain and used to describe the type of service input; $Interest\_based\ \_User\_Model$ is a knowledge concept in the Data-Brain and used to describe the type of service output. Similarly, the wisdom service $WS{:}LM$ can be described as $(WS{:}LM, \{\text{``}User\_Vector", \text{``}Semantic\_Literature\_Informa-tion"\}, \text{``}Literature\ \_Weight\ \_Vector")$ and the wisdom service $WS{:}Sim$ can be described as $(WS{:}Sim, \{\text{``}User\_Weight\_Vector", \text{``}Literature\ \_Weight\ \_Vector"\}, \text{``}Similarity\ \_Degrees\ \_of\ \_Literatures")$.

Furthermore, the goal of this example, i.e., "recommending literatures on PubMed for Professor Wang who is a psychiatrist" can also be described based on the Data-Brain: $SR = (\{user.name = \text{``}Wang\ Gan"\}, \text{``}Similarity\ \_Degrees\ \_of\ \_Literatures")$.

Based on these descriptions, the service workflow shown in Fig. 7.4 can be obtained by performing Algorithm 1. As stated above, the "matching" among services is not limited to the "same". The sub-class, sub-attribute and containment relationships can also be regarded as the "matching". For example, because the interest-based

Table 7.1 The 10 literatures with the highest similarity values

ID	Similarity degree	Literature title
1	0.9242911920248688	Assessing quality of life in Parkinson's disease using the PDQ-39. A pilot study
2	0.891631697505084	Screening psychiatric morbidity after miscarriage: application of the 30-item General Health Questionnaire and the Edinburgh Postnatal Depression Scale
3	0.891631697505084	The psychological symptoms of conjugal bereavement in elderly men over the first 13 months
4	0.891631697505084	A quality assurance instrument at ambulatory health centers. A scale for identification of depression among the elderly
5	0.891631697505084	MDMA (Ecstasy) use—an overview of psychiatric and medical sequelae
6	0.891631697505084	Aggressive behaviour in schizophrenia: the role of psychopathology
7	0.891631697505084	Subarachnoid meperidine-morphine combination. An effective perioperative analgesic adjunct for cesarean delivery
8	0.891631697505084	Inattentive and hyperactive behaviors and driving offenses in adolescence
9	0.891631697505084	Hopelessness and suicidal behavior
10	0.891631697505084	Maternity blues in Brazilian women

user model is a two-tuple including a user vector and a user weight vector, there is a containment relationship between the concepts "Interest-based User Model" and "User Vector" in the Data-Brain. Therefore, the wisdom service $WS{:}UM$ whose output is $Interest\_based\_User\_Model$ can be connected to the $WS{:}LM(U, L)$ where the input is "$User\_Vector$", as shown in Fig. 7.4.

Performing this workflow, similarity degrees of literatures can be obtained as the recommendation criteria. The higher similarity value means that the literature is more similar to user's research interests and has the higher recommendation worth. Table 7.1 gives the 10 literatures with the highest similarity degrees.

Our experiments are based on the PubMed semantic data set in which literatures are involved with broad research domains. For the user Professor Wang, many literatures cannot effectively match his interests. When a literature only matches a user interest aspect, its literature weight vector will only include a nonzero element. The corresponding cosine similarity formula is as follows:

$$Sim(U, L) = (w_{uj} * w_{lj})/(\sqrt{\sum_{i=1}^{n} w_{ui}^2} * w_{lj}) = w_{uj}/\sqrt{\sum_{i=1}^{n} w_{ui}^2}$$

where w_{lj} is the nonzero element in the literature weight vector W_l. This means that, if the similarity degrees are calculated between Professor Wang's user weight vector W_u and this kind of literature weight vectors, the same result will be obtained even if literature weight vectors are different. Hence, most of literatures have the same similarity degree in Table 7.1. The domain knowledge-driven document selection technology [48] can be used to solve this problem. It can be constructed as a wisdom service and added into the beginning of the workflow shown in Fig. 7.4.

In summary, the above example illustrates that, the WaaS architecture makes it possible to integrated multi-levels mental health big data from a perspective of systematic studies and construct different levels of big data services by a unified mode. Furthermore, automatic service planning can be performing to obtain service workflows, i.e., solutions of the target tasks, for any intelligent application demand based on mental health big data. Hence, it is possible to develop an open and extendable platform by using the proposed WaaS architecture and provide multi-level data services of mental health big data in a pay-as-you-go manner, for supporting large-scale research cooperation, achievement promotion and industrialization. This is the most important value of WaaS.

7.7 Conclusions

Systematic BI studies on mental disorders have led to multi-level and multi-aspect of mental health big data and bring new requirements of developing brain data center, from the data level to the wisdom level. It is necessary to develop a brain and health big data to effectively integrating multi-level mental health big data and provide multi-level content-oriented data services for different types of users by an open and extendable mode. The core issue is to realize a content-oriented cloud service architecture for mental health care, called WaaS. In this chapter, a global content integrating mechanism is proposed to realize a top-down integration of mental health big data. Based on it, service definition, description, discovery and planning are designed to realize the WaaS architecture on the cloud computing platform.

By the proposed approach, the brain and health big data center becomes an open and extendable platform to gather more and more data sources and services. It will become a collaborative research platform of mental health care for the BI community. Each researcher will use it to define research strategies and aims, design and manage experiments, collect and interpret results, incorporate the findings of others, disseminate observations, and extend observations in directions completely unanticipated, as stated in Bower et al.'s works [2]. It will also become an individual treatment platform [34] where patients, physicians, and researchers collect and analyze mental health big data from every patient, and use these results to individualize therapies. Furthermore, data contents will be updated continually to benefit subsequent patients.

Developing such a brain and health big data center is a large and complex project. Much work still needs to be done. For example, it is necessary to develop new technologies for the "Interactions + Adaptive Judgement" component of the WaaS layer. In this study, the semantic-based service discovery and planning is used to realize an adaptive rational judgement. However, interaction in complex systems needs to realize both intuitive and rational judgements. This can be realized by using interactive rough-granular computing [31, 32].

Acknowledgments The work is supported by National Basic Research Program of China (2014CB744600), China Postdoctoral Science Foundation (2013M540096), International Science & Technology Cooperation Program of China (2013DFA32180), National Natural Science Foundation of China (61272345), Research Supported by the CAS/SAFEA International Partnership Program for Creative Research Teams, Open Foundation of Key Laboratory of Multimedia and Intelligent Software (Beijing University of Technology), Beijing, the Japan Society for the Promotion of Science Grants-in-Aid for Scientific Research (25330270), and Support Center for Advanced Telecommunications Technology Research, Foundation (SCAT), Japan.

References

1. M. Armbrust, A. Fox, R. Griffith, A.D. Joseph, R.H. Katz, A. Konwinski, G. Lee, D.A. Patterson, A. Rabkin, I. Stoica, M. Zaharia, *Above the Clouds: A Berkeley View of Cloud Computing* (Technical report, EECS Department, University of California, Berkeley, 2009)
2. J.M. Bower, H. Bolouri (eds.), *Computational Modeling of Genetic and Biochemical Networks* (MIT Press, Cambridge, MA, 2001)
3. BrainMap, http://brainmap.org
4. H. Chaouchi, *The Internet of Things-connecting Objects to the Web* (ISTE Ltd., Wiley, New York, 2010)
5. J.H. Chen, N. Zhong, Data-brain modeling based on brain informatics methodology, in *Proceedings of 2008 IEEE/WIC/ACM International Conference on Web Intelligence (WI'08)* (2008), pp. 41–47
6. J.H. Chen, N. Zhong, Data-brain modeling for systematic brain informatics, in *Proceedings of 2009 International Conference on Brain Informatics (BI 2009)* (2009), pp. 182–193
7. J.H. Chen, N. Zhong, Toward the data-brain driven systematic brain data analysis. IEEE Trans. Syst. Man Cybernet. Syst. **43**(1), 222–228 (2013)
8. J.H. Chen, J.H. Ma, N. Zhong, Y.Y. Yao, J.M. Liu, R.H. Huang, W.B. Li, Z.S. Huang, Y. Gao, J.P. Cao, WaaS-wisdom as a service. IEEE Intell. Syst. **29**(6), 2–9 (2014)
9. C.A. Cocosco, V. Kollokian, R.K.S. Kwan, A.C. Evans, BrainWeb: online interface to a 3D MRI simulated brain database. NeuroImage **5**(4, part 2/4), S425 (1997)
10. O. Cure, On the design of a self-medication web application built on linked open data. J. Web Sem. **24**, 27–32 (2014)
11. T. Dillon, A. Talevski, V. Potdar, E. Chang, Web of things as a framework for ubiquitous intelligence and computing, in *Proceedings of the 6th International Conference on Ubiquitous Intelligence and Computing* (2009), pp. 1–10
12. P.L. Elkin, S.H. Brown, C.S. Husser, B.A. Bauer, D. Wahner-Roedler, S.T. Rosenbloom, T. Speroff, Evaluation of the content coverage of SNOMED CT: ability of SNOMED clinical terms to represent clinical problem lists. Mayo Clin. Proc. **81**(6), 741–748 (2006)
13. J. Han, J.H. Chen, H. Zhong, N. Zhong, A brain informatics research recommendation system, in *Proceedings of the 2014 International Conference on Brain Informatics and Health (BIH 2014)* (Springer, LNAI 8609, 2014), pp. 208–217
14. B. Hayes, Cloud computing. Commun. ACM **51**(7), 9–11 (2008)
15. J.D. Van Horn, A.W. Toga, Is it time to re-prioritize neuroimaging databases and digital repositories? NeuroImage **47**(4), 1720–1734 (2009)

16. D. Howe, M. Costanzo, P. Fey, T. Gojobori, L. Hannick, W. Hide, D.P. Hill, R. Kania, M. Schaeffer, S. St. Pierre, S. Twigger, O. White, S.Y. Rhee, Big data: the future of biocuration. Nature **455**, 47–50 (2008)
17. M. Hunter, R.L.L. Smith, W. Hyslop, O.A. Rosso, R. Gerlach, J.A.P. Rostas, D.B. Williams, F. Henskens, The Australian EEG database. Clin. EEG Neurosci. **36**(2), 76–81 (2005)
18. A. Jankowski, A. Skowron, and R.W. Swiniarski, Interactive rough-granular computing in wisdom technology, in *Proceedings of 2013 International Conference on Active Media Technology (AMT 2013)* (2013), pp. 1–13
19. P.D. Kaur, I. Chana, Cloud based intelligent system for delivering health care as a service. Comput. Methods Prog. Biomed. **113**(1), 346–359 (2014)
20. C. Knox, V. Law, T. Jewison, P. Liu, S. Ly, A. Frolkis, A. Pon, K. Banco, C. Mak, V. Neveu, Y. Djoumbou, R. Eisner, A.C. Guo, D.S. Wishart, DrugBank 3.0: a comprehensive resource for omics research on drugs. Nucleic Acids Res. **39**(suppl 1), D1035–D1041 (2011)
21. Z.Z. Liao, H.Y. Zhou, C. Li, J. Zhou, Y.L. Qin, Y. Feng, L. Feng, G. Wang, N. Zhong, The change of resting EEG in depressive disorders, in *Proceedings of the 2013 International Conference on Brain and Health Informatics* (Springer, LNAI 8211, 2013), pp. 52–61
22. P.F. Liu, M. Li, S.F. Lu, J. Wang, Y. Zhou, X.Y. Su, N. Zhong, Impairments of working memory for object-location associations in depression. Appl. Mech. Mater. **590**, 828–832 (2014)
23. N. Mazzocca, R.A. Micillo, S. Venticinque, Automatic and dynamic composition of web services using ontologies, in *Proceedings of 5th Atlantic Web Intelligence Conference (AWIC 2007)* (2007), pp. 230–235
24. NIF. http://nif.nih.gov/
25. NMDB. http://microcircuit.epfl.ch
26. ORDB. http://senselab.med.yale.edu/ORDB/default.asp
27. M. Paolucci, T. Kawamura, T.R. Payne, K. Sycara, Semantic matching of web services capabilities. Pro. ISWC **2002**, 333–347 (2002)
28. http://pubmed.gov/
29. C.P. Shen, W.Z. Zhou, F.S. Lin, H.Y. Sung, Y.Y. Lam, W. Chen, J.W. Lin, M.K. Pan, M.J. Chiu, F.P. Lai, Epilepsy analytic system with cloud computing, in *Proceedings of 35th Annual International Conference of the IEEE EMBS* (2013), pp. 1644–1647
30. Y.L. Simmhan, B. Plale, D. Gannon, A survey of data provenance in e-science. Sigmod Record **34**(3), 31–36 (2005)
31. A. Skowron, M. Szczuka, Toward interactive computations: a rough-granular approach. Adv. Mach. Learn. II, SCI **263**, 23–42 (2010)
32. A. Skowron, A. Jankowski, Interactive computations: toward risk management in interactive intelligent systems. Nat. Comput. (2015). doi:10.1007/s11047-015-9486-5
33. V. Stirbu, Towards a RESTful plug and play experience in the web of things, in *Proceedings of the 2008 IEEE International Conference on Semantic Computing* (2008), pp. 512–517
34. J.M. Tenenbaum, J. Shrager, Cancer: a computational disease that AI can cure. AI Mag. **32**(2), 14–26 (2011)
35. P.E. Turkeltaub, G.F. Eden, K.M. Jones, T.A. Zeffiro, Meta-analysis of the functional neuroanatomy of single-word reading: method and validation. Neuroimage **16**, 765–780
36. J.D. Van Horn, J.S. Grethe, P. Kostelec, J.B. Woodward, J.A. Aslam, D. Rus, D. Rockmore, M.S. Gazzaniga, The functional magnetic resonance imaging data center (fMRIDC): the challenges and rewards of large-scale databasing of neuroimaging studies. Philos. Trans. R. Soc. B: Biol. Sci. **356**(1412), 1323–1339 (2001)
37. E. Welbourne, L. Battle, G. Cole, K. Gould, K. Rector, S. Raymer, M. Balazinska, G. Borriello, Building the internet of things using RFID. IEEE Internet Comput. **33**(3), 48–55 (2009)
38. Y.Y. Yao, N. Zhong, J. Liu, S. Ohsuga, Web intelligence (WI): research challenges and trends in the new information age, in N. Zhong, Y.Y. Yao, J. Liu, S. Ohsuga (eds.) *Web Intelligence: Research and Development* (Springer, LNAI 2198, 2001), pp. 1–17
39. Y. Zeng, Y.Y. Yao, N. Zhong, Dblp-sse: a dblp search support engine, in *The 2009 IEEE/WIC/ACM International Conference on Web Intelligence(WI'09)* (2009), pp. 626–630

40. Y. Zeng, N. Zhong, Y. Wang, Y.L. Qin, Z.S. Huang, H.Y. Zhou, User-centric query refinement and processing using granularity based strategies. Knowl. Inf. Syst. **27**(3), 419–450 (2010)
41. N. Zhong, J.M. Liu, Y.Y. Yao, S. Ohsuga, Web intelligence (WI), in *Proceedings of the 24th IEEE Computer Society International Computer Software and Applications Conference (COMPSAC 2000)* (2000), pp. 469–470
42. N. Zhong, Impending brain informatics research from web intelligence perspective. Int. J. Inf. Technol. Decis. Mak. **5**(4), 713–727 (2006)
43. N. Zhong, J.M. Liu, Y.Y. Yao, J.L. Wu, S.F. Lu, Y.L. Qin, K.C. Li, B. Wah, Web intelligence meets brain informatics, in *Proceedings of the first WICI international workshop on web intelligence meets brain informatics (WImBI 2006)* (2006), pp. 1–31
44. N. Zhong, S. Motomura, Agent-enriched data mining: a case study in brain informatics. IEEE Intell. Syst. **24**(3), 38–45 (2009)
45. N. Zhong, J.H. Chen, Constructing a new-style conceptual model of brain data for systematic brain informatics. IEEE Trans. Knowl. Data Eng. **24**(12), 2127–2142 (2012)
46. N. Zhong, J.H. Ma, R.H. Huang, J.M. Liu, Y.Y. Yao, Y.X. Zhang, J.H. Chen, Research challenges and perspectives on wisdom web of things (W2T). J. Supercomput. **64**(3), 862–882 (2013)
47. H. Zhong, J.H. Chen, T. Kotake, J. Han, N. Zhong, Z.S. Huang, Developing a brain informatics provenance model, in *Proceedings of the 2013 International Conference on Brain and Health Informatics (BHI 2013)* (Springer, LNAI 8211, 2013), pp. 439–449
48. H. Zhong, N. Zhong, J.H. Chen, J. Han, Document selection for the data-brain ontology and related information. J. Guangxi Normal Univ. (Natural Science Edition) **32**(4), 45–51 (2014)

Chapter 8
Leveraging Neurodata to Support Web User Behavior Analysis

Pablo Loyola, Enzo Brunetti, Gustavo Martinez, Juan D. Velásquez and Pedro Maldonado

Abstract Given its complexity, understanding the behavior of users on the Web has been one of the most challenging tasks for data mining-related fields. Historically, most of the approaches have considered web logs as the main source of data. This has led to several successful cases, both in industry and academia, but has also presented several issues and limitations. Given the new challenges and the need for personalization, improvement is required in the overall understanding of the processes that lie behind web browsing decision making. The use of neurodata to support this analysis represents a huge opportunity in terms of understanding the actions taken by the user on the web in a more comprehensive way. Techniques such as eye tracking, pupil dilation and EEG analysis could provide valuable information to craft more robust models. This chapter overviews the current state of the art of the use of neurodata for web-based analysis, providing a description and analysis in terms of the feasibility and effectiveness of each strategy given a specific problem.

P. Loyola · G. Martinez · J.D. Velásquez (✉)
Web Intelligence Centre, Industrial Engineering Department,
University of Chile, Santiago, Chile
e-mail: jvelasqu@dii.uchile.cl

P. Loyola
e-mail: ployola@ing.uchile.cl

G. Martinez
e-mail: gumartin@ing.uchile.cl

E. Brunetti · P. Maldonado
Neurosystems Laboratory, Institute of Biomedical Sciences,
Faculty of Medicine, University of Chile, Santiago, Chile
e-mail: enzo@neuro.med.uchile.cl

P. Maldonado
e-mail: pedro@neuro.med.uchile.cl

N. Zhong et al. (eds.), *Wisdom Web of Things*, Web Information
Systems Engineering and Internet Technologies Book Series,
DOI 10.1007/978-3-319-44198-6_8

8.1 Introduction

The ubiquity of the Internet and the development of the Web represent two of the most critical technological advances in recent years. Services based on these two technologies have been integrated into most human activities and their presence has changed the way in which people behave and interact [74].

The amount of data and information generated on the Web every day surpasses any other human-generated system and represents a valuable opportunity in terms of understanding human behavior. First, from an academic point of view, the Web is seen as a source for visualizing a *human consciousness*, which is usually associated with the concepts of *collective intelligence* or *wisdom of the crowd*, where methods for pattern recognition and data aggregation are used to solve complex problems. Second, from a private point of view, processing data from the Web is essential in order to provide better services and maximize monetary utility through a personalization process [70].

Thus, as the understanding of Web user behavior is transversely considered a relevant task, several models have been proposed. Most of them are focused on the issue of user preference identification, which means the capture of which elements the user is searching for while he traverses a web site. With that information, service providers can improve the user's experience or offer custom services in a more effective way [71].

The majority of the methodologies developed use as a primary source of information the set of *web logs*, which are documents that store each action a given user generated during his visit, in a standardized way. This source and several techniques from the data-mining field are combined to perform standard tasks such as classification or prediction [58].

Although web logs represent an important source of data, there are several limitations that threaten the validity and degree of generalization of the results [67].

First, from the preprocessing of the data, there is no reliable way to extract the user sessions, which are the successive steps a user followed during a visit to a web site. There is a high dependency on how each web browser presents the data to the server and most of the approaches are based on heuristics.

Second, web logs do not provide an explicit way to capture a user's interest in certain elements of the web pages [97]. While the time spent on each web page has been used as a proxy for user preference, it does not show strong correlation results that could lead to solid conclusions. Additionally, and specifically in problems related to recommender systems, the use of web logs does not provide solutions to key problems such as the *cold start problem* [85].

Finally, in terms of the identification of relevant objects [91], most of the approaches perform a validation using qualitative techniques such as surveys, which limits the level of generalization and the overall reliability.

Given the limitations of the state of the art and the increasing demand for a more comprehensive analysis that could improve the results, our main hypothesis resides in the idea that the combination of Web data and neurodata in a KDD framework could perform synergistically and boost the effectiveness of the analysis.

The rationale of the previous statement underlies the nature of the neurodata. As it comes directly from the user, it provides a purely biological and quantitative measure of the changes perceived in a visitor given a certain stimulus presented on a web page. Thus, this new kind of data could be incorporated with the standard models where previously there were only assumptions or restrictions.

The remainder of this chapter is as follows. Section 8.2 presents an overview of the Web data, focusing on the different types of elements that can be extracted. Section 8.3 represents an introduction to the neurodata, specifically related to eye tracking and EEG techniques. Section 8.4 overviews the different approaches to modeling web user behavior and how neurodata can be included as a critical component. Section 8.5 present a discussion section, analyzing the main characteristics and limitations. Section. Finally, Sect. 8.6 presents a summary.

8.2 Web Data

Web data corresponds to the set of data sources that can be extracted from Web-based systems. Two main categories can be identified. First, from the web system point of view, a web site can be decomposed in terms of its content and structure. By analyzing these sources, a comprehensive view of what the user was exposed to in a given sequence of visits can be obtained. Second, from the data stored as logs on the server, the paths and patterns the visitor followed can be extracted [75].

8.2.1 Web Structure Data

Web structure data corresponds to the hyperlink network that can be formed within the page set of a web site. Based on this representation, nodes are web pages and edges are the links between them, generating a directed graph. Initially, when web activity was low, this graph was categorized as a static entity. The subsequent increase in development and usage showed the need to consider a time-dependent approach [6].

Several studies have reported a power law distribution in the hyperlink structure. Topological measures have been used to categorize pages in terms of their link degree, leading to concepts such as *hubs* and *authorities* [28, 83].

8.2.2 Web Content Data

Web content data represents all the humanly comprehensible content that can be stored on a web page. Initially, mainly text-based content was considered and several approaches from Information Retrieval and Text Mining were implemented, such as the Bag of Words and the Vector Space models. Other types of content such as images and video have been relegated given the complexity of extracting a standardized way for representing them. The Semantic Web initiative could provide a new framework in which all types of content could be identified beyond a simple meta-data centric approach [14].

Regarding text-based content, considerable progress have been made in order to capture a more comprehensive understanding of the meaning [40]. Natural Language Processing methodologies along with machine learning have been used to improve the analysis, especially in terms of identifying the context. Additionally, given the current user-generated nature of the content of the Web, disciplines such as Sentiment Analysis have gained popularity.

The text contained on the Web follows the same characteristics observed in other resources. In terms of the distribution of words, the Zipf Law is confirmed by several studies. The underlying cause for this phenomenon is the recurrent simplification of communication by reducing the set of words used in order to optimize memory functions [41, 50].

8.2.3 Web Usage Data

The key element from which all usage analyses have been developed is the *user session* [12, 84], which is the trail of web pages that a user follows during a visit to a web site. This data can be collected in several ways, including the storage of web logs on the server side and the use of Javascript-based client-side applications to track page transitions.

The extraction of web usage data has been challenging since the early days of the Web, given the lack of standardization and the constant evolution of the technologies used. The main points of concern can be summarized as follows:

- Web browser functionalities have contributed to enriching the visitor experience, giving the users several options and tools such as multiple page visualization, back button and collaborative navigation. These have represented a challenge in terms of identifying a pure session for analysis [87].
- From a performance point of view, as the main goal of web browsers is to provide better navigation through faster page load, several content caching and pre-loading techniques have been implemented, resulting in noisy logs which are difficult to process.
- The combination between client and server side technologies led to the widespread use of AJAX, which allows asynchronous calls to be performed. Although it has improved the overall usability, the concept of *user session* becomes diffuse and it is hard to distinguish transitions.
- The explosive increase in the use of new platforms such as smart phones and tablets has forced the web development process to generate adaptive solutions. Responsive designs have been implemented in order to provide a unified solution for all platforms, but it does not consider tools for understanding the context.

Given the above, using only a click-stream-based data source, such as web logs, does not necessary reflect web user behavior [99]. Both academia and industry have addressed this issue and have put efforts into finding new sources that could support and improve the analysis. In that sense, eye-tracking techniques and pointer tracking have been implemented during the last few years.

Regarding the statistical analysis of web user behavior, one of the most significant advances was the Law of Surfing, which states that the distribution of the length of the sessions follows an inverse Gaussian distribution. Additionally, the time spent on each page was found to be correlated to the interest the user had in the content [64].

The process of sessionization consists of the reconstruction and retrieval of web user sessions based on all the feasible data that could be captured. This involves mainly web logs stored on the server, but additionally other types of data can be collected, depending on the sessionization method selected and the depth required [103].

Regarding the types of sessionization methods, two main categories can be recognized:

8.2.3.1 Proactive Sessionization

These methods attempt to capture user information at the same time it is being generated. Historically, there have been three main ways to achieve this goal.

The first involves the use of *cookies*, which automatically store user information and activity and can be requested and updated by the system on the web page visited.

The second approach is to deploy a client-side tracking system. This could be implemented on top of a Javascript set of methods. Additionally, functionalities provided by the HTML 5 API, such as *local storage*, could improve the performance and accuracy. The main issue of this approach is the lack of standardization among web browsers, which reduces the reliability in terms of the support and handling of Javascript functionalities.

The third method consists of capturing user behavior under explicit agreement. This is usually presented as a *win-win* formula for the user; the web site benefits from the rich source of data, which can be used to optimize several processes. On the other hand, the user gets benefits as the service can be completely personalized. This schema is questionable and several information asymmetries arise.

In general, proactive sessionization methods suffer from privacy issues. Certain strategies have collided with the legislation in several countries, provoking changes in the delivery of the services [39].

8.2.3.2 Reactive Sessionization

Reactive sessionization means the reconstruction of the user session using previously stored data, in which web server logs play an important role.

Web server logs are a set of files which contain every HTTP request sent to the server in the form of a string of text. In this string there are several pieces of information about the machine that performed the request, such as the IP address, user agent, the requested file and a timestamp, among others.

One key step in reactive sessionization is the pre-processing of the web logs. As the server registers every request, it is necessary to select only the ones that correspond to a valid user, removing the activity of bots and crawlers from the registry. After that process, a grouping procedure needs to be performed in other to recognize unique visits. Usually, valid logs are grouped by IP address and then divided by a time threshold. This is clearly a simplification that could threaten the validity of the sessionization process.

8.2.3.3 Methods for Capturing the Web User Trail

Having collected the data by means of either reactive or proactive strategies, the central part is how to identify a real session. Methods for identifying the web user trail are mainly part of proactive sessionization, as the data is less complete.

- **Time-based identification:** After grouping by IP address and user agent, the resulting sequences are sliced considering an arbitrary accumulated time. Historically, researchers have set up a threshold in 30 min, which is based on empirical evidence [95].
- **Web site topology-based identification:** This technique assumes the user strictly follows the hyperlink structure of the web site. Thus, if there is a transition between two pages but there is no actual link between them, that represents the end of a session and the beginning of a new one [12].
- **Ontology-based identification:** This approach considers the use of the content from the visited web pages. From this, a semantic distance is computed between pages. Then, sessions are constructed by grouping pages that have the lowest semantic distance. The main assumption is that since a web session reflects the user purpose, there should be a natural connection between the content explored [45].
- **Integer programming-based identification:** This approach considers the formulation of the session reconstruction as an optimization problem. Given that, the set of constraints involves the grouping of logs by IP Address and user agent and the sequences follow the hyperlink structure of the web site, for a given time. The process consists of solving a bipartite cardinality matching problem (BMC), which in this case means finding the minimum number of feasible sessions from a bipartite network of *from* and *to* nodes [25].

8.3 Neurodata

8.3.1 Eye Tracking

Contrary to our continuous visual experience, eyes discretely move to different locations in the surrounding world at an average of three to four times per second. This biological characteristic is a consequence of the anatomical organization of the retina: the photoreceptors making the largest contribution to the information going to deeper brain centers -thus providing most of the fine-grained spatial resolvability of the visual system, concentrate in the central area of the retina. Whereas the entire visual field is roughly defined by an ellipsoid with the horizontal major axis subtending 180 ° visual angle, the diameter of the highest acuity circular region (fovea) subtends 2 °, the parafovea (zone of high acuity) extends to about 4 ° or 5 °, and acuity drops off sharply beyond. At 5 °, acuity is only 50 % [42]. The so- called "useful" visual field extends to about 30 °. The rest of the visual field has very poor resolvable power and is mostly used for perception of ambient motion.

Because of the previous fact, the oculo-motor behavior displayed in almost all exploratory conditions consists of a series of rapid ocular movements (*saccades*) intermingled with periods in which the eye manifests little or null change of its position (*fixations*). Saccades serve to direct the foveal position of eyes to regions of interest in the visual field, and are assumed to be periods of blindness for the visual system. By contrast, fixations are periods in which new sensory information can get into the brain, thus allowing for updating the visual scene.

Research centered on the definition of perceptual preferences during the exploration of different types of visual material have focused primarily on the quantification of fixations' parameters across time, assuming that the number and duration of fixations over specific parts of the scene reflect the subjective interest manifested by an observer. While this could be true in some circumstances, the specific pattern of ocular movements is highly non linear and determined by numerous aspects of the visual information examined, many of which depending on the specific task engaged [20, 88, 101].

The notion of a parallel between the fixations' spatial and temporal parameters allocation and the subjective individual interest for specific aspects of the scene fits well with original psychological models of attention. Indeed, as originally proposed, attention was conceived as a filter for perceptual information [44], which, in the case of the visual system, would be achieved by restricting the high resolution processing just to limited portions of the surrounding ambient. Because of its limited capacity, the brain processes sensory input by concentrating on specific components of the entire sensory realm so that interesting aspects may be examined with greater attention to detail than peripheral stimuli. Thus, we would may presume that if we can track fixational movements, we can follow along the path of attention deployed by the observer [27].

Despite general agreement exist in that attention is used to focus our mental capacities on selections of the sensory input so that the mind can successfully process the stimulus of interest, some modern theories of attention do not equate attentional resources with ocular fixations. The concept of attention as a " spotlight" proposed by Posner [73] dissociate that spotlight from foveal vision and consider it as an attentional mechanism independent of eye movements. Posner et al. identified two aspects of visual attention: the orienting and the detecting of attention. Orienting may be an entirely central (covert or mental) aspect of attention, whereas detecting is context-sensitive, requiring contact between the attentional beam and the input signal. The orienting of attention is not always dependent on the movement of the eyes; that is, it is possible to attend to an object while maintaining gaze elsewhere.

The discussion of the relation between attentional resources and fixational behavior is highly relevant because attention is included in almost all models of *visual exploration*, *decision making* and *choice*. Thus, at this point of the current knowledge, two main issues must be addressed and disambiguated to make of eye tracking a confident tool to evaluate users' preference in the context of visual exploration [53]. The first of them relates to the question discussed in the paragraphs above. That is, how and when we can really equate fixational' parameters with users' attention? Some authors argue for a strong coupling between eye fixations and visual attention [26, 36, 48]. These authors show that decoupling normally only occurs prior to a saccade, when attention moves to a new location that is subsequently fixated [77, 82]. However, these studies have been conducted in very controlled conditions, and we know that not all fixated visual material is finally selected in a decision task.

The second question relates to the definition of the specific role that attention plays within visual exploration, decision making and choice, which is again a matter of debate between different models. In the case of visual exploration models, the discussion centers in what is the type of attention that primarily define the individual interest in specific stimuli and, in turn, influence eye guidance. From a psychological perspective, there are two types of attention operating by different ways: " bottom-up" attention, which is triggered by stimulus attributes (salience) and " top-down" attention, which is driven by controlled, conscious and innerly generated processes. There have been a long standing debate about the contribution of each type of attention during eye guidance [88].

The earliest work on viewing complex scenes found that there were certain locations in scenes that were consistently looked at by most observers [20]. Buswell called these locations "centers of interest" and asked what it was about these locations that made them "interesting". He considered that there were two possibilities: that it was something external in the stimulus that attracted the viewers' eyes; or that it was something more internal to the viewer that reflected higher level cognitive "interest". Buswell favoured the latter explanation, and he famously showed that presenting the same image but with different instructions fundamentally changed the places that a viewer fixated; an observation that was confirmed by [101].

Despite some authors have maintained the discussion about the role visual salience (bottom up) in attention capture [30, 43, 69, 81], several factors have been identified that override attention capture by visual saliency, such as semantic or contextual cues about a visual scene, feature based attention, object representations, task demands, and rewards for task performance [47].

The top-down attention has been clearly favoured and corroborated by many contemporary studies, and some authors have proposed that saliency plays little or no role in human gaze allocation outside the laboratory [54, 89]. Nevertheless, the interaction effect between top down and bottom up processes has not yet received much attention, and it seems plausible that a large part of our attentional control consists of mixed top down/bottom up processes [24, 98], depending on specific task requirements.

The previous findings have clear implications in the Web context, considering that many efforts have been traditionally put in defining the specific characteristics of the visual scene that capture the user attention, ignoring the users' internal goals. Objects' location is one of them. In recent years, more complex models have been developed to deal with top down/bottom up interactions. Torralba, Oliva, Castelhano, and Henderson's [90] have developed a model that incorporated the notion of contextual guidance to narrow down searching for objects in scenes to locations we have learnt are likely to contain the objects we are looking for. For example, we will look at walls to find paintings and surfaces to find mugs. Ehinger, Hidalgo-Sotelo, Torralba, and Oliva [29] extend this model in the context of searching for people to include an object-detector. They found that a model that incorporates some notion of image salience, where observers expect to find people, and a person-detector does a rather good job of accounting for where observers fixate in images of natural scenes.

In the context of decision making and choice, classical models of decision making have gave to attention a rather secondary role, assuming that it serves the decision maker by passively acquiring the information needed to make decision. This has been strongly criticized recently by some authors, who argue that attention processes play an active role in constructing decisions (for a review see Orquin and Loose, 2013 [66]). Orquin and Loose focus this discussion evaluating evidence derived precisely from eye tracking studies in the context of decision making and choice.

Some recent studies, attempting to predict, rather than explain decisions, have incorporated fixation measures in their models. Overall, they show that modeling down-stream effects of attention can improve predictive validity [34, 49].

One of the main fields of study where the influence of attention on fixational behavior has been addressed is in the *goal-oriented attention*. As predicted by several decision theories, goal-oriented attention plays a significant role in decision making. Five major factors have been observed: task instructions, utility effects, heuristics, attention phases, and learning effects [66]. The effect of task instructions stems from direct experimental manipulations (which is also true for the effect of heuristics in most cases), and results in increased attention to goal-relevant stimuli. Utility effects refer to the observation that participants overwhelmingly attend to important or high utility information. The only way in which utility effects differ from the effect of task instructions and heuristics, is that utility effects are attributable to individual differences, whereas task instructions and heuristics are caused by experimental manipulations.

Observations on attention phases indicate that specific task demands often change during the decision task. Thus, a decision maker can begin the decision task with one top down goal, such as scanning alternatives, and later proceed to another goal, such as comparing alternatives based on relevant attributes.

Furthermore, findings on learning effects show that practicing a decision task increases top down control (e.g., the utility effect). Learning also increases processing efficiency, thereby diminishing the total number of fixations [66].

As pointed by Orquin and Loose, any theory that aims to describe decision making, in which visual information play a central role, must reflect the following assumptions:

- Eye movements in decision making are partially driven by task demands, i.e. by describing the attention and decision processes as segregated process streams sees the former being dependent on the latter.
- Eye movements in decision making are partially driven by stimulus properties that bias information uptake in favor of visually salient stimuli.
- Eye movements do not have a causal effect on preference formation; however through properties inherent to the visual system, such as stimulus-driven attention, eye movements do lead to down-stream effects on decision making.
- Decision makers optimize eye movements to reduce the demand on working memory and, in some cases, to reduce the number of fixations and length of saccades needed to complete the decision task.
- The drivers of eye movements in decision making change dynamically within tasks, such as in attention phases, and across time, such as through learning effects.

The previous evidence show that careful assumptions must be taken when deciding the objective measures to be extracted from eye-tracking information to evaluate behavior, particularly decision making and choice. This is especially important in dynamic contexts, like the interaction of users with the Web information.

The integration of complementary information to the ocular behavior, derived from different neuro-technologies seems to be a promising field of research in the attempt to create a more unified scenario of decision making and choice in the context of Web usage.

8.3.2 EEG

Our brain produces and works primarily by means of electrical activity. Is this electrical activity that recruits and coordinates specific brain regions to generate different levels of cognitive phenomena, from perception to decision making [21, 78, 79].

Its was shown early in the 20th Century that the electric fields generated by populations of neurons in the brain can be recorded non-invasively from electrodes placed on the scalp [13]. This technique, named Electroencephalography (EEG), was massively used during the last century, but it was not until recently that the physical principles and the functional role of the activity recorded began to be disentangled [22, 63].

Early applications of EEG were primarily restricted to clinical assessments. In this context, analysis of EEG signals was reduced to the coarse observation of gross patterns with the naked eye. It was not until the advent of digitalization techniques and the development of analysis tools allowing the manipulation of recorded signals that EEG was extensively introduced in the arena of basic research.

One of the earlier techniques introduced for the analysis of the EEG signal was the measurement of the average time series across many trials of exposition to sensory stimuli, in an attempt to increase the signal to noise ratio. As this method allows the quantification of the electrical activity triggered by specific events of sensorial stimulation, the average electrical activity obtained was originally called *evoked potentials* (EPs) -as opposed to the spontaneous EEG rhythms- and later *event related potentials* (ERPs) [55].

Obtaining ERP curves involve several steps of processing and analysis, which today are relatively well standardized [72]. Roughly, recorded digital EEG signals must be first "cleaned" from artifacts, applying different types of temporal and spatial filters. Some of these filters include the subtraction of an estimate of the artifactual activity, and one of the more widely utilized methods today includes the Independent Component Analysis (ICA). After that, averaging procedures are necessary to extract the ERPs from the overall EEG. Digital filters are then applied to isolate specific ERP components. The size and timing of the ERP components are then computed and subjected to statistical analyses.

ERPs consist of typical deflections in the voltage signal having conserved polarity, latency and topography. Typically, ERPs show the appearance of voltage changes after stimulus presentation taking the form of curves that are called "components", which are specific of the sensory modality evoking the perturbation. While earlier the latency of the specific component studied, greater is its relation with the processing in early sensory areas. Thus, after 250–300 ms, almost all evoked components can be considered a product of multi sensory integration processes.

Studies of the evoked components have remained until now, and much information is available today about the conditions that trigger and modulate the parameters (amplitude and latency) of the specific components. In the visual system, ERP components (usually called visual evoked potentials, *VEP*) are commonly labeled P1, N1, P2, N2, and P3. P and N are traditionally used to indicate positive-going and negative-going peaks, respectively, and the number simply indicates a peak's position within the waveform. The sequence of ERP components reflects the flow of information through the brain.

An operational distinction is made about the contribution of specific factors to the appearance of ERP components. The early sensory responses are called exogenous components to indicate their dependence on external rather than internal factors. For example, the initial peak (P1) is an obligatory sensory response that is elicited by visual stimuli no matter what task the subject is doing and its internal state during this (no particular task other than stimuli presentation is necessary to elicit a P1 wave).The P3 wave, in contrast, depends entirely on the task performed by the subject and is not directly influenced by the physical properties of the eliciting stimulus. The P3 wave is therefore termed an endogenous component to indicate its dependence on internal rather than external factors.

Despite the early sensory responses (like P1 and N2) are called exogenous components, some endogenous factors influence as well their parameters (particularly its amplitude), like the attentional resources destined to the specific task. It has been shown that P1 is sensitive to the direction of spatial attention (see review by Hillyard et al. 1998 [35]). That is, when subjects are required to attend to a spatial location (without looking at) within the visual field, stimuli appearing in or near that location elicited a P1 with greater amplitude compared with those appearing in another non attended location. P1 amplitude is also influenced by the subject's state of arousal [96]. Similarly, the N2pc that is observed at posterior scalp sites (over visual areas) contralateral to the position of the target item (N2 *posterior-contralateral*), is considered an attention-related component. This is typically elicited by visual search arrays containing targets. Luck and Hillyard [56, 57] had shown that this component reflects the focusing of attention onto a potential target item, which include information about color, orientation and motion.

The previous findings are relevant because imply that early and late components are susceptible to be modulated by the internal state, including goals, of subjects doing a task. This characteristic makes ERPs well suited as a complementary measure of the oculo-motor behavior during exploratory conditions. This is because, while fixational parameters inform about items that have been observed (and probably attended) during visual exploration, they are not highly confident by themselves to evaluate choice and decision making, one the main goals in the Web context. ERP components' amplitude, on the other hand, inform specifically about perceptual processes and the cognitive resources directed to a specific target.

Nevertheless, classical paradigms utilized to elicit ERPs including that showing attentional modulations are applied in very controlled conditions, normally eliminating the possibility for visual exploration. That is, stimulus are presented in different locations of the visual field while subjects are required to fix their gaze in a specific point (generally the center of the display). In these conditions, results about perceptual modulations produced by top-down cognitive phenomena are not directly applicable to the study of the Web use.

In recent years, more fine-grained tools have been developed for the analysis of ERPs in the context of visual exploration. These techniques make use of the information given by eye-tracking signals recorded in parallel to EEG. The result of these analyses has been called *Eye-fixation related potentials* (EFRP) or *fixation-event related potentials* (fERP). EFRPs are computed using traditional averaging procedures of the EEG signal across trials, but in contrast to conventional event-related potential (ERP) technique the averaged waveforms are time-locked to the onset and offset of eye-fixation, not to the onset of stimulus events. EFRPs have shown to be an useful technique, in addition to eye-movement recordings, to investigate early visual processes and for establishing a timeline of these processes during cognitive activities. Moreover, the technique permits to analyze the EEGs in a natural condition allowing the investigation of complex visual stimuli [4].

It has been shown that EFRPs exhibit equivalent components to traditional ERPs, that is P1, N1, P2, N2, and P3 [5, 33, 46]. This fact demonstrate that across exploration, each time a subject makes a fixation in the context of free viewing, similar perceptual processes take place in the brain as the originals occurred immediately after stimulus appearance. The fact that they do not appear in traditional ERPs as a train of potentials during the whole period of exploration is because fixations have a temporal jitter across trials, thus producing a mutual cancelation of potentials as a consequence of averaging across those trials.

In addition to repeat the perceptual activity after each fixation, the brain can also modulate this activity (and then EFRP amplitude) depending on the cognitive resources destined to each perceptual act. This fact allows the evaluation of the effect of goal directed top down phenomena like attention, target detection and choice, but now in the context of free visual exploration. The amplitude of EFRP can change across the sequence of fixations during object identification tasks [76], showing that they provide a useful tool to study temporal dynamics of visual perception. Also, the amplitude of the early positive component is modulated (decreased) by error rate, decline of task performance, and is inversely correlated with the score of fatigue during a task [86]. This fact shows that EFRP would reflect decline of mental concentration across a specific task.

In the context of visual search tasks, it has been shown that EFRP can extend the usage of P3 to drive an image search, or labeling task where images can be ranked by examining the presence of such ERP signals, to the context of free viewing [33]. Also, Kamienkowski observed a relatively early EFRP component ($\sim$150 ms) that distinguished between targets and distractors only in a freeviewing condition [46], in contrast to more controlled conditions. Because classical P3 component of ERP can be used to infer whether an observer is looking at a target or not, Brouwer [16] recently evaluated the possibility to differentiate between single target and nontarget fixations in a target search task involving eye movements. They showed an EFRP component consistent with the P3 that reliably distinguished between target and nontarget fixations.

During free viewing of dynamical visual material, encoding of change detection results very relevant. However, the objective identification of success or failure of encoding have been a major challenge. Nikolaev [62] evaluated the possibility to measure that by means of EFRP. They found a difference in EFRP between correct detection and failure. Overall, correspondence between EFRP amplitude and the size of the saccade predicted successful detection of change; lack of correspondence was followed by change blindness. Interestingly, behavioral parameters measured as saccade sizes and fixation durations around the target region were unrelated to subsequent change detection, showing the importance of complementing eye-tracking information with EEG parameters.

In the specific field of Web usage, Frey and cols. addressed the possibility to isolate the process of decision making embedded in the continuous reading of text [31]. They conducted an experiment in which participants had to decide as fast as possible whether the text was related or not to the semantic goal given at a prior stage.

The found that late components (P3b and N400) of the obtained EFRP reflected the decision to stop information searching.

Previous findings show that EEG activity is well suited as a fundamental tool in the exploration of human cognitive processes developed during visual exploration, which can be clearly applied to the analysis of subjects' Web usage. The possibility to evaluate complex cognitive phenomena, like the attention and choice manifested by users during Web interaction makes that the combination of eye-tracking and EEG becomes a promising and widely used tool for objective assessment, particularly in the context of increasingly complex and dynamic Web material. Future research will need to focus in the cognitive aspects generated and modulated during the human-computer interaction, and how Web material can dynamically adapt to the individual behavior displayed during exploration.

8.4 Improving Web Usage Analysis with Neurodata

The starting point of the proposed analysis framework resides in the fact that human behavior on the Web is the result of a brain-based neural information process [102]. This process is captured, from a conventional data mining point of view, through the set of web logs that are registered by the server. This source represents the main element that has been used by disciplines such as Web Usage Mining. In order to go further, the main limitations of the current approach are exposed. Subsequently, a set of requirements is proposed for structuring the addition of neurodata. Finally, how neurodata techniques could be used in order to improve the analysis of the users is studied, showing current solutions available in literature.

8.4.1 Current Limitations of Web Usage Analysis Systems

Two main limitations can be perceived while developing analytical systems based on the sole use of web logs. They can be classified as follows:

- **Parameter-Dependent Modeling:** Most of the standard machine learning techniques that involve prediction or classification, and that have been applied in the Web domain, require the generation of the so called *training set*, which allows to set a group of parameters and coefficients that provide the rules that will be applied to the data. This set of rules is tightly related to the training set, which undermines the generalization capabilities of the models. Thus, the models need to be constantly tweaked and adjusted when data with different characteristics is presented [2].

  For instance, if it is needed to analyze the response of the users to a specific content of a Web site, a common task could be to build an a classifier with existing historical usage data. But, how does this model perform when the data that needs to be analyzed suddenly suffer changes in its characteristics is a relevant issue. Although there are several techniques that allow to improve the support and avoid over-fitting, such as Regularization [60], the lack of an automated or formal way to achieve these kind of tasks make them more like an art than a pure technical procedure.

- **Black Box Nature:** The set of rules that standard machine learning algorithms generate follows a frequentist paradigm in terms of a successive comparison between observed and estimated values [10]. For instance, in a common linear regression model, a cost function is usually defined which is associated with the distance between the outputs of the model and the observed data. Thus, the entire training process consists of finding a minimum value, hopefully globally, for this function. At the same time, machine learning does not take into account the underlying reasons that lead to the observed phenomena, it only provides quantitative artifacts that are capable of estimating, for an unknown point, the corresponding value that fits a given configuration better.
  There are several ways to formulate interpretations and infer causality based on the results obtained from the training process, but that is not the main goal. The usefulness of these techniques cannot be denied, there are several successful cases in which a black box approach has contributed to solving complex problems, such as handwritten digit recognition, but it is still unclear how these models help to understand the underlying factors that drive the behavior of the studied phenomena [52].

8.4.2 Requirements

The main goal of incorporating neurodata is to understand the underlying mechanisms that lead to a specific user action, in terms of the decision-making process he needs to conduct in order to fulfill a Web-related task.

The main hypothesis behind this rationale is that the value that neurodata provides can contribute to the generation of more robust models which are not conditioned by the changes of peripheral conditions and that combine a black box nature with a solid rationale that is based on empirical evidence.

Thus, when designing analysis frameworks that incorporate neurodata, the following requirements need to be taken into consideration:

- **Considering new constraints:** It needs to be considered that adding a new source of data, such as eye-gaze trails, may add several new parameters to the standard models. In that scenario, researchers should take into account that tuning those parameters could be difficult and sometimes finding the appropriate values becomes a time-consuming task. In that sense, the real benefits that neurodata could provide must be addressed and their cost effectiveness analyzed.
- **Level of generalization:** The process of collecting the data from neural sources implies the use of a set of instruments and an idealized environment, in which

subjects perform given tasks, such as navigational or information foraging. This represents a challenge that is related to the real usefulness of the data, regarding whether this data could reflect a standard user behavior and if this data can interact in a synergistic way with standard sources of web usage such as web logs.
For example, consider a scenario in which eye-tracking data was used to infer certain user preference vectors. Assuming that this data was collected based on a controlled experiment, is it feasible to associate these preferences to a set of sessions that were collected via anonymous web log mining? [3] There are several threats to its validity regarding not considering the context and the different dimension from which neurodata is collected.
This is an issue that is caused by the current nature of neurodata, in the sense that it is impossible to conduct an unbiased recollection of data, since the devices needed are highly invasive. The ideal scenario could be to have a system that collects neurodata from the user without realizing that he is being tracked, but current technology does not provide such an advance. Thus, it is extremely important to acknowledge the limitations and set up a desired level of generalization in order to measure the quality of the results.

8.4.3 Current Approaches

Literature provides several examples on how neurodata has been applied to enrich web user analysis. The following is a summary of the most important cases, based on the level of generalization and the novelty provided.

8.4.3.1 Neurodata for salient web element identification

One of the most remarkable lines of research has been developed by Buscher et al. The main motivation comes from the need for understanding how people allocate visual attention on web pages, taking into account the relevance of this for both web developers and advertisers.

A study from 2009 performed an eye tracking-based analysis in which 20 users were shown 361 pages while performing information foraging and inspection tasks [17]. The main assumption was that gaze data could represent a proxy of attention. From that, an analysis framework was developed by first generating a tool that allows DOM elements to be characterized and a mapping performed between gaze data and the DOM elements. The second part involves the use of machine learning techniques to predict salient elements on a web page.

In this study, the concept of *fixation impact* is introduced. It allows the identification of which elements are under the gaze of the user at a certain time. It follows empirical studies that show that human vision is characterized by a narrow window of high acuity along with the standard gaze area. Thus, when visualizing an element, it also means that other elements in the surroundings are being considered. Therefore,

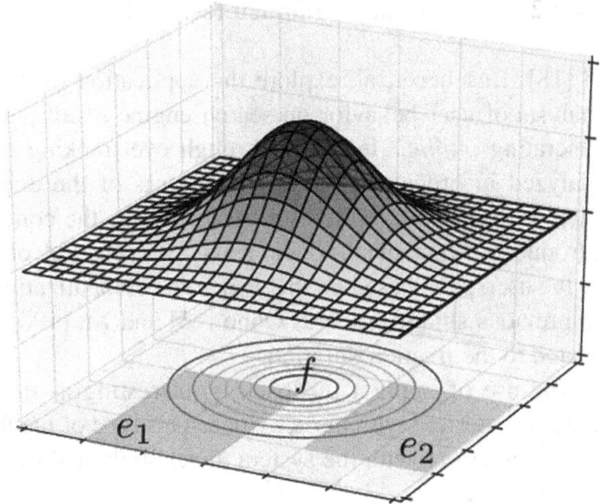

Fig. 8.1 Fixation impact example

given a fixation point, a DOM area is selected in order to identify every element under it. A distance score is given to each element based on its coverage, assuming a Gaussian distribution. The fixation impact is computed using this distance and also incorporating a time dimension, which means the fixation duration. An example can be seen in Fig. 8.1.

The information obtained in the previous step is used to predict salient elements. After performing a selection of the ten features that provide the highest information gain, Linear Regression was used in order to identify the measures that most influence the fixation impact scores. The results showed that positional features obtained the highest weights.

Another line of research has been developed by Velasquez et al., where the main goal is to identify the most relevant elements on a web site by using the concept of Website Keyobjects [94]. A web site object is considered as any group of words having some kind of structure, and in the same way, multimedia files which are shown on the web site pages, including all kinds of pictures, images, sound and animations. Objects based on word structure need to be inside delimitations such as paragraphs, tables or other kinds of tag separation.

Then, from the definition of Website object, a Web site Keyobject is derived as follows: *One or a group of website objects that attract the user attention and characterize the content of a page or website.* This definition states which web objects get more attention and are more interesting to the user and therefore, identify which object types would help to improve the presentation, usability and content of the web site. The identification of the Keyobjects involved primarily the analysis of web logs and a measure of time spent. In order to validate the findings, surveys were conducted, which do not provide a strong level of confidence for the results. The authors addressed this issue, and in [92] they incorporated eye-tracking methodologies to replace the use of surveys. With this, they were able to validate the approach by having an objective measure of the user attention.

8.4.3.2 Neurodata for implicit feedback

In [18], Buscher et al. explore the application of eye-tracking techniques for the analysis of user behavior on search engine result pages. In this work, the idea of generating *implicit* feedback through eye tracking is explored. Eye gaze data is analyzed in order to capture which parts of the document were read and which ones were relevant to the user. Additionally, the concept of *attentive documents* is introduced, which means documents that keep track of how they are being consumed by the users, and based on that generate personalization tasks. This concept is based on previous studies, such as Ohno [65] and Xu [100] where the idea of *intensity* is related to the fixation duration.

The use of implicit feedback is interesting as it does not burden the user and does not interfere with his activities. This type of feedback is captured by analyzing user interactions with the system under study and then analyzed to perform certain assistive action.

8.4.3.3 Neurodata for Ad Influence Identification in Search Result Pages

A study from 2010 [19] focuses on user behavior on search engines. The main motivation was to study the interaction between the users and the search results pages from a search engine, examining which variables influence the user gaze to a higher degree. In order to generate a practical analysis approach, the authors focused on the *sponsored links*, usually called *ads*, that appear along with the search results.

The key findings of the study are related to the influence of the tasks in which the user is involved while browsing, the quality of the ads and the sequence in which those ads appear along with the search results. In that sense, they found quantitative evidence of bias of user attention towards result entries which are located on the top of the lists. The influence of the quality of the ads represents the most interesting finding. The ad quality was measured in terms of the semantic distance to the search query. Based on the experimental results, users give less attention to organic results when the quality of the ads was good.

8.4.3.4 EEG in Web-Based Systems

EEG systems have not been used directly to support web user behavior. The approaches available in the literature deal with the development of tools to support navigation for disabled people, such as the work by Bensch et al. [11], where they developed an EEG-controlled web browser, in which the graphical interface was modified to process different brain responses corresponding to different frame colors associated with actions, such as link clicking.

Another study was performed by Anderson et al. [1], in which they analyze the effectiveness of data visualizations using EEG. This is an interesting problem since the way in which the information is presented to the users impacts the way they process it. This chapter proposes several metrics that involve EEG to quantify the cognitive load required. Several comparisons between different visualization techniques are performed, where the goal is to capture the burden they produce on the user's cognitive resources.

The above idea could be the starting point for the analysis of web-based advertisements, as usually, ads are presented to the user along with the organic content of the web site. Thus, there is an inherent competition between different elements in order to capture the viewer's attention. In this case, the cognitive load could be used to infer whether the user is noticing a given ad and additionally, what his level of comprehension of the information that is offered is, given that a web page presents several elements at a time.

8.4.4 Remarks

As seen above, neurodata has been applied to the Web analysis domain [80], but the scope has so far been limited. Most of the approaches have focused on identifying and classifying elements from the web sites, such as salient objects [51], but there is a lack of use in relation to improving the user modeling, which means incorporating these new sources of data into an understanding of the underlying mechanisms that lead to a specific behavior. In that sense, some possible extensions in which the use of neurodata could be explored are:

- **Sentiment Analysis:** The main flaw of the state of the art in Sentiment Analysis is related to the fact that most of the techniques depend on the use of a corpus, which is considered a gold standard, and from which the polarity of the sentences is computed [68]. One idea that could be explored is to use EEG techniques to identify emotions when users are writing a document. From that action, several inferences could be obtained, which could lead to improving the generalization of the predictions.
- **Decision-Making Modeling:** Eye tracking and pupil dilation could be used to test the effectiveness of ads in Web environments, since the correlation of neural activity and the likelihood of clicking can be studied. Classifiers could then be trained using the obtained data in order to test the user response a priori given the configuration of an ad.
- **Mobile Web:** Devices such as smart phones and tablets provide feasible eye-tracking capabilities given the current high quality of the embodied cameras [15]. Although their accuracy cannot be compared to a real eye-tracking device, there are two advantages that could be considered. First, tracking on a mobile-based system is less intrusive, which could generate more realistic data. Second, other sources of data could be combined, such as geographical data and context, which could enrich the explanatory power of the analysis as it could be possible to analyze the user response to different types of stimulus based on an aggregated data collection. But there are issues to tackle, as privacy concerns could arise.

8.5 Discussion

In this section, a general description of some aspects that should be considered when designing neurodata-centric systems is provided.

8.5.1 *Technical Feasibility*

The use of neurodata to improve web mining techniques involves certain entry barriers. While performing a standard data analysis requires simple computing resources, which can be local or cloud-based systems, neurodata represents a challenge in two main aspects.

First, the set of instruments required to extract the data from the subjects are usually expensive and demand a considerable learning curve. As seen in previous sections, eye-tracking systems are composed of several parts which work together, requiring time and training to set up correctly.

The second aspect is that, given the high amount of time required to perform an experiment, the number of subjects that can be inspected is limited. This represents a relevant threat to the validity of the results, as the level of generalization that can be obtained with a small sample is reduced.

Additionally, one of the advantages of the standard web log-based analysis is that the captured data, although not completely accurate, is not biased in the sense that the users did not know their usage was going to be analyzed, thus they could not modify their behavior based on privacy assumptions. In the case of neurodata-based analysis, all the gathered data comes from users that perform given tasks (such as specific information foraging tasks) in controlled environments.

8.5.2 *Mouse Cursor as a Proxy for Visual Gaze*

Although eye-tracking is considered the most reliable way to study gaze behavior in Web environments, certain studies have been conducted in order to find other ways to infer user attention [23].

As most people use a mouse to interact with web systems, researchers have focused on studying whether the behavior of a mouse cursor could also provide a reliable measure of what the user is doing. If that is the case, several advantages could be exploited, as it should be cheaper and more scalable than current eye-tracking devices [38].

There have been several studies showing a positive correlation between gaze and cursor with varying degrees of success. The variance in the results is caused by the lack of sophistication, as the cursor behavior is assumed to be a homogeneous phenomenon. But a recent study by Huang et al. [37] has tackled this issue by first identifying cursor interactions such as reading, hesitating, highlighting, scrolling and clicking. From this fragmentation, a more robust model was developed by applying linear regression. Therefore, the main goal is to use cursor features to predict eye gaze. The overall results show promising opportunities, but further research is required to generate a feasible tool [61].

The general consensus among researchers is that although cursor tracking cannot replace eye tracking, there is room for improvement that could lead to use it as a reliable proxy for user attention. Thus, in terms of choosing between eye tracker and cursor tracker there is a trade-off that needs to be acknowledged, considering several aspects such as cost, quality required and available time [32].

8.5.3 Representation Learning-Based Alternatives

As previously noted, one of the main motivations for extending the current approaches for Web user behavior analysis was due to the limitations of the standard machine learning techniques involved. As stated by Bengio et al. [8], the performance of machine learning algorithms is heavily dependent on the choice of data representation.

While incorporating a neurodata perspective to the analysis could contribute to improving the *explanatory power* of the resulting tools, the level of adaptability and flexibility that could be achieved is still unclear. In that sense, the sole use of an additional data source could lead to an ad-hoc analysis, which could provide more accuracy, but it will still be hard to extend for further research [9].

Currently, *Representation learning*, a relatively new field in machine learning, has gained a high amount of attention along with several successful cases in both academia and industry. This approach consists of discovering multiple levels of features by using deep hierarchical artifacts. The nonlinear transformations that these kinds of structures provide, could help to disentangle the underlying factors that produce the variation in the data, and at the same time, give a level of flexibility to make useful for a wide range of problems [7].

Given the above, researchers should take into account the advantages that this new paradigm could provide. Instead of adding new sources of data such as neurodata, which can be expensive to collect, and process them with standard machine learning techniques, a new way could be to use current data, which is cheap in terms of capturing and storage, and use more advanced methods to process it.

8.5.4 Privacy Issues

The analysis of web data has always been restricted by the legitimate desire of protection of privacy. Large amounts of joint interdisciplinary work have been conducted in order to design a common language from which regulations could be implemented.

The use of neurodata represents a new challenge in terms of the level of detail that this technology could provide and how this new source of data could threaten anonymity [93].

Current deployment of eye-tracking techniques requires an idealized environment, in which the user is aware that he is being tracked, thus the capturing of data has an explicit agreement. But the question still remains in the sense that with the advance in technology, how a future non-invasive eye-tracking technique could be handled and how the user could be protected. Mobile interfaces, such as smart phones and tablets are of special interest given the monitoring capabilities and increasing processing capacity [59].

8.5.5 *Relationship with Wisdom Web of Things*

We consider neuro based systems a central part in the Wisdom Web of Things framework, as they allow to obtain unique knowledge from the users which can be used to improve any service or even personalize the configuration or network of services. Neuro data provides a way to obtain in a objective way the real preferences from the users and the underlying factors that explain their behavior and decision processes. Additionally, our vision is that in the future, systems will be able to capture brain activity in real time, such as current research on Brain Computer Interaction allows to do, therefore, understanding this type of data could allow to improve the level of adaptation. This represents an enormous opportunity in fields such as education, where any Web based service that provides online classes could be able to monitor the cognitive or emotional response from the users, and use the captured data to improve the teaching strategies.

8.6 Summary

This study presents an overview of the use of neurodata for Web user analysis. Neurodata represents new opportunities in order to improve the current state of the art of Web usage mining, but at the same time it imposes certain challenges, both technical and methodological.

Literature review shows that most of the work has been done using eye-tracking devices trying to estimate user attention and interests based on eye gaze analysis. Most approaches take advantage of the new sources of data to enrich standard analysis, but their contribution is still limited, given the costs and difficulties of the implementation. EEG also represents an alternative, but has not been tested extensively in Web environments, basically due to technical challenges. It could a good opportunity to enrich models that incorporate decision making and emotional components.

Acknowledgments The authors would like to acknowledge the continuous support of the Chilean Millennium Institute of Complex Engineering Systems (ICM: P-05-004-F, CONICYT: FBO16), the Fondecyt Project 1160117, and the FONDEF-CONICYT CA12I10061 - AKORI project.

References

1. E.W. Anderson, K.C. Potter, L.E. Matzen, J.F. Shepherd, G. Preston, C.T. Silva. A user study of visualization effectiveness using eeg and cognitive load, in *Computer Graphics Forum*, vol. 30 (Wiley Online Library, 2011), pp. 791–800
2. J.R. Anderson, R.S. Michalski, R.S. Michalski, T.M. Mitchell, et al. *Machine Learning: An Artificial Intelligence Approach*, vol. 2 (Morgan Kaufmann, 1986)
3. T. Arce, P.E. Román, J. Velásquez, V. Parada, Identifying web sessions with simulated annealing. Expert Syst. Appl. **41**(4, Part 2), 1593–1600 (2014)
4. T. Baccino, *Eye Movements and Concurrent Event-Related Potentials: Eye Fixation-Related Potential Investigations in Reading* (Oxford University Press, New York, NY, USA, 2011)
5. T. Baccino, V. Drai-Zerbib, A new cognitive engineering technique: eye-fixation-related potentials, in *The 5th PSU-UNS International Conference on Engineering and Technology (ICET-2011)* (2011)
6. R. Baeza-Yates, C. Castillo, E.N. Efthimiadis, Characterization of national web domains. ACM Trans. Internet Technol. (TOIT) **7**(2), 9 (2007)
7. Y. Bengio, Learning deep architectures for ai. Found. Trends Mach. Learn. **2**(1), 1–127 (2009)
8. Y. Bengio, A. Courville, P. Vincent, Representation learning: a review and new perspectives. IEEE Trans. Pattern Anal. Mach. Intell. **35**(8), 1798–1828 (2013)
9. Y. Bengio, Y. LeCun, et al. Scaling learning algorithms towards ai. Large-scale Kernel Mach. **34**(5) (2007)
10. J.M. Benítez, J.L. Castro, I. Requena, Are artificial neural networks black boxes? IEEE Trans. Neural Netw. **8**(5), 1156–1164 (1997)
11. M. Bensch, A.A. Karim, J. Mellinger, T. Hinterberger, M. Tangermann, M. Bogdan, W. Rosenstiel, N. Birbaumer, Nessi: an eeg-controlled web browser for severely paralyzed patients. Comput. Intell. Neurosci. (2007)
12. B. Berendt, B. Mobasher, M. Nakagawa, M. Spiliopoulou. The impact of site structure and user environment on session reconstruction in web usage analysis, in *WEBKDD 2002—Mining Web Data for Discovering Usage Patterns and Profiles* (Springer, 2003), pp. 159–179
13. H. Berger, Uber das Elektrenkephalogramm des Menschen. Archiv fur Psychiatrie und Nervenkrankheiten **17**(6–7), 777–789 (2009). Aug
14. T. Berners-Lee, J. Hendler, O. Lassila et al., The semantic web. Sci. Am. **284**(5), 28–37 (2001)
15. G. Boening, K. Bartl, T. Dera, S. Bardins, E. Schneider, T. Brandt. Mobile eye tracking as a basis for real-time control of a gaze driven head-mounted video camera, in *Proceedings of the 2006 Symposium on Eye Tracking Research & Applications* (ACM, 2006), p. 56
16. A.M. Brouwer, B. Reuderink, J. Vincent, M.A. van Gerven, J.B. van Erp, Distinguishing between target and nontarget fixations in a visual search task using fixation-related potentials. J Vis **13**(3), 17 (2013)
17. G. Buscher, E. Cutrell, M.R. Morris, What do you see when you're surfing?: Using eye tracking to predict salient regions of web pages, in *Proceedings of the SIGCHI Conference on Human Factors in Computing Systems*, CHI'09, New York, NY, USA (ACM, 2009), pp. 21–30
18. G. Buscher, A. Dengel, R. Biedert, L.V. Elst, Attentive documents: eye tracking as implicit feedback for information retrieval and beyond. ACM Trans. Interact. Intell. Syst. **1**(2), 9:1–9:30 (2012)
19. G. Buscher, S.T. Dumais, E. Cutrell, The good, the bad, and the random: an eye-tracking study of ad quality in web search, in *Proceedings of the 33rd International ACM SIGIR Conference*

on Research and Development in Information Retrieval, SIGIR'10, New York, NY, USA (ACM, 2010), pp. 42–49
20. G.T. Buswell, *How People Look at Pictures: A Study of the Psychology of Perception in Art* (University of Chicago Press, Chicago, USA, 1935)
21. G. Buzsaki, *Rhythms of the Brain* (Oxford University Press, New York, NY, USA, 2006)
22. G. Buzsaki, A. Draguhn, Neuronal oscillations in cortical networks. Science **304**(5679), 1926–1929 (2004)
23. M.C. Chen, J.R. Anderson, M.H. Sohn. What can a mouse cursor tell us more?: correlation of eye/mouse movements on web browsing, in *CHI'01 extended abstracts on Human factors in computing systems* (ACM, 2001), pp. 281–282
24. M. Corbetta, G.L. Shulman, Control of goal-directed and stimulus-driven attention in the brain. Nat. Rev. Neurosci. **3**(3), 201–215 (2002)
25. R.F. Dell, P.E. Román, J.D. Velásquez. Web user session reconstruction using integer programming, in *IEEE/WIC/ACM International Conference on Web Intelligence and Intelligent Agent Technology, 2008. WI-IAT'08*, vol. 1 (IEEE, 2008), pp. 385–388
26. H. Deubel, W.X. Schneider, Saccade target selection and object recognition: evidence for a common attentional mechanism. Vis. Res. **36**(12), 1827–1837 (1996)
27. D.T. Duchowski, *Eye Tracking Methodology* (Springer, London, UK, 2006)
28. D. Easley, J. Kleinberg, *Networks, Crowds, and Markets*, vol. 8 (Cambridge Univ Press, 2010)
29. K.A. Ehinger, B. Hidalgo-Sotelo, A. Torralba, A. Oliva, Modeling search for people in 900 scenes: a combined source model of eye guidance. Vis. Cogn. **17**(6–7), 945–978 (2009)
30. T. Foulsham, G. Underwood, What can saliency models predict about eye movements? Spatial and sequential aspects of fixations during encoding and recognition. J. Vis. **8**(2), 1–17 (2008)
31. A. Frey, G. Ionescu, B. Lemaire, F. Lopez-Orozco, T. Baccino, A. Guerin-Dugue, Decision-making in information seeking on texts: an eye-fixation-related potentials investigation. Front Syst. Neurosci. **7**, 39 (2013)
32. Q. Guo, E. Agichtein, Towards predicting web searcher gaze position from mouse movements, in *CHI'10 Extended Abstracts on Human Factors in Computing Systems* (ACM, 2010)
33. G. Healy, A.F. Smeaton, Eye fixation related potentials in a target search task. Conf. Proc. IEEE Eng. Med. Biol. Soc. 4203–4206 (2011)
34. D.A. Hensher, *Atribute Processing, Heuristics, and Preference Construction in Choice Analysis* (Bingley, Emerald, UK, 2010)
35. S.A. Hillyard, E.K. Vogel, S.J. Luck, Sensory gain control (amplification) as a mechanism of selective attention: electrophysiological and neuroimaging evidence. Philos. Trans. R. Soc. Lond., B, Biol. Sci. **353**(1373), 1257–1270 (1998)
36. J.E. Hoffman, B. Subramaniam, The role of visual attention in saccadic eye movements. Percept. Psychophys. **57**(6), 787–795 (1995)
37. J. Huang, R. White, G. Buscher, User see, user point: gaze and cursor alignment in web search, in *Proceedings of the SIGCHI Conference on Human Factors in Computing Systems*, CHI'12, New York, NY, USA (ACM, 2012), pp. 1341–1350
38. J. Huang, R.W. White, G.Buscher, K. Wang, Improving searcher models using mouse cursor activity, in *Proceedings of the 35th International ACM SIGIR Conference on Research and Development in Information Retrieval*, SIGIR'12, New York, NY, USA (ACM, 2012), pp. 195–204
39. G. Iachello, J. Hong, End-user privacy in human-computer interaction. Found. Trends Human-Comput. Interact. **1**(1), 1–137 (2007)
40. N. Indurkhya, F.J. Damerau, *Handbook of Natural Language Processing*, vol. 2 (CRC Press, 2010)
41. P.G. Ipeirotis, L. Gravano, When one sample is not enough: improving text database selection using shrinkage, in *Proceedings of the 2004 ACM SIGMOD International Conference on Management of Data* (ACM, 2004), pp. 767–778
42. D.E. Irwin, *Visual Memory Within and Across Fixations* (Springer, New York, NY, USA, 1992)

43. L. Itti, C. Koch, A saliency-based search mechanism for overt and covert shifts of visual attention. Vis. Res. **40**(10–12), 1489–1506 (2000)
44. W. James, *The Principles of Psychology*, vol. I (Harvard University Press, Cambridge, MA, USA, 1981)
45. S. Janzen, W. Maass, Ontology-based natural language processing for in-store shopping situations, in *IEEE International Conference on Semantic Computing, 2009, ICSC'09* (IEEE, 2009), pp. 361–366
46. J.E. Kamienkowski, M.J. Ison, R.Q. Quiroga, M. Sigman, Fixation-related potentials in visual search: a combined EEG and eye tracking study. J. Vis. **12**(7), 4 (2012)
47. E. Kowler, Eye movements: the past 25 years. Vis. Res. **51**(13), 1457–1483 (2011)
48. E. Kowler, E. Anderson, B. Dosher, E. Blaser, The role of attention in the programming of saccades. Vis. Res. **35**(13), 1897–1916 (1995)
49. I. Krajbich, C. Armel, A. Rangel, Visual fixations and the computation and comparison of value in simple choice. Nat. Neurosci. **13**(10), 1292–1298 (2010)
50. V.V. Kryssanov, K. Kakusho, E.L. Kuleshov, M. Minoh, Modeling hypermedia-based communication. Inf. Sci. **174**(1), 37–53 (2005)
51. M. Kudelka, V. Snasel, Z. Horak, A. Ella Hassanien, A. Abraham, J.D. Velásquez, A novel approach for comparing web sites by using microgenres. Eng. Appl. Artif. Intell. **35**, 187–198 (2014)
52. Y. Lee, Handwritten digit recognition using k nearest-neighbor, radial-basis function, and backpropagation neural networks. Neural Comput. **3**(3), 440–449 (1991)
53. P. Loyola, G. Martínez, K. Muñoz, J.D. Velásquez, P. Maldonado, A. Couve, Combining eye tracking and pupillary dilation analysis to identify website key objects. Neurocomputing **168**, 179–189 (2015)
54. P. Loyola, J.D. Velásquez, Characterizing web user visual gaze patterns: A graph theory inspired approach, in *Brain Informatics and Health* (Springer International Publishing, 2014), pp. 586–594
55. S.J. Luck, *An Introduction to the Event-Related Potential Technique* (MIT Press, Cambridge, MA, USA, 2005)
56. S.J. Luck, S.A. Hillyard, Electrophysiological correlates of feature analysis during visual search. Psychophysiology **31**(3), 291–308 (1994)
57. S.J. Luck, S.A. Hillyard, Spatial filtering during visual search: evidence from human electrophysiology. J. Exp. Psychol. Hum. Percept. Perform. **20**(5), 1000–1014 (1994)
58. H. B. McMahan, G. Holt, D. Sculley, M. Young, D. Ebner, J. Grady, L. Nie, T. Phillips, E. Davydov, D. Golovin, S. Chikkerur, D. Liu, M. Wattenberg, A.M. Hrafnkelsson, T. Boulos, J. Kubica, Ad click prediction: a view from the trenches, in *Proceedings of the 19th ACM SIGKDD International Conference on Knowledge Discovery and Data Mining*, KDD'13, New York, NY, USA (ACM, 2013), pp. 1222–1230
59. M. Moloney, F. Bannister, A privacy control theory for online environments, in *42nd Hawaii International Conference on System Sciences, 2009. HICSS'09* (IEEE, 2009), pp. 1–10
60. K.P. Murphy, *Machine Learning: A Probabilistic Perspective* (The MIT Press, 2012)
61. V. Navalpakkam, L. Jentzsch, R. Sayres, S. Ravi, A. Ahmed, A. Smola, Measurement and modeling of eye-mouse behavior in the presence of nonlinear page layouts, in *Proceedings of the 22nd International Conference on World Wide Web*, WWW'13, Republic and Canton of Geneva, Switzerland (International World Wide Web Conferences Steering Committee, 2013), pp. 953–964
62. A.R. Nikolaev, C. Nakatani, G. Plomp, P. Jurica, C. van Leeuwen, Eye fixation-related potentials in free viewing identify encoding failures in change detection. Neuroimage **56**, 1598–1607 (2011)
63. P. Nunez, R. Srinivasan, *Electric Fields of the Brain* (Oxford University Press, New York, NY, USA, 2006)
64. H. Obendorf, H. Weinreich, E. Herder, M. Mayer, Web page revisitation revisited: implications of a long-term click-stream study of browser usage, in *Proceedings of the SIGCHI Conference on Human Factors in Computing Systems* (ACM, 2007), pp. 597–606

65. T. Ohno, Eyeprint: support of document browsing with eye gaze trace, in *Proceedings of the 6th International Conference on Multimodal Interfaces* (ACM, 2004), pp. 16–23
66. J.L. Orquin, S. Mueller Loose, Attention and choice: a review on eye movements in decision making. Acta. Psychol. (Amst) **144**(1), 190–206 (2013)
67. S.K. Pal, V. Talwar, P. Mitra, Web mining in soft computing framework: relevance, state of the art and future directions. IEEE Trans. Neural Netw. **13**(5), 1163–1177 (2002)
68. B. Pang, L. Lee, Opinion mining and sentiment analysis. Foundations and trends in information retrieval **2**(1–2), 1–135 (2008)
69. D. Parkhurst, K. Law, E. Niebur, Modeling the role of salience in the allocation of overt visual attention. Vis. Res. **42**(1), 107–123 (2002)
70. R. Peña-Ortiz, J. Sahuquillo, A. Pont, J.A. Gil, Dweb model: representing web 2.0 dynamism. Comput. Commun. **32**(6), 1118–1128 (2009)
71. M. Perkowitz, O. Etzioni, Towards adaptive web sites: conceptual framework and case study. Artif. intell. **118**(1), 245–275 (2000)
72. T.W. Picton, S. Bentin, P. Berg, E. Donchin, S.A. Hillyard, R. Johnson, G.A. Miller, W. Ritter, D.S. Ruchkin, M.D. Rugg, M.J. Taylor, Guidelines for using human event-related potentials to study cognition: recording standards and publication criteria. Psychophysiology **37**(2), 127–152 (2000)
73. M.I. Posner, C.R. Snyder, B.J. Davidson, Attention and the detection of signals. J. Exp. Psychol. **109**(2), 160–174 (1980)
74. D. Quah. *Digital Goods and the New Economy* (LSE Economics Department, 2002)
75. A. Rajaraman, J.D. Ullman, *Mining of Massive Datasets* (Cambridge University Press, New York, NY, USA, 2011)
76. P. Rama, T. Baccino, Eye fixationrelated potentials (EFRPs) during object identification. Vis. Neurosci. **27**, 187–192 (2010)
77. K. Rayner, G.W. McConkie, S. Ehrlich, Eye movements and integrating information across fixations. J. Exp. Psychol. Hum. Percept. Perform. **4**(4), 529–544 (1978)
78. P.E. Román, J.D. Velásquez, Cognitive science forweb usage analysis, in *Advanced Techniques in Web Intelligence-2* (Springer Berlin Heidelberg, 2013), pp. 35–73
79. P.E. Román, J.D. Velásquez, A web browsing cognitive model, in *Knowledge Engineering, Machine Learning and Lattice Computing with Applications* (Springer, Berlin Heidelberg, 2013), pp. 31–40
80. P.E. Román, J.D. Velásquez, A neurology-inspired model of web usage. Neurocomputing **131**, 300–311 (2014)
81. U. Rutishauser, C. Koch, Probabilistic modeling of eye movement data during conjunction search via feature-based attention. J. Vis. **7**(6), 5 (2007)
82. M. Shepherd, J.M. Findlay, R.J. Hockey, The relationship between eye movements and spatial attention. Q. J. Exp. Psychol. A **38**(3), 475–491 (1986)
83. M. Spaniol, D. Denev, A. Mazeika, G. Weikum, P. Senellart, Data quality in web archiving, in *Proceedings of the 3rd Workshop on Information Credibility on the Web* (ACM, 2009), pp. 19–26
84. J. Srivastava, R. Cooley, M. Deshpande, P.-N. Tan, Web usage mining: Discovery and applications of usage patterns from web data. ACM SIGKDD Explorations Newsletter **1**(2), 12–23 (2000)
85. G. Takács, I. Pilászy, B. Németh, D. Tikk, Major components of the gravity recommendation system. ACM SIGKDD Explor. Newsl. **9**(2), 80–83 (2007)
86. Y. Takeda, M. Sugai, A. Yagi, Eye fixation related potentials in a proof reading task. Int. J. Psychophysiol. **40**, 181–186 (2001)
87. Y.-H. Tao, T.-P. Hong, W.-Y. Lin, W.-Y. Chiu, A practical extension of web usage mining with intentional browsing data toward usage. Expert Syst. Appl. **36**(2), 3937–3945 (2009)
88. B.W. Tatler, Current understanding of eye guidance. Vis. Cogn. **17**(6–7), 777–789 (2009)
89. B.W. Tatler, M.M. Hayhoe, M.F. Land, D.H. Ballard, Eye guidance in natural vision: reinterpreting salience. J. Vis. **11**(5), 5 (2011)

90. A. Torralba, A. Oliva, M.S. Castelhano, J.M. Henderson, Contextual guidance of eye movements and attention in real-world scenes: the role of global features in object search. Psychol. Rev. **113**(4), 766–786 (2006)
91. J.D. Velásquez, Web site keywords: a methodology for improving gradually the web site text content. Intell. Data Anal. **16**(2), 327–348 (2012)
92. J.D. Velásquez, Combining eye-tracking technologies with web usage mining for identifying website keyobjects. Eng. Appl. Artif. Intell. **26**(56), 1469–1478 (2013)
93. J.D. Velásquez, Web mining and privacy concerns: some important legal issues to be consider before applying any data and information extraction technique in web-based environments. Expert Syst. Appl. **40**(13), 5228–5239 (2013)
94. J.D. Velásquez, L.E. Dujovne, G. L'Huillier, Extracting significant website key objects: a semantic web mining approach. Eng. Appl. Artif. Intell. **24**(8), 1532–1541 (2011)
95. J.D. Velásquez, V. Palade, Adaptive web sitesa knowledge extraction from web data approach, in *Proceedings of the 2008 Conference on Adaptive Web Sites: A Knowledge Extraction from Web Data Approach* (Ios Press, 2008), pp. 1–272
96. E.K. Vogel, S.J. Luck, The visual N1 component as an index of a discrimination process. Psychophysiology **37**(2), 190–203 (2000)
97. R.W. White, S.M. Drucker, Investigating behavioral variability in web search, in *Proceedings of the 16th International Conference on World Wide Web* (ACM, 2007), pp. 21–30
98. M. Wischnewski, A. Belardinelli, W. Schneider, J. Steil, Where to look next? Combining static and dynamic proto-objects in a TVA-based model of visual attention. Cogn. Comput. **2**(4), 326–343 (2010)
99. S.S. Won, J. Jin, J.I. Hong, Contextual web history: using visual and contextual cues to improve web browser history, in *Proceedings of the SIGCHI Conference on Human Factors in Computing Systems* (ACM, 2009), pp. 1457–1466
100. S. Xu, H. Jiang, F. Lau. User-oriented document summarization through vision-based eye-tracking, in *Proceedings of the 14th International Conference on Intelligent User Interfaces* (ACM, 2009), pp. 7–16
101. A.L. Yarbus, *Eye Movements and Vision* (Plenum Press, New York, NY, USA, 1967)
102. N. Zhong, Impending brain informatics research from web intelligence perspective. Int. J. Inf. Technol. Decis. Mak. **5**(04), 713–727 (2006)
103. Y. Zhou, H. Leung, P. Winoto, Mnav: a markov model-based web site navigability measure. IEEE Trans. Softw. Eng. **33**(12), 869–890 (2007)

Chapter 9
W2T Framework Based U-Pillbox System Towards U-Healthcare for the Elderly

Jianhua Ma, Neil Y. Yen, Runhe Huang and Xin Zhao

Abstract Healthcare is a challenging issue for persons with physical disabilities (e.g., the elderly). One significant issue refers to non-adherence of medication regimens in geriatric healthcare, particularly among elderly patients who live alone. To address this problem, thousands of ubiquitous hardware (e.g., smart objects) and software (e.g., u-pillbox, etc.) have been developed. Although partial solutions were given, it is important to have a comprehensive understanding to medication adherence. This requires a framework expected to host healthcare devices, execute related applications, and provide an open platform for accessing and interacting with other healthcare systems (e.g., hospital and pharmacy). This chapter proposes a W2T data cycle based holistic elderly healthcare framework and demonstrates its functionality with a u-pillbox system for the elderly. The u-pillbox system consists of three main processes: data acquisition of the elderly situation and medicine taking state; data analysis and elderly model enhancement; and provision of empathetic services to the elderly, in which cyber-I, human model, data cycle for the spiral quality of model enhancement, knowledge fusion towards wisdom for providing smart services are our critical concepts and techniques. Although this system is designated for geriatric healthcare, it has a potential extension to general health monitoring and care at home.

J. Ma · R. Huang · X. Zhao
Faculty of Computer and Information Science, Hosei University, Tokyo 184-8584, Japan
e-mail: jianhua@hosei.ac.jp

R. Huang
e-mail: rhuang@hosei.ac.jp

N.Y. Yen (✉)
School of Computer Science and Engineering,
The University of Aizu, Fukushima, Japan
e-mail: neilyyen@u-aizu.ac.jp

N. Zhong et al. (eds.), *Wisdom Web of Things*, Web Information Systems Engineering and Internet Technologies Book Series,
DOI 10.1007/978-3-319-44198-6_9

9.1 Background

Healthcare is an increasingly-important issue nowadays, which widely considers a basic human right in economically advanced countries and as an essential concomitant of economic development in less economically developed countries. According to a report by the international Organization for Economic Co-operation and Development (OECD), almost 10 % of GDP in Japan and the United Kingdom was spent on healthcare in 2012. In the major western European economies this figure was slightly higher, and in the United States 17.6 % of GDP was spent on healthcare [1]. A significant proportion of healthcare expenditure, and one which is increasing at a rate greater than the GDPs of these countries, is that of providing healthcare to the elderly. The pressing problems caused by the provision of efficient and quality healthcare to the elderly and the ongoing continuous nature of their healthcare needs cannot be ignored as health care expenditure directed at the population 65 years and older has been rising year on year. According to an OECD Economic Department report of 2010 [2], the percentage of health care expenditure on the elderly to GDP reached 3.98 % in Japan, 3.73 % in Germany, and 6.48 % in USA. Moreover, the demographic problem of a graying population creates another big problem in the form of a shortage of nursing staff and caregivers. The Japanese Health Ministry has stated that the number of nurses, midwives and other medical staff needed to fulfill its needs reached about 1.4 million in 2011, but according to one current investigation, there will be a shortfall of nearly 56,000 people. This problem is particularly acute in geriatric healthcare.

One answer to spiraling costs and staff shortages, and also to the proliferation of paper-based patient health records, is e-healthcare systems [3, 4]. These apply advanced Information and Communications Technology (ICT) to the sharing of patient data among healthcare professionals and even envisage network-based health consultation and medication provision. Whilst these developments may provide overall improvements in healthcare system efficiency [5], they have a limited impact on the quality of care experienced by patients as this would require a more detailed and timely picture of patients' health situations. These deficiencies in combating the healthcare situation described above have led to the appearance of proposed u-healthcare systems for the elderly. A u-healthcare system, u-health meaning ubiquitous healthcare, is envisaged as overcoming the deficiencies of e-healthcare systems. Stemming from the vision of Mark Weiser [6], the concept of u-healthcare refers to the application of ubiquitous technology with ICT to gather continuous pertinent and timely information about a patient's situation to provide comprehensive non-intrusive healthcare. Among the ubiquitous technologies that could realize this vision are miniaturized smart devices, wireless sensor networks, and seamless interfaces. These would acquire data on a patient and their environment. Developments in ubiquitous intelligence computing, in particular AI, machine learning, large scale data mining and other related technologies would enable a u-healthcare system to process and analyze the data acquired, and in tandem with the expertise of health professionals, ensure healthcare of the highest quality. Moreover, a u-health system would empower patients to take a more active role in their personal health management and illness prevention.

A huge numbers of healthcare systems [7–9], especially those ubiquitous- and/or pervasive-empowered ones, have been proposed to provide efficient and effective supports and, the most important of all, to ensure the quality of healthcare services. As Web of Things (W2T) gives an original view on data processing, researchers come to agree that the ultimate goal is expected to be providing right service to right person with right context and at right timing. Although it is obvious that W2T refers a wide range of issues related to the Web, we look at its fundamental, which is the data itself, and concentrates on the way the data is being processed, namely from things to data, information, knowledge, wisdom, services, humans, and then back to things. Thus in this chapter, an framework, which is designed based on the concept of data cycle in W2T, is proposed. It is expected to be one of the promising framework that prompts the ubiquitous healthcare service provision by understanding the needs of subjects (i.e., elderly in this chapter).

9.2 Reviews of the Present Situation in U-Healthcare

9.2.1 WaaS (Wisdom as a Service)

Pervasive sensing can collect huge amount of data. How to analyze them, and discover knowledge so as to provide smart services is another challenge. In the u-pillbox system, we adopt a from-data-to-wisdom data analysis and knowledge fusion platform called Wisdom as a Service (WaaS) to mine knowledge which leads to the wisdom for providing services from huge amounts of data. In this platform, there are three layers: structured data, information, and knowledge, and each layer can provide services as: data as a service (DaaS), information as a service (InaaS), knowledge as a service (KaaS), and wisdom as a service (WaaS) on the whole. Each layer is to provide services based on the lower layer and is the basis for the upper layer to provide services shown in Fig. 9.1.

- **From big data to structured data**
  Pre-processing, cleansing and formatting are examples performed in this process for reducing the volume and complexity of the recorded huge data. Data are organized and structured via further filtering and clustering. The structured data can be packaged according to specific data request for provision of data service.
- **From structured data to information**
  Information is a collection of organized and interpreted data which is meaningful to questions like "who", "whose", "what", "which", "where", and "when", etc. in an application. A set of interpretable data being meaningful to and binding with a specific application according to its syntax and semantics can be as an information service to a request from a user or an application.

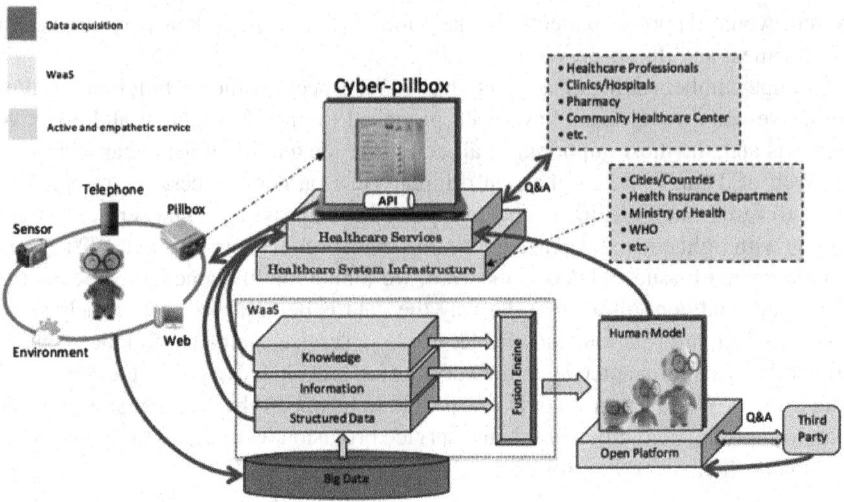

Fig. 9.1 The framework of the u-pillbox system

- **From information to knowledge**
  Knowledge is a collection of appropriate information such as facts, common sense truths, derived rules, etc. which are logical and rational to a specific task or domain problem solving. A set of facts, rules in a specific representation to an application domain can be structured as a knowledge service corresponding to a problem solving request.
- **From data, information, and knowledge to wisdom by a fusion engine**
  Wisdom is a resulting fusion of available data, information, knowledge, which is able to achieve a deep and comprehensive understanding of people, things, situations, and the ability to make decisions which can receive the maximal benefit and reward referring to a goal. The outcome from the fusion engine can provide the holistic integration of intelligence as a wisdom service.

9.2.2 *Wearable Devices*

Combining ubiquitous computing devices such as sensors or actuators, wearable technologies hold great promise in expanding the capabilities of healthcare systems by improving monitoring and maximizing the independence and participation of individuals. Wearable wireless sensors are no longer science fiction. A Body sensor network (BSN), a term coined to harness several allied technologies that underpin the development of pervasive sensing, enables ubiquitous, pervasive and remote health monitoring of physical, physiological, and biochemical parameters [10]. It can gauge walking speed, stride, step width, and body sway for activity monitoring, physical therapy, and even detect warning signs that a person might be at risk of falling [11]. Using rapidly improving wireless communication technology, working together with other equipment, the u-pillbox device can provide a well-thought out service and have many more functions than simply giving medication reminders.

Blood pressure and heartbeat are the representative crucial physical signs of human beings. For healthcare service provision, especially for the elderly, recording these physical signs intermittently or even continuously is helpful in monitoring and nursing in daily life. Thanks to advanced developing sensor and network technology, it is possible to acquire the bodys physical signs outside hospital and transmit the measured results to the data storage directly. Most somatometric measurement sensors or devices need to touch the body for a while to get results. To make the measurement simple and convenient, there are some companies and research centers creating wearable sensors and sensing fiber for healthcare such as blood pressure monitors, hematology analyzers, inertial sensors, electrocardiography, electromyography, etc. Other frontier research is devoted to embedding sensors in the body and recording inner physical signs. Connecting all the sensors and devices around the body to form a body sensor network, it is easy to acquire body information, transmit this to the data center automatically and share it with others.

9.2.3 Environment Sensing

To provide empathetic and active healthcare service, it is essential to be aware of a persons activity and to acquire environmental information such as temperature, humidity and illumination, which affect a persons emotions and activity. Environment monitoring sensors for temperature, humidity and illumination are small and may not need to be deployed in a special place, instead, deploying them in the u-pillbox device may be a good design idea to save space and for easy management.

Being aware of the location and activity of the elderly in the room is an auxiliary function of providing empathetic healthcare service. An indoor personnel tracking system uses a wireless sensor network which integrates varieties of sensors at home to monitor and calculate a persons location. Radio Frequency Identification (SENSOR), Bluetooth, Wi-Fi AP, and ZigBee are the current technologies that are applied to indoor positioning. ZigBee has the property of low cost, small size and large sensing range comparing to other technologies, so that it is a better choice for indoor tracking. From the research in [12], the deviation between default parameter results and actual location are at least 0.5 m, which is acceptable in a home healthcare system. Sensors deployed to monitor the household appliances, bed, toilet/showers and so on can assist in ascertaining the information of a persons current location and activity. This is used to create a persons activity pattern and detect abnormal activity, which is important in a geriatric healthcare system.

9.2.4 Essentials in User Understanding

Current service creation trends in telecommunications and web worlds are revealing the convergence towards a future Internet of user-centric services. In fact, several previous works [13] already provide user-oriented creation/execution environments, but these are usually tied to specific scopes and still lack on the capability to adapt to the heterogeneity of devices, technologies and the specificity of each individual user. Based on these limitations, the research in [14] identifies flexibility and personalization as the foundation for users satisfaction, where the demand for different types of awareness needs to be present across the entire value of chain of a service.

Independently from the technology, all systems should allow user related data to be queried, subscribed or syndicated and ideally through web service interfaces. However, standardization, interoperability, flexibility and management are not the only challenges. To improve the degree of services personalization it is important to generate new information from the existing one. In this sense, social networks, user modeling and reality mining techniques can be empowered to study patterns and predict future behaviors. Consequently, all the adjacent data necessary to perform such operations must be managed within the scope of a user/human profile. Nevertheless, due to the sensitiveness of the information we are referring to, it is important to efficiently control the way this information is stored, accessed and distributed, preserving user privacy, security and trust.

Real world situations usually have to be derived from a complex set of features. Thus, context or behavior aware systems have to capture a set of features from heterogeneous and distributed sources and process them to derive the overall situation. Therefore, recent approaches are intended to be comprehensive, i.e. comprise all components and processing steps necessary to capture a complex situation, starting with the access and management of sensing devices, up to the recognition of a complex situation based on multiple reasoning steps and schemes. To handle complex situations, the concept of decomposition is applied to the situation into a hierarchy of sub-situations. These sub-situations can be handled autonomously with respect to sensing and reasoning. In this way, the handling of complex situations can be simplified by decomposition [15]. Another similar perspective is called layered reasoning, where the first stage involves feature extraction and grouping (i.e., resulting in low-level context), the second event, state and activity recognition (i.e., originating mid-level context), while the last stage is dedicated to prediction and inference of new knowledge [16]. In what concerns social networks, research usually focuses on quantifying or qualifying the relationship between peers, where algorithms such as centrality and prestige can be used to calculate the proximity, influence or importance of a node in a network [17], while clustering and classification can be applied to similarity computation, respectively [18]. In addition, when user related data is associated with time and space dimensions, by empowering data mining techniques it is possible to find hidden patterns that can be used in any of the previously identified stages of reasoning. In this sense, combining all of pre-enunciated concepts with ontologies and semantic technologies, we present a generic framework for managing user related data, which, together with a specific methodology will pave the way to understanding and predicting future human behavior within social communities.

9.2.5 *Emerging Techniques, Applications and Services*

In rapidly-changing information society, the pace of life has rapidly accelerated, resulting in improper diet over a long period of time that could harm our health gradually. Long-term negligence of health is likely to lead to the onset of modern civilization related diseases such as stroke, heart disease, diabetes, and hypertension, of which heart diseases is the number one killer in the world. The World Health Organization even forecasted that nearly 23.6 million people will die from cardiovascular diseases by 2030 [19]. Cardiovascular diseases have become the greatest health concern for the modern people.

Generally, the conditions of patients with cardiovascular diseases can be placed under control through medication and surgery. At present, clinical surgery is divided into coronary artery bypass surgery, angioplasty, heart transplantation etc. In order to ensure a seamless integration of health care system for postoperative patients with cardiovascular disease and hospital care, doctors will recommend a healthcare mode outside the hospital based on the evaluation of patients conditions. Patients can choose a healthcare mode outside the hospital including home care, subacute care, and nursing home care that best suits their needs. Subacute care is a comprehensive inpatient care and is designed for patients with acute illness, injuries, or aggravated diseases. It is a type of target-oriented treatment aimed at assisting patients through the stage of disease to recovery. Patients can return home or be admitted to nursing home when their conditions are stabilized. Nursing homes offer care to patients with chronic diseases that require follow-up care after discharge from hospitals. In general, patients of this type whose conditions have been stabilized still require technical care and need care in daily life [20].

Accompanied by the rising needs of mobile hospital and home nursing, the concept of Telecare arises. The origin of this concept can be traced back to the term of eHealth that use Internet technology to support and advance the quality of healthcare practice in the field of public health and medical informatics. In the broader sense of healthcare practice, eHealth is not only a fruit of the development of technology but also a globalized thinking, attitude, and obligation. Nowadays, equipment used in Telecare adopt wireless sensor that enables users to collect vital signs including heart beat, pulse, glucose, and blood pressure and to transmit these information through mobile devices to medical institutions where doctors can grasp patients current condition based on received information [21, 22]. In the field of Telecare, researches related to the study of vital signs monitoring propose the alarm mechanism that warnings users when their health condition appears abnormal phenomenon and inform them their health require extra attention. Besides the alarm mechanism to users, other researches apply the alarm mechanism on mobile devices used by nursing staff to assist their work of nursing [23].

Regarding the development of the platform for home care back-end operation, researches develop a platform for personal health information that users can manage such as medical examination report and prescription [24]. Studies [17, 25, 26] investigated the applications of service platform on medical practice to assist healthcare at anytime, anywhere, and with right context.

The development of cloud computing has evolved the development of professional medical technology. For example, the sharing of medical knowledge and professional experience is not restrained within the same institution. Medical units such as hospital, clinical station, nursing center, even home care institution from different areas can cooperate with each other remotely. Cloud service can be applied to the field medical care and can assist the management of data center in the way of united data collection that can expand software and workflow and make full use of available software and hardware resources. It also provides consistent services and safety [27–29]. Thus, based on cloud computing, the wireless homecare supporting mechanism proposed in this chapter seems to be simple but actually requires several intelligent mechanisms working together to accomplish the goal of customer-oriented concept delivering the easiest to users while leaving the most difficult to the cloud.

Some researches dedicated themselves to the development of point-of-care data delivery based on sensor technology. Staff badges, medication packaging and patients identity bracelets contain sensor technology [30]. This facilitates identification of a patient by caregivers, who are thus able to submit orders in real-time at the very point of care, instead of being handwritten and sent off for future input. This kind of system saves time, and reduces the chances of human error [31, 32]. Moreover, sensor technology can be applied on asset tracking and locating. Some position-based indoor tracking systems have been used in hospitals, where expensive equipment needs to be tracked to avoid being stolen, and the patients can get guidance to efficiently use limited medical resources inside complex environments of the hospital. For instance, surgical instruments and other devices must be properly cleaned and packaged between uses. Tags on the instruments and readers on the sterilization chambers and storage cabinets can validate proper cleaning and help locate needed instruments. SENSOR can also facilitate better management of medical equipment, medicine, and storage which leads to a more efficient and less medical error environment [33–35].

Sensor technology can also be applied on patient location: tracking the location of patients in case of long-term care, mentally challenged patients, and newborns. It has the ability to determine the location of a patient within a hospital and facilitate the delivery of health care. For example, when a patient arrives in a lab for a radiology exam, medical staff is instantly alerted via the tag [36], and the transfer of records can be affected immediately. Patient tracking mechanism can manage patients efficiently to provide a better health care service [37].

Being aware of situations, aware of the needs of the elderly, the maximum benefits to the elderly services are the points of the u-pillbox system. Being able to provide wisdom services to the elderly is the supreme goal of the u-pillbox system. Therefore, the three service layers and the fusion engine within the WaaS platform are the core techniques of the proposed u-pillbox system.

9.3 A Data Cycle-Based Framework for U-Healthcare

To achieve the goal stated above, we propose a framework for a humanistic and empathetic service system as given in Fig. 9.1, which includes four important parts: data acquisition; WaaS (Wisdom as a Service); the Cyber-pillbox; and a human model enhanced empathetic service. Under this framework, the u-pillbox system is developed. As shown in Fig. 9.1, the u-pillbox device has a twofold function: one is as a sensing device for acquiring the elderly dynamic data and information, and the other is as an active interface for interacting with and providing services to the elderly. The Cyber-pillbox is the mirror system of the u-pillbox device. It has a twofold role: one is as a back-end support of the u-pillbox device for undertaking all related software implementations, and the other is as a gateway for accessing and exploiting opened or collaborative resources from the public healthcare platform and authorized healthcare system infrastructure. Both the u-pillbox device and the Cyber-pillbox work in tandem to provide efficient and effective healthcare services to the elderly under the support of a public open healthcare platform and authorized healthcare system infrastructure.

9.3.1 The U-Pillbox System

Understanding humans is the key to building a human-centric system. Continuously monitoring data of users body functions, their context and environmental parameters can be seen as analogous to a mirror in front of a human subject. The collected data are mainly from the u-pillbox device, wearable devices, and sensors in the environment around the elderly.

Due to the size limitations and complexity in maintenance, the u-pillbox device is conceptually designed based on the principle of being as compact as possible. It mainly collects the health and medicine-taking related state of the elderly and environmental monitoring data with the essential embedded sensors or plugin-able sensing devices as given in Table 9.1. Although only a limited number of sensors are embedded in the u-pillbox device, it leaves a space for plugging in some

Table 9.1 U-pillbox device embedded sensors and plugin-able devices

U-pillbox device		
Body state sensor	Ambient sensing	Plug-in device
Pillbox state	Environment temperature	Blood glucose meter
Skin temperature	Humidity information	Blood analyzer
Blood information	Illumination information	Pedometer
Pulse information etc.	Air pressure etc.	Urine analyzer etc.
Application/device interface		

external sensors or devices with the application or device interface so as to enhance its capability and functionality in its compact size.

- **Body state sensor**
  The basic functions of the u-pillbox device are managing medication dispensation, reminding the user to take their medicine when necessary. The u-pillbox device records the medicine name, the time taken, and the dosage taken. The record is organized in the u-pillbox device and sent to the upper layer platform for use in monitoring the treatment process and analyzing the medicinal efficacy.
  Some small health state test devices for measuring physical signs like a thermometer, pulse ox meter, blood analyzer, urine analyzer, etc. can be embedded into or plugin-able to the u-pillbox to provide a convenient test service since they are often used or even used daily. Furthermore, via the u-pillbox, data from the test devices can be sent directly to the upper layer Cyber-pillbox system for further analysis, processing, and integration.
- **Ambient sensing**
  The environment or context persons are exposed to can affect their physical and mental health. Temperature, humidity, illumination, air pressure, etc. are the basic observed values of an environment. Integrated sensors feed context information into the u-pillbox device via which the collected data are sent to the cyber pillbox system. The u-pillbox links the actual world with the virtual cyber world as a bridge and provides a clear vision of the actual world in the virtual cyber world.
  Although some sensors for monitoring environmental condition can be embedded in the u-pillbox device, most of sensors are distributed in the environment to monitor the activities and physical signs of the elderly. Some are fixed and some are portable. Human activity and behavior oriented sensors have been receiving increasing attention from companies, universities and research centers. These sensors data are transmitted via wired or wireless sensor network to the cyber u-pillbox system for analysis and processing and the results are merged with other results of to support the elderly healthcare.
- **Plugin-able devices and application/device interfaces**
  There are lots of electronic healthcare products and healthcare application being sold in the market. In Apple App Store and Google Play, healthcare related applications and accessories have become a big sector and sell well. Extended devices give smart phone applications much more functions, such as measuring heartbeat, tracking sleep, tracking daily activity and even tracking food and drink consumption, such as UP by Jawbone [38], Fitbit OneTM Wireless Activity + Sleep Tracker [39], sold in Apple Store, sensing the information that helps users better understand their sleep, movement and eating. These extended devices are small and stylishly designed and their data can be transmitted to smart phones or PADs using Bluetooth or other wireless networks. The u-pillbox device is designed to have an application/device interface so that it can support these extended devices by being directly plugged in via the device interface or receiving collected data via the application interface. This function gives the u-pillbox device great potential for extending its capability and functionality.

9.3.2 Human Model and Empathetic Service

Providing active and empathetic services is the emphasized objective of the u-pillbox system. Apart from the core techniques of the WaaS platform, the human individual model is another critical highlight to the whole vision of delivering the elderly active and empathetic services. To enable this requires an understanding of users activities and intentions, awareness of their environment or context, and subsequently a response to the users according to their preferences. Therefore, capturing the patient's physical and psychological reactions is helpful for understanding how favorable or antipathetic they will be to the service provided. Affective computing, which is devoted to the detection and recognition of emotions aroused by specific trigger events, is one technology competent to accomplish this challenging task [31]. In addition, the resulting data from this technology will provide further input to the emotion model of the u-pillbox system.

However, the dynamic stream data in real time from the real world provides limited awareness of a user, and the understanding of the user is a long term accumulating process of understanding from different angles and aspects. The u-pillbox device and system alone is insufficient. An elderly individual model, a digital clone in the digital world, inspired from Cyber-I [32] with an open platform provides the space for different parties and applications to make contributions to the understanding of a user and enhancement of the human model and by sharing the resulting model, the comprehensive digital description of a human in the real world. As for the u-pillbox system, it has a twofold role, one is contributing to the model and the other is benefiting from the model. Like any other health service system, it, unexceptionally, has to work or cooperate with other healthcare systems or organizations for which the Cyber-pillbox system plays an important role as a gateway for accessing open and public resources and enabling various levels of collaboration. The u-pillbox system can be both a query subject benefiting from public resources and a query object to possibly provide third parties valuable information or resources. The benefits are mutual and bilateral to all collaborators.

The provision of active and empathetic services to the elderly is emphasized as the basis of the continuing understanding of the elderly within the u-pillbox system, contributions about the elderly from third parties, and the publicly available shared information and resources from the open platform and infrastructure.

9.3.3 Cyber-Pillbox System

The Cyber-pillbox system simulates the physical u-pillbox device in the cyber world in the application layer, running on top of the public healthcare service platform, which further runs on top of the open healthcare system infrastructure.

Analogous to entities in the real world, the Cyber-pillbox is the virtual mirror of the u-pillbox device with an ancillary information network in the computing virtual world. It is a reflection of the physical world and facilitates empathetic services after computer processing. The Cyber-pillbox runs in the home healthcare server and has a browser interface to users which can be accessed from a terminal like computer, PDA, or even smart phone, from which the elderly or a patient can interact with the system.

Its basic functions include showing users medicine taking agenda and the u-pillbox device filling real-time state; keeping the record of medicine-taking diary, body signs, and environmental information; and displaying the stored record in visualized tables, curves, and figures. Besides this, there are other four featured additional real-time functions, they are

- a social group formation that enables elderly or patients, doctors, caregivers, recovered patients to share state-of-affairs information, testimonials, advices and encouragement;
- a pill information system accessing and downloading from which users are aware of what medicine they are taking and what they should pay attention to;
- doctor and pharmacist-shared interface with which they can edit a patients medicine taking agenda under authentication and send the change notification to users; and
- medicine taking agenda updating to the u-pillbox device when having changes or after the u-pillbox device refilling.

9.4 Features and Viewpoints

Compared with existing pillbox systems, the proposed u-pillbox system has its own seven significant features employing advanced technologies so as to enable the provision of empathetic and active healthcare services. These significant features include a humanistic approach, personalized healthcare, human individual model based, emotion model embedded, W2T cycle for spiraling enhancement of a human model, data/information/knowledge fusion towards wisdom, and Internet-empowered transparent and smart healthcare service. These are realized not only through fundamental technologies like ubiquitous computing, body sensor networking, the Internet of Things, and the Web of Things, but also the concepts of Cyber-I [32], W2T [9], WaaS and their associated advanced technologies such as the W2T cycle, a WaaS platform, a data mining engine, a data/information/knowledge fusion engine, human modeling, an Internet-empowered transparent healthcare service framework, and the fusion of these technologies.

9.4.1 A Humanistic Approach

Humanistic medical care, the fundamental principles of which are open communication, mutual respect, and emotional connection between physicians (via the u-pillbox device) and their patients, is an important element of quality healthcare. Care of this type is termed "relationship-centered" or "patient-centered" care, in contrast to "case-centered" or "disease-centered" care. The process of humanistic medical care can build a relationship of trust between a u-pillbox device and a patient. The u-pillbox device knows and understands a patient and can give individual patients the attention they need. The crux of a humanistic u-pillbox system emphasizes "holistic healing" [40], which can encourage physical recovery through empathy, patience, and compassion.

9.4.2 Provision of Personalized U-Healthcare

In a patient-centered healthcare system, individual patients needs and preferences are two primary factors to be taken into consideration. There is increasing expectation that patients are the driving force of change in care delivery systems toward improved quality. With the growing burden of chronic disease and the need for continuous care, patients play important roles in the implementation of their care. Making them active participants in their care instead of conventional passive recipients is a significant trend in innovative healthcare systems. To achieve this, a patient-friendly, patient-accessible, and patient-centered health information and care system is necessary. The crux of a patient-centered health care system is to have an individual expandable model [41–43] for each individual patient from which a care system can elicit the patients needs and preferences and respond to them, and make a contribution to the growth of the model in the process of providing healthcare as well. On the one hand, with increasing comprehensive individual model, the quality of personalized health care services will be improved; on the other hand, in the course of receiving health care services, the individual model [41–43] will be growing. This is the so-called interdependence double-edged sword.

9.4.3 An Eco-Human Growing Model

In philosophy, essence is defined as the attribute or set of attributes that make an entity or substance what it fundamentally is, and which it has by necessity, and without which it loses its identity (from Wikipedia). The human essence is fundamental human nature which is unchanging and is conducive to a fulfilling, balanced, healthy, creative and growth-oriented human life [44]. It can be represented by a set of attributes in digital format, termed the human essence model.

Human beings are social creatures who are born into a wide variety of situations and have to adapt to the challenges in the environments in which they are living in order to survive and prosper, maintain health, and be able to continue a family line. These environmental constraints create limits on behaviors, beliefs, personalities, and so on, and define the range of acceptable conditions for life. Different people have different constraints in the varied environments in which they grow up, and which lead to their different behaviors, beliefs, personalities, and so on. The individual human model is based on the human essence model and continuously develops on top of the essence model and becomes more and more comprehensive through ones life.

9.4.4 Embedded Emotion Factors

A human individual model that approximates the mental processes of a real individual contains three levels: state, behavior, and mind from different angles/aspects. This is achieved through data mining, intelligent processing, and knowledge fusion mechanisms and methodologies. One aspect of this is the emotion model, modeling concurrent emotions and sequences of emotions of the elderly as they perform routine daily activities or which is triggered by a single event or multiple events. This is embedded in an elderly individual model currently at the behavior level. The emotion model, named PAEM (Personality-Associated Emotion Model) [45], is set out in our previous research work. This takes into consideration individual personality traits and a triggered main emotion point in the PAD space [46]. The embedded individual emotion model is extended from the event-driven PAEM model by combining the OCC model [36] and BDI agent theory. It not only takes into account personality traits but also a number of emotion points in the PAD space. It can simulate the sequence of the elderly patient's mixed emotions over time after these emotions are triggered by an event, multiple simultaneous events or a sequence of events.

With an embedded emotion model, the u-pillbox system can provide not only the elderly or patients' physical healthcare but also mental care so as to achieve truly empathetic healthcare and services. However, the proposed emotion model is still at an infant stage, much work remains to build a comprehensive computational emotion model.

9.4.5 W2T Spiraling Enhancement of Human Model

W2T stands for Wisdom Web of Things and the W2T cycle [9] refers to the data transformation from raw data acquired in the physical world to information, knowledge, and wisdom in the Cyber world, and the data circulation of "Things → Data → Information → Knowledge → Wisdom → Service → Human → Things" in the Hyperworld [47], combining the physical world and Cyber world.

Data acquisition, data mining and transformation in the data mining engine within the WaaS platform, and generation of wisdom for active and empathetic services in the fusion engine do not solely undergo one-time process tasks. In the u-pillbox system, the process of transforming data to services, providing services to the elderly, and updating data by monitoring the elderly and things in the real world form a data circulation which passes data and its analysis output from one step to next. Most original raw big data come from healthcare sensors and service-providing applications such as the u-pillbox device. These data are passed to the data mining engine and fusion engine and the generated results can be resources for healthcare services directly or be used to enhance a human model which is then handed over to healthcare services. The healthcare service applications are not only providing services, but also collecting usage tracks, physical signs and environment or context data. Therefore, new data generated in employment is seen as a raw source put into WaaS framework. It forms a cycle which brings the system spiraling performance. The human model becomes more and more comprehensive and healthcare services to the human become more and more empathetic.

9.4.6 Data/Information/Knowledge Fusion Towards Wisdom

Analyzing the huge amounts of multidimensional data generated by continuous healthcare monitoring sensors and contained within medical records submitted by third party healthcare bodies, is a big challenge in implementing the u-pillbox system. The data to be processed in our u-pillbox system have the "4V" features of Volume, Velocity, Variety, and Value. In this context, volume refers to relevant patient healthcare data with time stamps continuously collected from sensors and their networks, comprising overwhelmingly huge amounts of data; velocity refers to the processing of this huge amount of data which the healthcare services must perform in real-time; variety refers to the multifarious formatting of the data, from structured tables such as medical records, half- or un-structured documents, and medical images to video and sound formats; and value refers to information being detailed enough about patients daily lives to be advantageous in individualizing medical treatment, organizing preventive treatment, and arriving at therapeutic solutions.

Due to these features, the processing involved in healthcare data mining and knowledge discovery is extremely onerous. From data storage, pre-processing, algorithm selection, feature extraction, knowledge discovery, and prediction to visualization, the vast amount of data involved can't simply be processed using relational databases and desktop statistics. A comprehensive set of data mining techniques like our proposed data mining engine is urgently required together with powerful parallel software running on tens, hundreds, or even thousands of servers may be required to process data within tolerable time limits [48]. Therefore, the u-pillbox healthcare system adopts an infrastructure built on top of its cloud computing architecture with an implementation model of "X as a Service (XaaS)" [49] such as Software as a Service (SaaS), Platform as a Service (PaaS), and Infrastructure as a Service (IaaS).

The u-pillbox device as a lightweight front-end device is not equipped with computational power or involved with infrastructure system features such as servers and data centers; they are simply accessible and sharable from the clouds in the cloud computing sky via the Internet and networks.

Data/information/knowledge fusion towards wisdom derived from this overwhelming data is quite complex and difficult. The u-pillbox system exploits the WaaS platform and the fusion engine which are the task-oriented data mining and knowledge discovery mechanisms on the W2T data cyclic circulation platform [9] and provides application protocol interfaces for three layers; structured data, information and knowledge. Complex or comprehensive knowledge is composed by fusing data, information, and/or atomic knowledge from each layer according to the specific task. After continued data cyclic circulation of data acquisition, WaaS and active healthcare services, a virtuous spiral is created, and a clear human model is provided to the upper layer applications, the basis for providing empathetic healthcare services to individual patients.

9.4.7 Internet-Empowered U-Healthcare Service Provision

The Internet is an increasingly important source of health-related information for patients. Healthcare is traditionally a field characterized by a high degree of specialized knowledge and expert intervention in the life of patients. With the wide use of the Internet and rapidly developing network and communication technologies, patients are being continuously empowered in many aspects of healthcare; access to health records and medical diagnosis results, online counseling with doctors or healthcare givers, discussion of health issues on social network systems, etc. Patients are becoming more active participants in the healthcare process, contrasting with the traditionally passive role they played. Better resourced and smarter healthcare services for treating illness and maintaining health have become available and are being enhanced with the use of Internet and communication network infrastructure.

The proposed Cyber-pillbox, as the mirror of the u-pillbox device, is laid on top of the Healthcare Service platform carried out under the Healthcare System Infrastructure. As a front-end device, the u-pillbox device should be light, stylish, user-friendly, and all its functions and services transparent to a user. Conventional processes of human-computer interaction that employ hardware input devices, e.g., keyboard, mouse, etc. no longer meet the increasing needs of individuals. Communication between humans is diverse in nature, expressed not only through speech, but also body language, eye contact and so on. The u-pillbox system demonstrates an example of instant responses captured from individuals, implicit data analysis, and valuable services provided via multiple devices (i.e., sensors, wearable devices) in the environment. A wide spectrum of sensing devices (or u-Things) [50] is applied such as bio-inspired body sensors [51], Zigbee, SENSOR, and related sensors already existing in the environment. The sensing process, which is the most significant aspect of the U-pillbox device, identifies procedures of which users are not conscious, concentrating on the provision of an organized flow of services to individuals anytime, anywhere, and in the right context (i.e. medical services in this study).

As the back-end, the Cyber-pillbox system is not only Internet-empowered but also acts as a gateway to ancillary intelligent processing and healthcare resources in the transparent computing infrastructure [52], with which the front-end pillbox device can see every cloud in the cloud computing sky, and is able to access resources from any cloud environment under the relevant policy or agreement. Active healthcare services are provided to patients with the strong backing of the Internet empowered healthcare services platform, and system infrastructure.

9.5 Implementation at a Glance

The u-pillbox system consists of three main modules: data acquisition, context awareness, and service provision. Figure 9.2 shows the overview of its prototype implementation. The data acquisition module provides all necessary functions for collecting various types of data from real world devices including the u-pillbox device, Web sites, and the environmental context. The collected data is the input of the context awareness module and its outputs are the patients situation. The module draws a conclusion of the current understanding about the patient together with the human model and the conclusion is passed to the service provision module. The context awareness module can be implemented by a back-end big data mining and knowledge discovery supporting system which can be placed in a cloud computing environment. The service provision module is implemented in a three-layer architecture: a healthcare application layer, a healthcare platform layer, and a healthcare infrastructure layer as shown in Fig. 9.2.

9.5.1 The Application Layer

In the healthcare application layer, Cyber-pillbox system emulates the u-pillbox device, enables interfaces to users and the healthcare service platform, and manages the necessary data and resources. The application layer implements the UI layer, the business layer, and the persistence layer in a combined framework Spring + Struts + Hibernate (SSH). Where, the persistence layer is for completing the transactions with the database in a Hibernate persistence framework. The Business layer uses a Spring framework as the inversion of the control container for completing all the logical and computing processes and Data Access Objects (DAO) classes for transmitting data with the persistence layer. The UI layer uses an Apache Struts web application framework to provide user interfaces and interacts with the business layer through a service locator (Fig. 9.3).

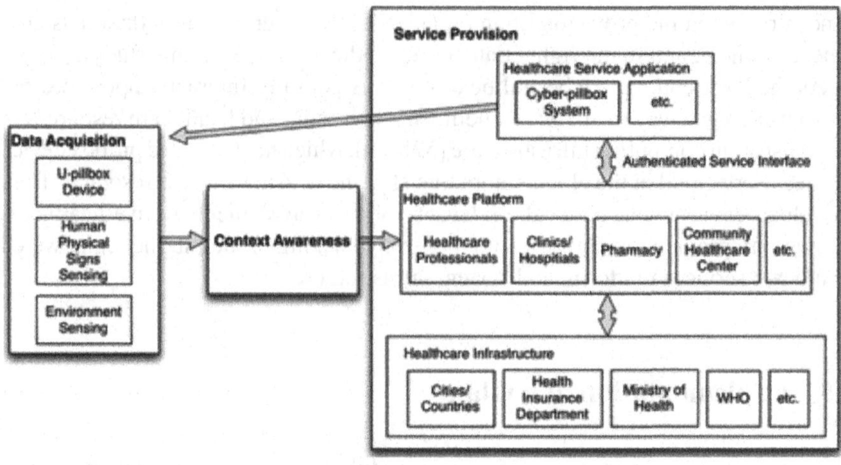

Fig. 9.2 The prototype implementation modules of u-pillbox system

9.5.2 The Service Platform

This platform is designed for coordinating healthcare professionals, hospitals, clinics, pharmacies, community centers, etc. to have a common platform to provide, share, exchange healthcare or health treatment information so as to provide high quality and patient satisfaction healthcare services. To facilitate the provision of healthcare services, a conventional service-oriented architecture, named SOA is adopted for this

Fig. 9.3 The implementation outline of the healthcare application layer

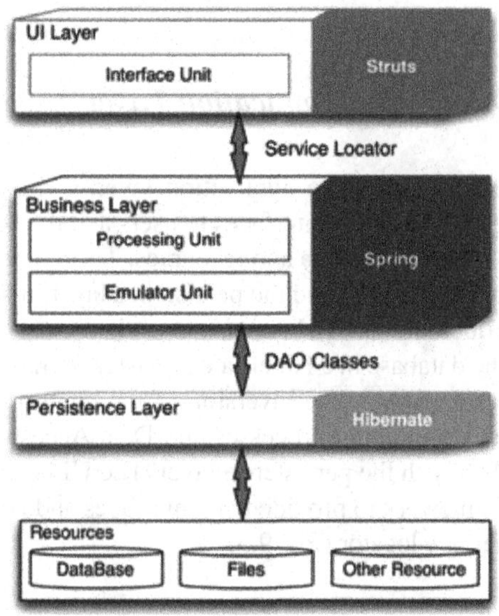

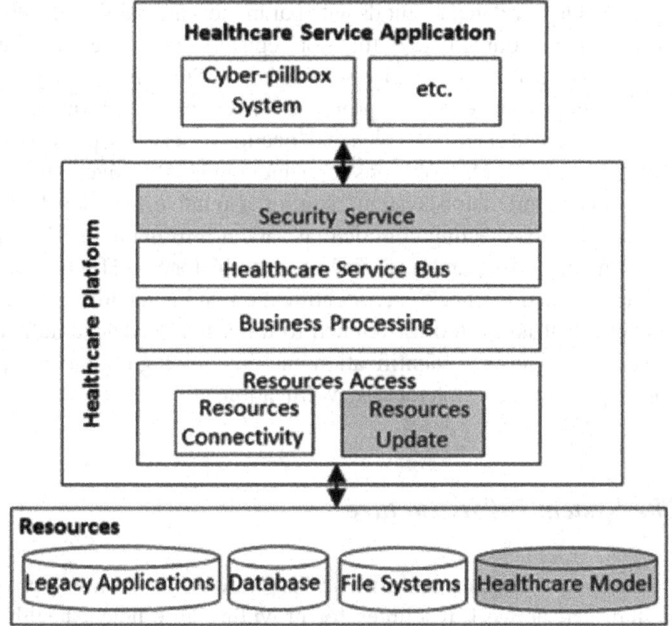

Fig. 9.4 Healthcare service-oriented architecture

platform together with the underlying enhancements based on the characteristics of healthcare services. The enhanced architecture is named, Healthcare Service-oriented Architecture (HSOA) as given in Fig. 9.4, in which the components, marked in grey, i.e. healthcare model, resources update and secure quality of service.

Resources are the basis for providing not only healthcare services but also all kinds of services. However, healthcare services are highly reliant on sufficient and high quality resources from professionals and richly experienced providers. The resources stored in the healthcare service provision system should not be limited to traditional databases, and a variety of new forms like healthcare models, medical case histories, and even surgery videos or rehabilitation recordings, etc. will be useful for supporting a "Q&A" service as a resource. HSOA provides a healthcare model database in the resources for simulation, prediction and estimation of the medical situation and disease recovery. One example of such a healthcare model is the human emotion model in [45], named PAEM (Personality-Associated Emotion Model). The model can be dynamically enhanced in the process of acquiring and mining patients' physiological data continuously so as to provide a dynamic and adaptive service. For different individuals, their models differ, and for different models, the system can provide differing personalized healthcare services.

To manage and access the healthcare models, the resource update function unit is added the conventional data persistence technology in the healthcare service platform. Its implementation is highly reliant on each healthcare model. Once there is a new incoming model, its related methods with parameters are published to the healthcare platform and the resource update function registers the updates. The healthcare service bus is the same as the enterprise service bus in SOA. It provides the service of reliable messaging, service access, protocol conversion, data format conversion, content-based routing and shields the physical location of services, protocols and data formats. It is the core of HSOA solutions for achieving HSOA governance platform.

Healthcare service provision system requires a relative high level of security due to the necessity of protecting confidential patient information such as personal information, clinical history, and medicine regimen history. In HSOA, the security service module is added to check user identification and authentication before any service is provided. It is not too far-fetched to think that advanced authentication technology such as fingerprint identification and facial recognition can replace the traditional user-password for this identity verification.

9.5.3 The System Infrastructure

The healthcare system infrastructure is the hardware and software support of the physical system and network resources for providing an efficient health services strategy to the healthcare service platform in the upper layers. Inspired by IBMs white paper [53] about cloud architecture, the healthcare system infrastructure adopts IBMs proven cloud reference architecture for building a unique private cloud. Under the umbrella of IBMs proven cloud reference architecture with effective security, resiliency, service management, governance, business planning and lifecycle management, it is expected that all other healthcare organizations such as WHO, Ministries of national healthcare, City Healthcare Departments, community healthcare centers, etc. could efficiently, effectively, and smoothly coordinate and collaborate in sharing and supporting of request-on-demand healthcare and computing resources. To illustrate, our healthcare cloud services built on the IBM reference architecture are shown in Fig. 9.5.

The armamentarium of medical practitioners, fundamental equipment and international, national and municipal healthcare entities can be connected to provide services to the upper layer under the management of the IBM cloud reference architecture. The common cloud management platform in the architecture manages and operates healthcare infrastructure resources in order to provide the required service to the cloud service layer. The connected organizations in the healthcare infrastructure provide equipment, platform, software services and healthcare processes. An extended information service concerning rules, certification, healthcare related criteria, legislation, etc., is provided so as to meet the special requirements of healthcare. For example, if WHO publishes diagnostic criteria for diabetes, healthcare professionals need to comply with them to guide patients diagnosis and treatment. That means concurrently, clinics, hospitals, pharmaceutical factories, community healthcare centers, etc. also need a healthcare infrastructure to participate in healthcare. When the upper layer discerns that this information is not applicable the current

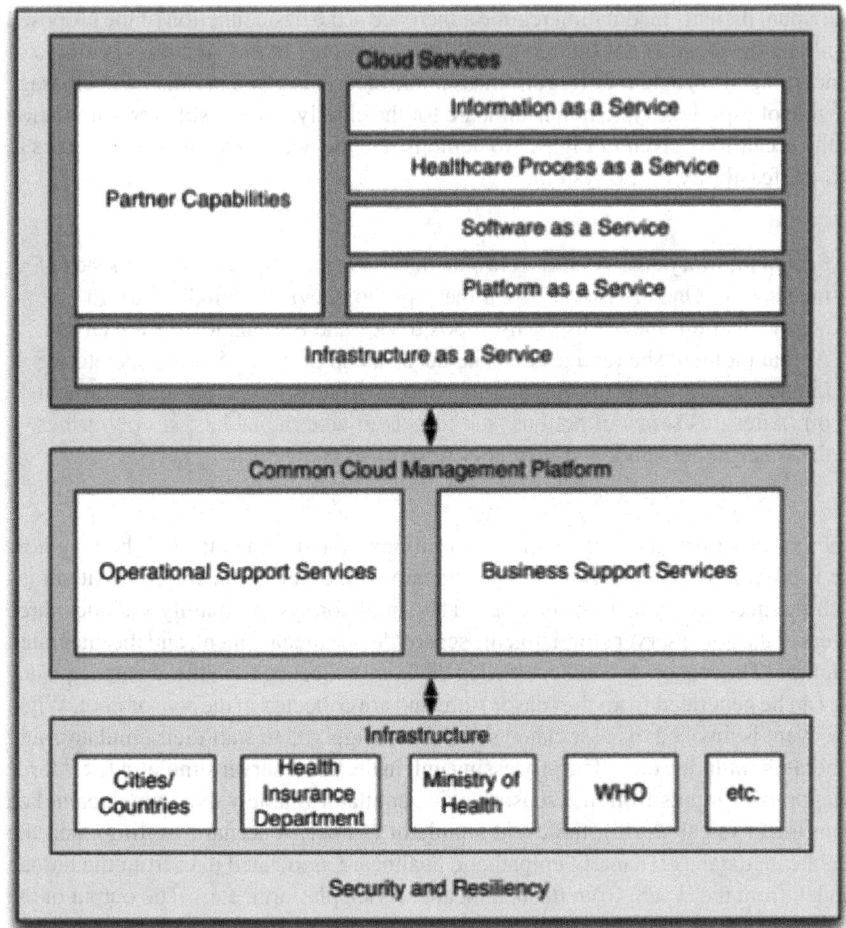

Fig. 9.5 Healthcare infrastructure architecture based on IBM cloud reference architecture

situation, it can submit changed advice for the correlative organization to consider. This is mutually beneficial to both sides and provides efficient services to patients and their relatives. Furthermore, the functions of security and resiliency in the cloud ensure the architecture encourages trust in and provides a flexible service to the upper layer.

9.6 Scenario and Practice

Poor medication adherence often risks preventable serious deterioration in the health of patients, particularly for elderly patients with chronic illnesses. Although tracking individual patients medication regime adherence is the basic function of the proposed u-pillbox device, it is not limited to this function alone. In this section, a scenario of concerning the problem of forgetfulness in the elderly is given in Fig. 9.6 to envisage the role of u-pillbox system in healthcare for the elderly, and the software simulation of the scenario is given in Fig. 9.7 to demonstrate the necessary function modules in and the feasibility of the system.

Scenario: Mary, age 70, has a chronic disease and has to take several kinds of medication. One afternoon, when the u-pillbox device reminds Mary to take her medication, she opens the u-pillbox device and is going to take the tablets. At that moment she realizes that she needs a cup of water. She walks into the kitchen to get water, finding that the smoke exhaust fan is on, so she turns it off. After this series of actions, she forgets to take the tablets, simply drinks the water in her hand, and then goes upstairs to take a rest.

Figure 9.7 gives an overview of the u-pillbox system simulator for showing how the u-pillbox system provides the healthcare to the elderly in different situations with the necessary function modules. The simulator system mainly includes three layers of the home server simulator, the sensor/device management, and the integrated database. The sensor objects specified in the event sequence from the events sequence file can be generated from the sensor store and are collected in the sensor pool. When any event is invoked, its associated sensors are triggered to start their emulators and generate simulation data. The processing unit in the home server simulator takes three categories of inputs from the sensor/device emulator (namely dynamic stream data from the physical world), the event simulator (namely a scenario setting), and the healthcare database (namely empathetic healthcare associated data from the human model, from the WaaS, from the healthcare service platform, etc.). The output of the processing unit is the effector on the sensors, devices, and environment for providing services to the users.

9.7 Conclusion

Concept of Web of Things (W2T) has prompted the development and integration of many related fields of studies (e.g., web intelligence, ubiquitous computing, brain informatics, etc.) and identifies a rather promising research direction in the post-Web era. Its original and unique point of view on data processing, a sustainable and computable lifecycle of data, inspires researchers who are in the related fields.

Considering the fundamental of data science and W2T, this chapter discusses a general framework for ubiquitous healthcare service provision. An empathetic u-pillbox system is instanced to address few significant and challenging issues in geriatric healthcare, and it shows the potential for the enhancement of existing care

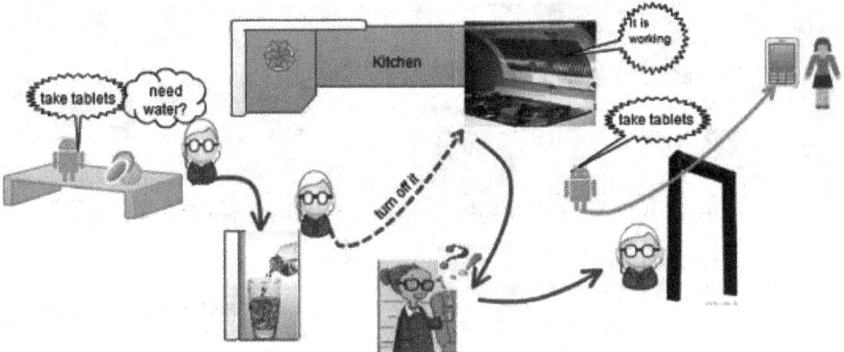

Fig. 9.6 Reminding the elderly to take medicine

arrangements for the elderly, and aid the development of more innovative care in the future. This framework consists of three layers: the u-pillbox system application layer running on a Web server; the healthcare service framework layer running on an HSOA; and a healthcare system infrastructure running on IBM cloud reference architecture. The system would be a significant advance on existing pillbox systems with features that extend beyond medication dispensation to utilize ubiquitous technologies to amass data on individual patients, and then process this data to provide the most appropriate care possible to individual patients based on wisdom as a service model and individual human modeling.

The u-pillbox system is considered the front-end with which services can be delivered to the elderly. Through integration with healthcare infrastructures, and with the individual human model generated by the u-pillbox system and third parties, improved healthcare strategies can be delivered to patients efficiently and targeted in the form most empathetically suited to each individual patient. Recognition by elderly patients of the extent to which healthcare services provided through the u-pillbox system are targeted specifically to their needs generates trust and acceptance of their treatment, and encourages efforts to reach better treatment outcomes by involving geriatric patients as active participants in their own treatment. A u-healthcare system, available everywhere, at anytime and to anyone, could become a preferred option among the elderly seeking advice on diet, exercise and health-related issues.

Throughout the world, demographic changes are placing ever greater pressure on resources available for geriatric healthcare, whilst at the same time making the need for more effective and responsive health care provision to the elderly ever more urgent. The need for innovative approaches that leverage the far-reaching development of ubiquitous technologies to address this demographic situation is an expanding field, ripe with opportunity to make a significant impact within geriatric healthcare.

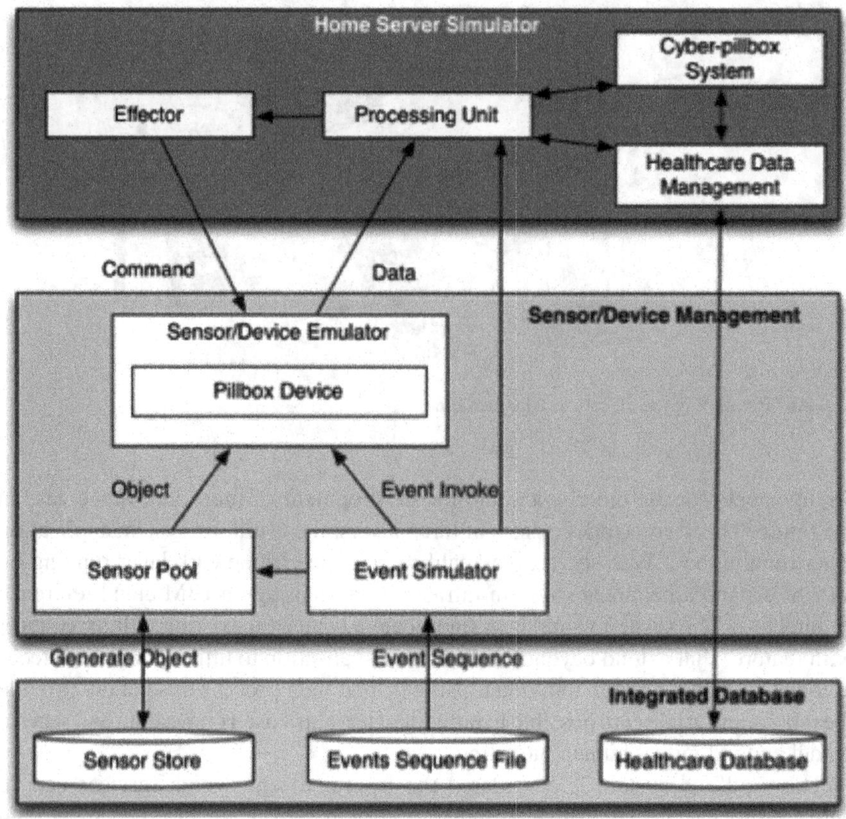

Fig. 9.7 U-pillbox system simulator

9.8 Challenges and Directions

This chapter discusses the principle design pattern of a general framework that facilitates the issues in the realm of geriatric healthcare. As a practical implementation, a promising prototype system, namely U-pillbox, for U-Healthcare support is developed. It is applied to outline realistic simulations and scenarios demonstrating the feasibility and performance of a W2T-empowered framework. Although significant results were obtained, however, challenges remain, which cover a wide range of research fields. Considering the main theme of this chapter and the book, some challenging issues are addressed:

Hardware/software design for U-pillbox: Usability and Reliability

Referring to the development of u-healthcare systems, the design matters. It is undoubtedly that most of subjects under the scope of u-healthcare are those elderly or persons who are physically-unavailable. Thus the design of u-healthcare system (i.e., u-pillbox) requires comprehensive understanding to its users. The design, for both hardware and software, needs to be attractive, light, portable/flexible and user-friendly to each generation especially those traditionally uncomfortable with technology. It is also considered feature-rich to generate accurate health data and derived contexts of individual. This need for relative complexity has also to be balanced against an absolute need for reliability. If the device cannot generate accurate data reliably, no reliable or trusted services can be delivered properly. The challenges related to the physical u-pillbox device may not be as complicated as those posed by the Cyber-pillbox system. However, the time by which we can envisage these challenges being met is still a long way off.

U-pillbox Applications: Complexity, Empathy and Integration

The issue in U-pillbox system is design and coordination of discrete applications, hosted on the system, that sufficiently innovative to address specific issues and conditions within geriatric healthcare. These applications have to work in concert and minimize conflicts with each other to provide holistic healthcare. The service is then delivered to the patient, regarding all aspects of their healthcare. It needs to be clear, easy-to-understand and precise. Another challenge is to ensure that applications are applicable to be delivered sensitively, and to create an empathetic effect. Though the patient receives the service through the u-pillbox device, the "bedside manner", often exists the metric by which doctors are judged by elderly patients. It needs to be created by applications within the U-pillbox system. Crucial to solving the problem of ensuring an empathetic service is the development of a comprehensive individual human model from every perspective and in all aspects through the tracing of the individual patients footprint and collection of their data in the real world and Cyberworlds.

The need for sensitivity within the healthcare environment is also complicated by the sheer variety and subtlety of health indicators between individual patients that need to be detected and then interpreted by applications within the cyber pillbox system. This will require a significant investment in a parallel processing infrastructure powerful enough to mine and process data, generate the Individual Human Model, and then deliver a service to the user of the u-pillbox device in the most suitable manner possible and with sufficient speed.

The final challenge concerning U-pillbox system is that the system cannot, or will not, provide healthcare services in a vacuum. The u-pillbox system requires all bodies involved in healthcare such as health ministries, hospitals and clinics, pharmaceutical companies and outlets, medical and nursing schools and so on. A seamless integration with third parties is strongly necessary to provide holistic healthcare. It will require a sophisticated platform working under the proposed infrastructure (and data framework as well). A consensus on a suit of protocols and a standard interface will have to be reached to guarantee delivery of a clear unified service to users and to deliver services to the institutions mentioned above to formulate more efficient healthcare policies and practices.

U-pillbox system: Verifiability of Effect

Except the above-mentioned issues, an emerging challenge is worth a mentioning. It is about an optimally-designed and mass-produced u-pillbox devices, and a sufficiently powerful infrastructure employing a wide range of innovative applications be built. How will we be able to judge whether the u-pillbox system has improved geriatric healthcare for the better? The answer probably lies in a balance of carefully designed longitudinal medical studies and clinical testing, requiring cooperation with a range of health bodies.

Acknowledgments Except the above-mentioned issues, an emerging challenge is worth a mentioning. It is about an optimally-designed and mass-produced u-pillbox devices, and a sufficiently powerful infrastructure employing a wide range of innovative applications be built. How will we be able to judge whether the u-pillbox system has improved geriatric healthcare for the better? The answer probably lies in a balance of carefully designed longitudinal medical studies and clinical testing, requiring cooperation with a range of health bodies.

References

1. Health. Growth in health spending grinds to a halt, http://www.oecd.org/health/healthgrowthinhealthspendinggrindstoahalt.htm
2. The organization for economic co-operation and development, OECD health data 2012—country notes. http://www.oecd.org/els/healthpoliciesanddata/oecdhealthdata2012-countrynotes.htm
3. F. Kart, G. Firat et al., A distributed e-healthcare system based on the service oriented architecture, in *Services Computing* (SCC, 2007), pp. 652–659 (2007)
4. B. Haynes, T.G. Weiser et al., A surgical safety checklist to reduce morbidity and mortality in a global population. New Engl. J. Med. **360**(5), 491–499 (2009)
5. M. Avinandan, J. McGinnis, E-healthcare: an analysis of key themes in research. Int. J. Pharma. Healthc. Market. **1**(4), 349–363 (2007)
6. M. Weiser, Some computer science issues in ubiquitous computing. Commun. ACM **36**(7), 75–84 (1993)
7. Y. Yamamoto, R. Huang, J. Ma, Medicine management and medicine taking assistance system for supporting elderly care at home, in *Aware Computing (ISAC)*, pp. 31–37 (2010)
8. T. Tamura, A. Sato, R. Huang, J. Ma, Recommendation engine based system towards creating a harmonious family living environment, in *2013 IEEE International Conference on Orange Technologies (ICOT)*, Tainan, Taiwan, Mar 12–16 (2013) (to be published)
9. N. Zhong, J. Ma, R. Huang et al., Research challenges and perspectives on wisdom web of things (W2T). J. Supercomput. **64**(3), 862–882 (2013). doi:10.1007/s11227-010-0518-8. Print ISSN 0920-8542, Online ISSN 1573-0484
10. G.Z. Yang, *Body Sensor Networks* (Springer, London, 2006)
11. Design world staff, Sensors advance medical and healthcare applications. http://www.designworldonline.com/sensors-advance-medical-and-healthcare-applications/
12. A. Gaddam, S.C. Mukhopadhyay, G.S. Gupta, Smart home for elderly care using optimized number of wireless sensors, in *4th International Conference on Computers and Devices for Communication, 2009, CODEC*, p. 14 (2009)
13. S. Parlak, A. Sarcevic, I. Marsic, R.S. Burd, Introducing RFID technology in dynamic and time-critical medical settings: requirements and challenges. J. Biomed. Inform. **45**(5), 958–974 (2012)
14. R. van der Togt, P.J.M. Bakker, M.W.M. Jaspers, A framework for performance and data quality assessment of Radio Frequency IDentification (RFID) systems in health care settings. J. Biomed. Inform. **44**(2), 372–383 (2011)
15. T. Teraoka, Organization and exploration of heterogeneous personal data collected in daily life. Human-centric Comput. Inf. Sci. **2**, 1 (2002)

16. F. Barigou, B. Atmani, B. Beldjilali, Using a cellular automaton to extract medical information from clinical reports. J. Inf. Process. **8**(1), 67–84 (2012)
17. J. Yao, R. Schmitz, S. Warren, A wearable point-of-care system for home use that incorporates plug-and-play and wireless standards. IEEE Trans. Inf. Technol. Biomed. **9**(3), 363–371 (2005)
18. F. Paganelli, D. Giuli, An ontology-based system for context-aware and configurable services to support home-based. IEEE Trans. Inf. Technol. Biomed. **15**(2), 324–333 (2011)
19. K. Sabine, Home telehealth—current state and future trends. Int. J. Med. Inform. **75**(8), 565–576 (2006)
20. R.G. Lee, C.C. Hsiao, C.C. Chen, H.M. Liu, A mobile-care system integrated with bluetooth blood pressure and pulse monitor, and cellular phone. IEICE Trans. Inf. Syst. 1 (E89-D), 1702–1711 (2006)
21. L.M. Kaufman, Data security in the world of cloud computing. IEEE Secur. Privacy **7**(4), 61–64 (2009)
22. A. Sitek, R.H. Huesman, G.T. Gullberg, Tomographic reconstruction using an adaptive tetrahedral mesh defined by a point cloud. IEEE Trans. Med. Imaging **25**(9), 1172–1179 (2006)
23. C.T. Lin, K.C. Chang, C.L. Lin, C.C. Chiang, S.W. Lu, S.S. Chang, B.C. Lin, H.Y. Liang, R.J. Chen, Y.T. Lee, L.W. Ko, An intelligent telecardiology system using a wearable and wireless EKG to detect atrial fibrillation. IEEE Trans. Inf. Technol. Biomed. **14**(3), 726–733 (2010)
24. Y. Gu, et al. A survey of indoor positioning systems for wireless personal networks. Commun. Surv. Tutorials IEEE **11**(1), 13–32 (2009)
25. K. Eleanna, K.W. Dickson, S.C. Cheung, K. Marina, Alerts in mobile healthcare applications: requirements and pilot study. IEEE Trans. Inf. Technol. Biomed. **8**(2), 173–181 (2004)
26. C.F. Juang, C.M. Chang, Human body posture classification by a neural fuzzy network and home care system application. IEEE Trans. Syst. Man Cybernet. Part A: Syst. Humans **37**(6), 984–994 (2007)
27. I. DSouza, et al., Real-time location systems for hospital emergency response. IT Prof. **13**(2), 37–43 (2011)
28. J.A. Fisher, T. Monahan, Tracking the social dimensions of RFID systems in hospitals. Int. J. Med. Inform. **77**(3), 176–183 (2008)
29. G. Gentili, et al. Dual-frequency active RFID solution for tracking patients in a children's hospital. Design method, test procedure, risk analysis, and technical solution. Proc. IEEE **98**(9), 1656–1662 (2010)
30. D.-H. Shih, H.-S. Chiang, B. Lin, S.-B. Lin, An embedded mobile ECG reasoning system for elderly patients. IEEE Trans. Inf. Technol. Biomed. **14**(3), 854–865 (2010)
31. M.B. Mollah, K.R. Islam, S.S. Islam, *Next Generation of Computing Through Cloud Computing Technology* (2012), p. 16
32. J. Ma, J. Wen, R. Huang et al., Cyber-individual meets brain informatics. IEEE Intell. Syst. **26**(5), 30–37 (2011)
33. R. Want, A. Hopper, V. Falcao, J. Gibbons, The active badge location system. ACM Trans. Inf. Syst. **10**(1), 91–102 (1992)
34. C.A. Thompson, Radio frequency tags for identifying legitimate drug products discussed by tech industry. Am. J. Health-Syst. Pharm. **16**(14), 1430–1431 (2004)
35. J.A. Fisher, T. Monahan, Tracking the social dimensions of RFID systems in hospitals. Int. J. Med. Inform. **77**, 176–183 (2008)
36. A. Ortony, G.L. Clore, A. Collins, *The Cognitive Structure of Emotions* (Cambridge University Press, Cambridge, UK, 1988)
37. Y. Gu, A. Lo, A survey of indoor positioning systems for wireless personal networks. IEEE Commun. Surv. Tutorials **11**(1), 13–32 (2009)
38. UP by Jawbone. http://store.apple.com/us/product/HA627LL/A/up-by-jawbone
39. Fitbit OneTM Wireless Activity Sleep Tracker. http://store.apple.com/us/product/HA523VC/A/fitbit-one-wireless-activity-sleep-tracker?fnode=76
40. S. Ventegodt, N.J. Andersen, J. Merrick, Holistic medicine III: the holistic process theory of healing. Sci. World J. **3**, 1138–1146 (2003)

41. J. Wen, et al., *Cyber-I: Vision of the Individual's Counterpart on Cyberspace, Dependable, Autonomic and Secure Computing* (DASC'09, 2009), pp. 295–302
42. J. Wen, J. Ma, R. Huang et al., A malicious behavior analysis based Cyber-I Birth. J. Intell. Manuf. **1–9** (2012)
43. O.P. Judson, The rise of the individual-based model in ecology. Trends Ecol. Evol. **9**(1), 9–14 (1994)
44. A model of human nature. http://eftsettings.com/chapters/model-of-human-nature
45. S. Yang, R. Huang, J. Ma, A computational personality-based and event-driven emotions model in PAD space, in *Sino-foreign-interchange Workshop on Intelligence Science & Intelligent Data Engineering*, Oct 15–17 (to be published LNCS, Springer, 2012)
46. A. Mehrabian, Analysis of the big-five personality factors in terms of the PAD temperament model. Aust. J. Psychol. **48**(2), 86–92 (1996)
47. J.H. Ma, R.H. Huang, Improving human interaction with a hyperworld, in *Proceedings of the Pacific Workshop on Distributed Multimedia Systems (DMS96)*, pp. 46–50 (1996)
48. Adam Jacobs, The Pathologies of Big Data. ACMQueue **6** (2009)
49. Y. Jadeja, K. Modi, Cloud Computing—Concepts, Architecture and Challenges (2012), pp. 877–880
50. J. Ma, Smart u-Things and ubiquitous intelligence, in *Proceedings of the 2nd International Conference on Embedded Software and Systems (ICESS 2005)*, p. 776 (2005)
51. Lo, S. Thiemjarus, A. Panousopoulou, G.Z. Yang, Bioinspired design for body sensor networks [Life Sciences]. IEEE Sign. Process. Mag. **30**(1), 165–170 (2013)
52. Y. Zhang and Y. Zhou, Transparent computing: a new paradigm for pervasive computing, in J. Ma, H. Jin, L.T. Yang, J.J.P. Tsai (eds.), *Ubiquitous Intelligence and Computing*, vol. 4159, Berlin, Heidelberg (Springer, Berlin Heidelberg, 2006), pp. 1–11
53. IBM, Getting cloud computing right—the key to business success in a cloud adoption is a robust, proven architecture. http://public.dhe.ibm.com/common/ssi/ecm/en/ciw03078usen/CIW03078USEN.PDF

Chapter 10
Hot Topic Detection in News Blog Based on W2T Methodology

Erzhong Zhou, Ning Zhong, Yuefeng Li and Jiajin Huang

Abstract A social event is often unlimitedly amplified and promptly spread in blogspace, and it is valuable to correctly detect blog hot topics for managing the cyberspace. Although hot topic detection techniques have a great improvement, it is more significant o find what determines the life span of a blog topic, because the online consensus brought by the topic unavoidably experiences the real life. The W2T (Wisdom Web of Things) methodology considers the information organization and management from the perspective of Web services, which contributes to a deep understanding of online phenomena such as users' behaviors and comments in e-commerce platforms and online social networks. This chapter first applies the W2T methodology to analyze the formation and evolution of a blog hot topic, and some influential factors which determine the development of the topic are identified to recognize hot topics. And then, the construction of a blog topic model considers information granularity in order to detect and track the evolution of the topic. Experimental results show that the proposed method for detecting the blog hot topic is feasible and effective.

E. Zhou · J. Huang
International WIC Institute, Beijing University of Technology,
Beijing 100124, China
e-mail: zez2008@emails.bjut.edu.cn

J. Huang
e-mail: hjj@emails.bjut.edu.cn

N. Zhong
Beijing Advanced Innovation Center for Future Internet Technology, The International WIC Institute, Beijing University of Technology, Beijing, China

N. Zhong (✉)
Department of Life Science and Informatics, Maebashi Institute of Technology,
460-1 Kamisadori-Cho, Maebashi 371-0816, Japan
e-mail: zhong@maebashi-it.ac.jp; zhongn@bjut.edu.cn

Y. Li
Faculty of Science and Technology, Queensland University of Technology,
Brisbane, QLD 4001, Australia
e-mail: y2.li@qut.edu.au

N. Zhong et al. (eds.), *Wisdom Web of Things*, Web Information Systems Engineering and Internet Technologies Book Series,
DOI 10.1007/978-3-319-44198-6_10

10.1 Introduction

The various kinds of social websites have constituted an important space for similar individuals to gather the strength, momentum and force. A blog is a typical platform for information share and communication. The hot topic and online consensus in blogspace are most valuable information for the business and social security. A Web hot topic is a topic that Web users pay more attention to or actively participate in. An online consensus is a representative online opinion that the majority of users own. When users have an agreement on a Web topic, the online consensus emerges.

How to provide the personalized service at the right time and place is a key issue in Web services. With the rapid development of Internet, Internet encounters an important carrier to store various information sources. As for the Internet of Things, it is essential to organize and manage the Web data for further knowing the different habits, characters and real demands of Web users. The W2T (Wisdom Web of Things) methodology is proposed to analyze and solve those problems oriented to the hyper world [29]. One of three key issues in W2T methodology is how to effectively combine the ideas of humans, networks and information granularity for problem solving in the hyper world [30]. As shown in Fig. 10.1, some definitions on the concepts related to W2T methodology are listed. The ideas of networks and information granularity simulate human information processing mechanism. For example, human beings often decrease the complexity of a task by separating the task into some subtasks. Hence, the granularity has a great impact on the effect of the problem solving. The arrangement of the related workflow is often based on relationships among subtasks. Hence, the idea of networks reflects the nature of a task.

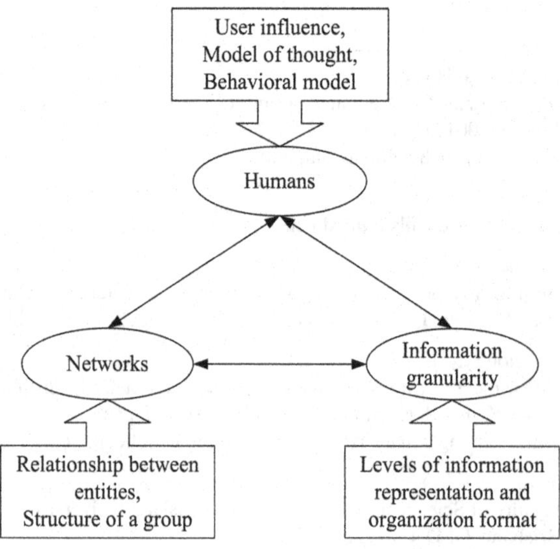

Fig. 10.1 Definitions on the ideas of humans, networks and information granularity

Text clustering algorithm [11, 12, 16] and hot word extraction [7, 15, 28] are often applied for online hot topic detection. The hot topic detection method based on text clustering first clusters the Web pages into different clusters that stand for different topics. Then user behavior record is extracted to evaluate the degree of user attention or participation for identifying hot topics. The hot topic detection method based on hot word extraction first counts the influence of each word according to its spatio-temporal feature, and hot topics are identified by hot word clustering. Although the methods mentioned above can be easily accomplished, they don't pay more attention to what on earth determines the formation or evolution of an online hot topic. Online topics are often derived from the real events that happened in the physical world or society world. It is valuable to detect the present online hot topics because of the unexpected feature of those real events. However, in comparison with the former, it is more important to predict the development of a topic to detect the forthcoming hot topic in advance. On the other hand, it is useful to study the characteristics of information diffusion in online network for observing the evolution of a hot topic. Some researchers found that the information diffusion is not only related to the structure of online social network and role of different codes, but also influenced by the external event [3, 10, 18]. Hence, it is necessary to take the human that creates and propagates information, networks that refer to external and internal conditions, and information granularity that reflects the form of information organization into consideration. The paper adopts the W2T methodology to identify the important factors that have a great impact on the formation or evolution of a blog topic in order to correctly detect hot topics. Meantime, the construction of a blog topic model considers information granularity in order to conveniently detect and track the evolution of the topic.

10.2 Problem Statements

The emergence of a hot topic in blogspace is strongly related to the user behavior and interests. As far as the user behavior is concerned, the behavior is liable to be influenced by surroundings and user mood. The change of the surrounding also influences the user interest. Hence, it is important to analyze the characteristics of blog topics that users frequently and recently comment on, and observe the information propagation in an online community by means of the W2T methodology.

10.2.1 Characteristics of a News Topic in Blogspace

The development of a topic is related to the characteristics of the related blog that attracts the special kind of users. Based on the norm of journalism, blogs can be categorized into three types according to the contents of blog posts, namely professional technique, individual life and temporal topics [19]. Topics in the professional blog mainly refer to professional techniques related information, but topics in the life blog are with respect to individual life affairs. Moreover, topics in the temporal blog are mainly related to news events. A news blog inherits the characteristics of the temporal topic blog. Compared with the professional blog topics, topics in the news blog often show burst and temporal features. Users visit different kinds of blogs with different motivations. For example, users share the specific knowledge and learn from each other in professional blogs. Users construct social networks or maintain their social contacts by means of individual life blogs. However, bloggers publish posts in news blogs with the purpose of revealing the truth of a news event or drawing other users' attention to the special event. Users with their own different backgrounds take part in topic interaction for the sake of knowing the truth of a news event or expressing their own personal feeling. The relationships among members in a topic group are weak because the group is mainly maintained by the user interest [23]. The topic group dissolves when users lose interests in the related topic. Hence, the user motivation determines the burst and temporal features of a news blog topic to a great extent.

10.2.2 Information Propagation in a Blog Community

A topic is the precondition that information communication arises from. There are two kinds of special text information during the information propagation. One is a post that reports an event related to a topic. The other is an emotional comment on the topic, namely, an online opinion. The focus on a topic during the information propagation often shifts from the event to the online opinion. Hence, a topic, opinion and user are three important entities for analyzing the information propagation in an online community.

The analysis of blogspace based on W2T methodology is shown in Fig. 10.2. Although the user is the most active entity in blogspace, a blog community which is composed of bloggers with similar interests is the main context for information propagation, and the characteristics of the community play an important role in the development and evolution of a hot topic. Hence, the analysis on the blog community from the perspective of the Web technique is useful to understand the process of information propagation in blogspace. The main characteristics of the blog community are as follows:

- The user is awarded more rights so that the decentration is the obvious phenomenon in the community.
- The open and anonymity policy makes users more active and braver in expressing their views.
- The quarrels between different groups often become more and more fierce, because there is no arbitrator.

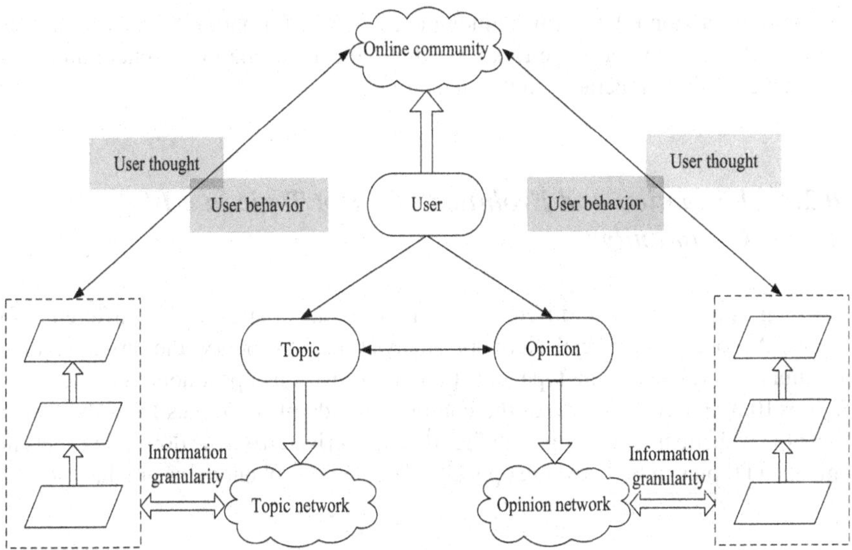

Fig. 10.2 Analysis of blogspace based on W2T methodology

- The structure of the blog community is dynamic. Users can publish their posts and comments within different time intervals, and freely join or quit the community according to their interests.

Users play the role of the information maker or transmitter. As far as the audience is concerned, the interest and confidence in the information transmitter determine if the audience can receive the information. If a topic is novel, interesting or disputable, and related to the personal life, users are more likely to be interested in the topic. On the other hand, if audiences have little social experience, they are easily susceptible to the guidance of media or community surroundings. As far as the information transmitter is concerned, the role of topical initiator often changes with the development of the given topic. Especially, the initiators have to rise to the challenges from opponents to maintain their legitimacy. The strength of the relationship between inner members also influences the process of information propagation. For example, when researchers take the blogosphere as a unit to observe the blog community, they find that the most communications among bloggers happen inside the group and the communication between groups seldom happens [6, 23]. Hence, the process of information propagation not only needs to carefully observe the evolution of the topic and related online opinions, but also needs to observe the changes of user roles.

As for the information, different topics pertain to different blogospheres, and users comment on the given topic in the given blogosphere. Hence, the process of information propagation can be observed from the equivalent topic network and opinion network. The topic network is composed of topics with different granularities and evolutionary relationships among topics. The opinion network is composed of opinions and interaction relationships among users. The information granularity stands for the different view or angle to know what happens in the blogosphere and why users have different reactions on the same topic.

10.2.3 Formation and Evolution of a Hot Topic in a Blog Community

The blog community has different structural characteristics within different life phases. According to Social Network Analysis (SNA) theory, the structure of a community is related to the type and strength of relationships among members [2]. Figures 10.3 and 10.4 show that the comment trends of hot topics from the China Sina blog website in 2011. Topics in Fig. 10.3 are derived from the domestic events in China, and topics in Fig. 10.4 are opposite. The obvious phenomena are that most of

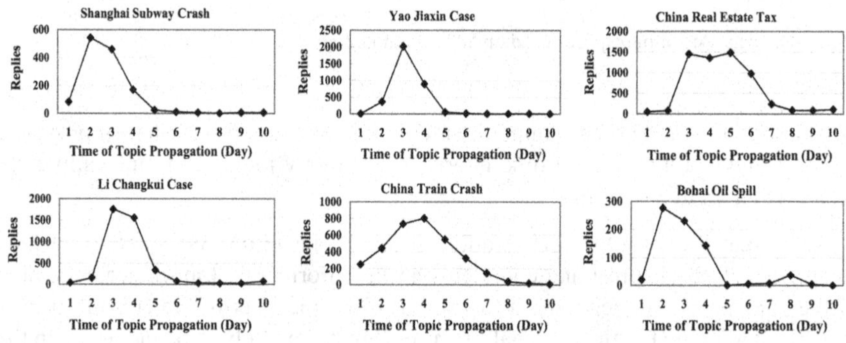

Fig. 10.3 Comment trends of the hot topics related to news events in China

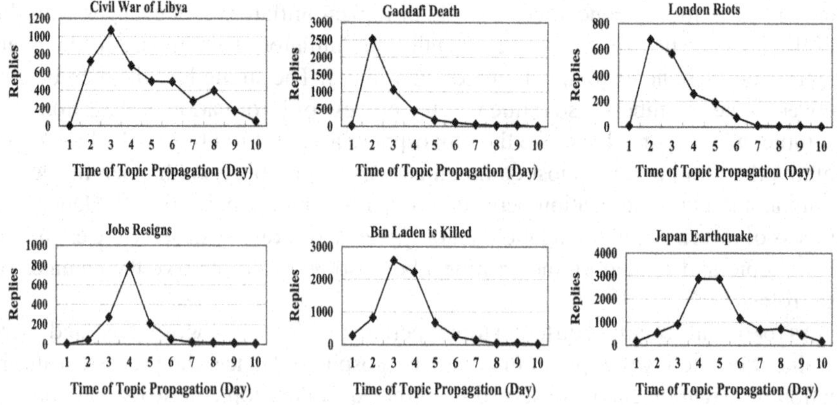

Fig. 10.4 Comment trends of the hot topics related to news events in other countries

the users are active in the early phase. The phenomena can be explained as follows. Users lack authoritative information and are very curious about the event in the early phase. Hence, the effect of sheep flock occurs in the community. When a public opinion comes into being, the spiral of silence emerges. Namely, users often keep silent when their opinions are in the minority. Moreover, the novelty of topics gets weaker and weaker with the lapse of time so that the behavior patterns of users have drastic changes. The structural change of a blog community can consequently reflect the development trend of a topic, and the behavior patterns of users also determine the burst and temporal features of blog topics. As far as the user role is concerned, users evolve into three categories, namely the opinion leader, active user and ordinary user. The opinion leader is influential during the evolution of a network opinion. An active user plays the role of a transmitter. However, the authority of such an active user is often weak in comparison with the opinion leader. Ordinary users often lurk after the public opinion emerges.

The change of the topic network also influences the development of a hot topic. Figures 10.5 and 10.6 show the distribution of 115 hot topics listed by Sina website in 2011 and 116 hot topics in 2012. Figure 10.5 shows that hot topics are unevenly distributed per month. Hence, the number of hot topics cannot be fixed. Figure 10.6 shows that the time interval between hot topics is very short. Hence, topics are competitive to attract other users' attention. Based on the analysis mentioned above, it is clear that the user behavior pattern, network opinion, opinion leader and timeliness determine the developmental trend or life of a blog topic.

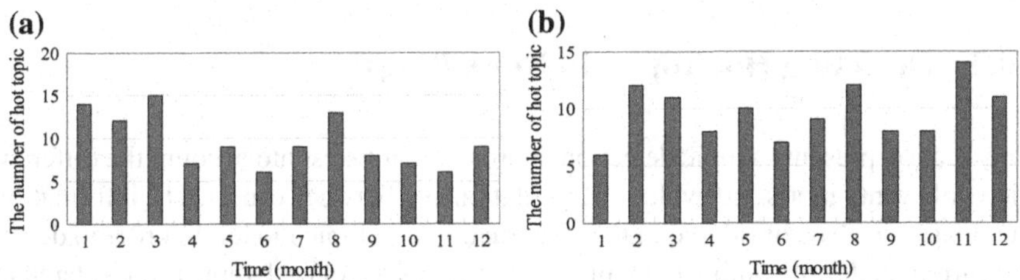

Fig. 10.5 Distribution of blog hot topics by the month in Sina websites. **a** 2011-1-1~2011-12-31. **b** 2012-1-1~2012-12-31

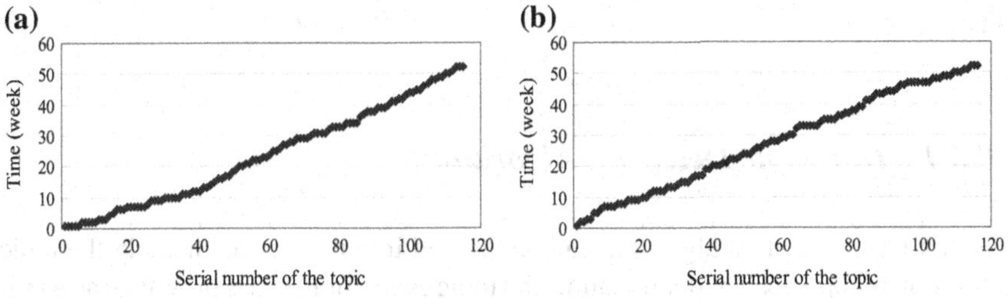

Fig. 10.6 Distribution of blog hot topics by the week in Sina websites. **a** 2011-1-1~2011-12-31. **b** 2012-1-1~2012-12-31

10.2.4 What Is an Opinion Leader?

A typical phenomenon during the evolution of network opinions is the emergence of opinion leaders. An opinion leader is the blog user who plays a crucial role in influencing opinion makings of other users. However, opinion leaders in blogspace are different from those in a physical community. The high popularity and recognition are the basic conditions of opinion leaders. At the same time, the ordinary users do not pay more attention to the opinion leader's social background in the physical world. Moreover, the diffusion speed of Web accelerates the formation of an opinion leader in blogspace. The burst feature of opinion leaders is very obvious in blogspace. According to the previous studies, the opinion leaders can be categorized into three types, namely fluctuant, long-term and transient opinion leaders [25, 27]. The fluctuant leader often changes his/her own personal role during the evolution of a network opinion. The long-term leader is active to participate in topic interaction in order to gain the better recognition and popularity. The transient opinion leaders often either voluntarily keep silent after they publish a special idea or passively lose the influence because of the opposition from surroundings. The publication number of high quality posts is a main difference between the long-term leader and the transient leader. The fluctuant leader is not interested in promoting the recognition and popularity in comparison with the long-term leader. For example, some public figures often take part in opinion interaction for controlling the moods of other users when network opinions are in issue.

10.3 Detecting Hot Topics in News Blogs

This section presents a topic detection approach that takes into account the different views of event reports and evolutionary relationship between events. The information granularity is also considered in the construction of a topic model. In order to detect the current and forthcoming hot topics, the growth state of each topic is considered in addition to user interests because the growth state not only indicates the development trend of the topic but also represents the vitality of topics. The topic is consequently evaluated by measuring the duration, topical novelty, attention degree of users and topical growth.

10.3.1 Hot Topic Detection Algorithm

The hot topic detection algorithm can be divided into three parts, namely the topic detection, opinion leader identification and topic evaluation, and is presented as Algorithm 2. The part corresponding to the blog topic detection is introduced from Steps 1–13 in Algorithm 2. The part corresponding to the opinion leader identification is described from Steps 14−17, and the rest of Algorithm 2 is oriented to the topic evaluation. The following three sections respectively detail the corresponding part.

Algorithm 2 Hot Topic Detection

Require: S is a post set, n is the number of time units, d is the threshold of topic evaluation.
Ensure: T_{set} is a hot topic set.
1. **for** each post i in S **do**
2.   Extract keywords from i;
3.   Construct the subtopic model of i;
4. **end for**
5. **for** time unit $j = 0$ to n **do**
6.   Identify the posts related to the event according to correlated keywords;
7.   Construct the event models based on single pass clustering algorithm;
8.   Add the event models into event list EL_j within j;
9.   **if** j is equal to 1 **then**
10.   Construct the topic models within j manually;
11.   **else**
12.   Construct a new topic model or update the previous topic model according to the related event model in EL_j;
13.   **end if**
14.   Analyze the structure of the community based on interaction relationships among users;
15.   Detect network opinions on each topic according to the topic models;
16.   Construct the opinion network within j on the basis of the blog community;
17.   Identify opinion leaders with respect to each topic;
18.   Count the changes of repliers, opinion leaders, replies and network opinions to measure the growth state of each topic within j;
19.   Evaluate all topics within j by measuring the duration, topical novelty, attention degree of users and topical growth;
20.   Select the topics whose value is more than d, and add new hot topics are into T_{set};
21. **end for**
22. Return T_{set}.

10.3.2 Topic Model Construction

As shown in Fig. 10.7, users can comment on one topic from different aspects and publish posts with different writing styles because of personalized management. Hence, a blog topic model represents multi-view or multi-center features in terms of temporal distributions of the topic. At the same time, the topic model represents multi-level features in terms of spatial distributions of the topic.

Considering information granularity in the semantic expression, a topic can be considered to be a cluster that is comprised of related events, and an event can be considered to be a cluster that is comprised of related subtopics. As for the literal expression of a subtopic, the subtopic can be expressed by a group of related keywords. Hence, as shown in Fig. 10.8, the topic can be divided into three layers. The models in three layers are as follows:

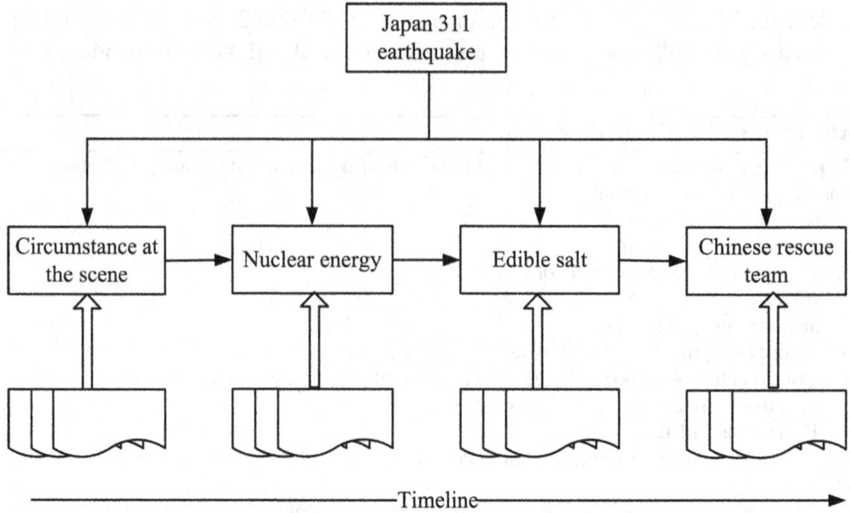

Fig. 10.7 Shift process of topical center

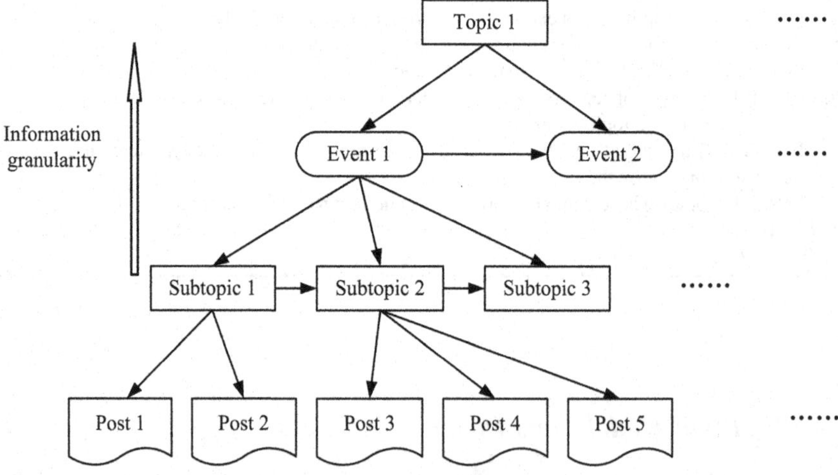

Fig. 10.8 Construction of a topic model based on information granularity

- A subtopic model is defined as $Subtopic_i = \{Keyword_1, Keyword_2, \ldots, Keyword_s\}$, where $Subtopic_i$ denotes the ith subtopic, $Keyword_i$ denotes the ith keyword of a post;
- An event model is defined as $Event_i = \{(Subtopic_1, wt_1), (Subtopic_2, wt_2), \ldots, (Subtopic_m, wt_m)\}$, where $Event_i$ denotes the ith event, wt_m is the weight of the mth subtopic with respect to the ith event;
- A topic model is defined as $Topic_i = \{Event_1, Event_2, \ldots, Event_n\}$, where $topic_i$ denotes the ith topic.

10.3.3 Topic Detection Based on the View of Event Reports

The event model is the key to constructing the topic model. News topic detection methods often rely on some studies of event detection and tracking. Two important tasks for the construction of a blog topic model are listed. One is how to arrange post themes (subtopics) with different information granularities to extract a news event. The other is how to track a news event by identifying the evolutionary relationship between events. The single pass clustering algorithm is widely used in event detection and tracking [8]. The topic detection based on the view of event reports first adopts the single pass clustering algorithm to extract the events which occur in a given time interval. Then the evolutionary relationship between events is identified by computing the content similarity between events and distribution of each event on different topics. At last, the topic model is created or updated by detecting the new event and tracking the previous event. The topic detection based on the view of event reports copes with the posts that are in the chronological order and refines different topic models.

10.3.3.1 Keyword Extraction and Keyword Correlation

A keyword is a basic element for the topic model. Nouns and verbs are selected from the title and the first paragraph of a blog post. Tags of a post are also picked as keywords. The keyword is identified according to the weight of the word. The weight of a word is evaluated by the following equation in the Term Frequency Inverse Document Frequency (TFIDF) method [20]:

$$Weight(t_k, r) = TF(t_k, r) * \log(\frac{N}{N_k + 0.5}) \tag{10.1}$$

where r is a blog post, t_k is a word, $Weight(t_k, r)$ is the weight of t_k in r, $TF(t_k, r)$ is the frequency of t_k in the text of r, N is the number of blog posts, and N_k is the number of blog posts where t_k appears.

In order to increase the precision of the single pass clustering algorithm, an information retrieval strategy is adopted to filter irrelevant posts in advance. Namely, the posts related to a special event are retrieved by the correlated keywords which can describe the event. If a keyword set includes at least two keywords, each possible keyword pair is extracted at random for the post retrieval. If users frequently publish and comment on an event, some keywords are highly correlated within a given time interval. The chi-square test that is successfully used to measure the correlation between keywords is presented as follows [4]:

$$\chi^2 = \frac{(E(uv) - A(uv))^2}{E(uv)} + \frac{(E(\bar{u}v) - A(\bar{u}v))^2}{E(\bar{u}v)} + \frac{(E(u\bar{v}) - A(u\bar{v}))^2}{E(u\bar{v})} + \frac{(E(\bar{u}\bar{v}) - A(\bar{u}\bar{v}))^2}{E(\bar{u}\bar{v})} \tag{10.2}$$

$$E(uv) = \frac{A(u) * A(v)}{N} \tag{10.3}$$

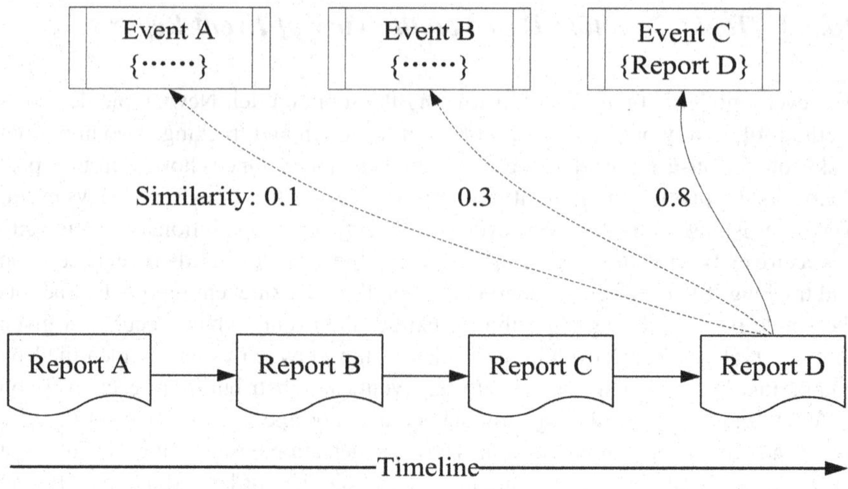

Fig. 10.9 Principle of single pass clustering algorithm

where $A(u)$ is the number of the posts which word u appears in, $A(\bar{u})$ is the number of the posts which word u does not appear in, $A(uv)$ is the number of the posts which both words u and v appear in, and N is the total number of posts.

10.3.3.2 Post Clustering

As shown in Fig. 10.9, the single pass clustering algorithm can be explained as follows. A report is merged into an event if the content similarity between two reports is above a threshold. Otherwise, the report is considered to be the first report of a new event. A post can be represented by its subtopic model, and the similarity between posts is consequently based on the similarity between subtopic models. However, different users often lay emphasis on different episodes or event attributions of a news event. Moreover, subtopic models abstracted from different posts can own different event attributions. Sometimes, one subtopic model can be a subset of the other subtopic model in terms of event attributes. Hence, the intersection of subtopic models is essential to compare the similarity between subtopic models. On the other hand, the size of a subtopic model has a great impact on the intersection of two subtopic models. When the size of one subtopic model is small, the intersection of two subtopic models is also small even if one subtopic model is the subset of the other one. As for that phenomenon, the minimum of two subtopic models is also taken into account. In order to correctly compare the similarity between subtopic models, the following equation based on the Jaccard coefficient [13, 24] is used:

$$Sim(d_i, d_j) = \alpha * \frac{|d_i \cap d_j|}{|d_i \cup d_j|} + \beta * \frac{|d_i \cap d_j|}{min(|d_i|, |d_j|)} \quad (10.4)$$

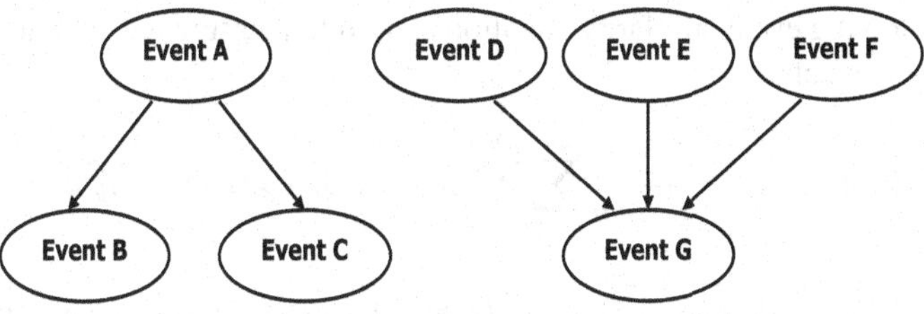

Fig. 10.10 Evolutionary relationship between events

where d_j denotes the keyword set of the jth subtopic, $Sim(d_i, d_j)$ is the similarity between the ith and the jth subtopics, $d_i \cap d_j$ is the intersection of sets d_i and d_j, $d_i \cup d_j$ is the union of sets d_i and d_j, $|d_i|$ is the size of set d_i, α and β are coefficients, and $min(y, z)$ is the minimum between y and z.

10.3.3.3 Identification of the Evolutionary Relationship Between Events

As shown in Fig. 10.10, one event may evolve into other events. The attributes of events sometimes change a lot so that the evolutionary relationship between events needs carefully considering. However, time is the key to the identification of the evolutionary relationship between events. If two events occur very closely and the content similarity between them is high, the events are likely to be correlated with each other. Moreover, if most of the similar events which occur before the target event belong to the same topic, the target event may evolve from those related events. On the other hand, the life spans of topics are different, and the length of the time span can influence the integrity of an event model. Hence, the evolutionary relationship between two events is identified by the following process:

1. The topic model $Topic_k$ which the original event $Event_i$ belongs to is identified;
2. The similarity event set $S_{ij}(i \neq j)$ within the former time unit is constructed for the target event $Event_j(j \neq i)$ according to the content similarity between events;
3. If S_{ij} is not empty and most of the events in S_{ij} belong to $Topic_k$, there exists an evolutionary relationship between $Event_i$ and $Event_j$;
4. If S_{ij} is empty, the similarity event set S'_{ij} in which similar events for $Event_j$ occur within the current time unit and are earlier than $Event_j$ is constructed;
5. The same strategy stated above for S'_{ij} is adopted.

If there is only one similar event for the target event and the content similarity is very high, the two events are considered to be the same event.

According to the definition of the event model, the subtopic model is the basis of the event model. Hence, the comparison of content similarity between events means that the related subtopic models need comparing. When two events are compared, each subtopic in one event model is compared with that in the other event model, and the following event similarity equation is used to measure the content similarity between two events:

$$Comp(e_i, e_j) = \frac{1}{cn * cm} \sum_{p=1}^{cn} \sum_{q=1}^{cm} Sim(d_{ip}, d_{jq}) * (wt_{ip} * wt_{jq}) \tag{10.5}$$

where $Comp(e_i, e_j)$ denotes the similarity between events e_i and e_j, cn is the number of the subtopics that belong to event e_i, cm is the number of the subtopics that belong to event e_j, d_{ip} denotes the pth subtopic of event e_i, d_{jq} denotes the qth subtopic of event e_j, wt_{ip} denotes the weight of the pth subtopic with respect to event e_i, and wt_{jq} denotes the weight of the qth subtopic with respect to event e_j. The weight of a given subtopic with respect to the related event is measured by the following equation:

$$WT(x) = \sum_{i=1}^{n} e^{-\Delta t_i(x)} \tag{10.6}$$

where x denotes one subtopic with respect to a given event, i denotes the ith subtopic that belongs to x, n is the number of subtopics that compose x, and $\Delta t_i(x)$ is the time distance between the date when the ith subtopic published and the current time.

10.3.4 Identification of Opinion Leaders

The identification of opinion leaders is important in evaluating the developmental trend of a blog topic. As for opinion leaders, the high popularity is beneficial to spread personal opinion and enhance the recognition. In order to gain the high popularity, a blog user has to actively take part in topic interaction. Individual popularity is often assessed according to user behavior pattern and position in the social network [1, 5]. As far as the structure of the social network is concerned, opinion leaders have a larger central degree than other users because the leaders have a group of followers. If one user has high recognition, his/her opinion can be widely accepted by other users and related posts are also widely cited. In order to gain the high recognition, the user must often publish high quality posts. Individual recognition is often assessed according to the user influence on neighbors [17]. The influence of a user on network opinions can be measured by counting the sentiment polarity distribution of neighbors' opinions and the quotation number of posts. Hence, if a user is active and famous in a community, owns many high quality posts, and holds the representative opinion, the user is more likely to be an opinion leader.

The degree of user participation, position in a social network, influence on neighbors' opinions and the number of high quality posts are used to recognize the opinion leader. Moreover, the user role during the evolution of network opinions needs carefully analyzing because the status of opinion leaders may be not stable. The influence evaluation equation for identifying the opinion leader is defined as follows:

$$Opind_n(b,x) = \sum_{i=1}^{n} \frac{nop_i(b,x)}{Tnop_i(x)} * (\psi * cen_i(b) + \varphi * \frac{nos_i(b,x)}{Tnos_i(x)} + \delta * \frac{bp_i(b,x)}{Tp_i(x)}) \tag{10.7}$$

where $Opind_n(b,x)$ is the influence of user b with respect to topic x within the nth time unit, i denotes the ith time unit, $nop_i(b,x)$ is the number of the opinions that user b publishes with respect to topic x within the ith time unit, $Tnop_i(x)$ is the total number of the opinions that all users publish with respect to topic x within the ith time unit, $cen_i(b)$ is the central degree of user b in the social network within the ith time unit, $nos_i(b,x)$ is the number of the users who have the same opinion as user b within the ith time unit, $Tnos_i(x)$ is the total number of the users who publish their opinions on topic x within the ith time unit, $bp_i(b,x)$ is the number of the high quality posts that user b publishes with respect to topic x within the ith time unit, $Tp_i(x)$ is the total number of the posts that all users publish with respect to topic x within the ith time unit, φ is the emotion coefficient, ψ is the location coefficient, and δ is the quotation coefficient.

10.3.5 Topic Evaluation

The interest degree of users and development trend of a topic are measured for detecting a hot topic. As far as user interests are concerned, the context of topic propagation can stimulate users to participate in the topic interaction. If a topic spreads a long time, the topic can have a great probability to attract users. If a topic is very new, the blog user is more likely to be interested in the topic. If the posts related to a topic have high quotation or a great number of replies, the topic is popular with users. Hence, if a topic meets all conditions mentioned above, user interests in the topic are undoubtedly high. User interests in a topic are consequently evaluated by measuring the duration of the topic, topical novelty and attention degree of users.

The changes of user replies or the number of users are the most direct representations for the vitality of a blog topic. However, it is difficult to discriminate between the growth and maturity phases according to those changes. Opinion leaders grow up in the growth phase, and really play a vital role in the maturity phase. If most opinion leaders quit the topic interaction in the maturity phase, the topic is likely to fade. Moreover, the emergence of a public opinion is an important signal for the development trend of a blog topic. If a previous public opinion is proven to be wrong by the authority, the short dormancy of a blog topic is over and the topic is likely to thrive again. As a result, the changes in the number of opinion leaders and network opinions can also contribute to measuring the development trend of a blog topic. The paper consequently integrates the above four factors that play a vital role in different phases to measure the development trend of the topic. When opinions are counted, repetitive opinions of which the same user publishes are ignored.

The topical growth can be evaluated by using the following equation:

$$Growth(x) = (\mu_1 * \sum_{i=1}^{n} f(m_i) + \mu_2 * \sum_{i=1}^{n} f(l_i) + \mu_3 * \sum_{i=1}^{n} f(c_i) + \mu_4 * \sum_{i=1}^{n} f(s_i)) * \frac{1}{n} \quad (10.8)$$

$$f(p_i) = \begin{cases} 1, & i = 1 \\ norm(\frac{p_i}{p_{i-1}+0.1}), & i > 1 \end{cases} \quad (10.9)$$

$$norm(y) = \begin{cases} 1, & y \geq 1 \\ y, & otherwise \end{cases} \quad (10.10)$$

$$\mu_1 + \mu_2 + \mu_3 + \mu_4 = 1 \quad (10.11)$$

where $Growth(x)$ is the growth degree of topic x, m_i is the number of repliers of topic x within the ith time unit, l_i is the number of opinion leaders of topic x within the ith time unit, c_i is the number of replies to topic x within the ith time unit, s_i is the number of opinions on topic x within the ith time unit, n is the total number of time units, μ_1 is the growth coefficient of a user, μ_2 is the growth coefficient of an opinion leader, μ_3 is the growth coefficient of a reply, and μ_4 is the growth coefficient of an opinion. The growth degree of a topic varies from 0.0 to 1.0, and the topic is at the maturity phase if the value is close to 1.

The topic is evaluated by using the following equation [31]:

$$Hotness(x) = \frac{cu}{n} * Growth(x) * (\lambda * sc(x) + \xi * qu(x)) * \Delta t(x)^{-k} \quad (10.12)$$

where $Hotness(x)$ denotes the evaluation value of topic x, n is the total number of time units, cu is the number of the consecutive time units in which topic x occurs, $Growth(x)$ is the growth degree of topic x, $sc(x)$ is the total number of replies to topic x, $qu(x)$ is the quotation number of the posts that belong to topic x, $\Delta t(x)$ is the time difference between the publication date of topic x and the current time, k is the decay coefficient, λ is the comment coefficient, and ξ is the quotation coefficient of a post.

10.4 Experiments and Discussions

Experiments are performed in order to validate the feasibility and effectiveness of the proposed method. At the same time, the influence of opinion leaders on topic propagation as well as their features is analyzed. The test sample set includes the 1520 posts and 202290 related replies published at the China Sina blog website. The publication dates of the test samples are between November 9, 2011 and January 18, 2012. The training sample set includes 17910 plain texts for the keyword extraction from the China Sogou laboratory [22], 14317 Web comments for the sentiment analysis, and the 12 blog hot topics that are listed at the China Sina blog website in 2011 and refer to the society, politics and economy [21]. The software ICTCLAS is applied for Chinese word segmentation [14]. In order to improve the precision of the named entity recognition of ICTCLAS, a user dictionary is constructed according to the tags of posts manually because such tags can be successfully used to detect the bursty event [26].

10.4.1 Performance of the Proposed Method

In order to validate the performance of the proposed method, three experiments were carried out. Experiment 1 evaluates the topic on the basis of the proposed method, but not takes the degree of topical growth into account. Experiment 2 uses the proposed method to evaluate the topic. Experiment 3 adopts the hot topic detection method based on the agglomerative hierarchical clustering algorithm [9], and the topic is evaluated by counting the total number of posts and replies. In order to select optimum parameters for the performance of the proposed method, the influence of parameter regulation on the performance is observed at first. As shown in Fig. 10.11, the comment coefficient λ is set as 0.1 and the quotation coefficient ξ is set as 0.5. As shown in Fig. 10.12, the performance of the proposed method is good.

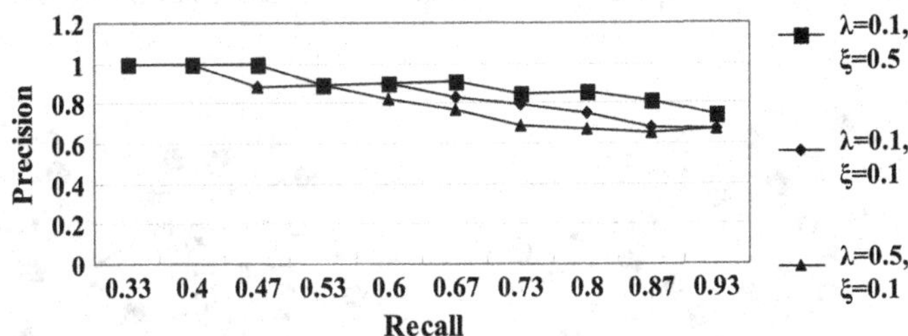

Fig. 10.11 Results of the proposed method under different parameters

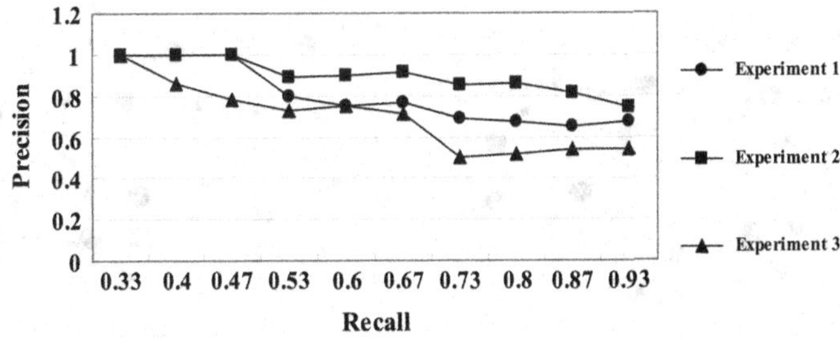

Fig. 10.12 Performance comparison of three experiments

The agglomerative hierarchical clustering algorithm is based on the vector space model, and most blog posts are not normalized so that the accuracy of the topic detection method based on the agglomerative hierarchical clustering algorithm is low. However, the topic detection based on the view of event reports focuses on keywords of a post. Hence, the posts that are not normalized do not cause a great impact on the proposed method. Moreover, the precision of hot topic detection is improved by measuring the growth state of a blog topic. On the other hand, the topics recommended at the blog website are all detected in three experiments. Hence, the influence of the blog service provider on topic propagation cannot be ignored. In other words, the reports of related media can direct the development trend of an online hot topic.

10.4.2 Analysis on the Features of Opinion Leaders

Famous bloggers in a given domain often have a number of followers and more advantages than ordinary users. In order to identify if the famous blogger is an opinion leader or not, an experiment is carried out by using the 1406 famous bloggers from 14 domains picked at the Sina blog website, and the opinion leaders who appear in the training sample set are identified by using the influence evaluation equation. The behavior of opinion leaders and famous bloggers in different time intervals are observed. Figure 10.13 represents the behavior patterns of opinion leaders and famous bloggers during the development of the topic related to the news that Bin Laden is

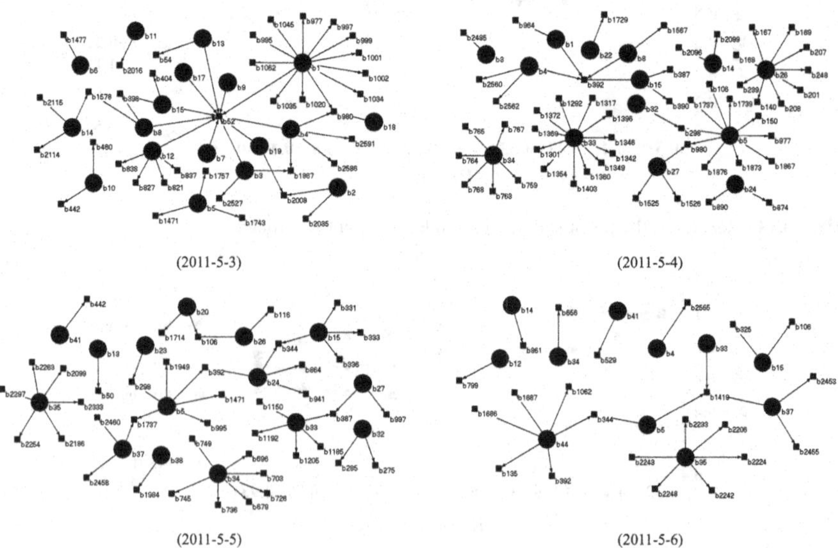

Fig. 10.13 Interaction among opinion leaders and famous bloggers within different time intervals

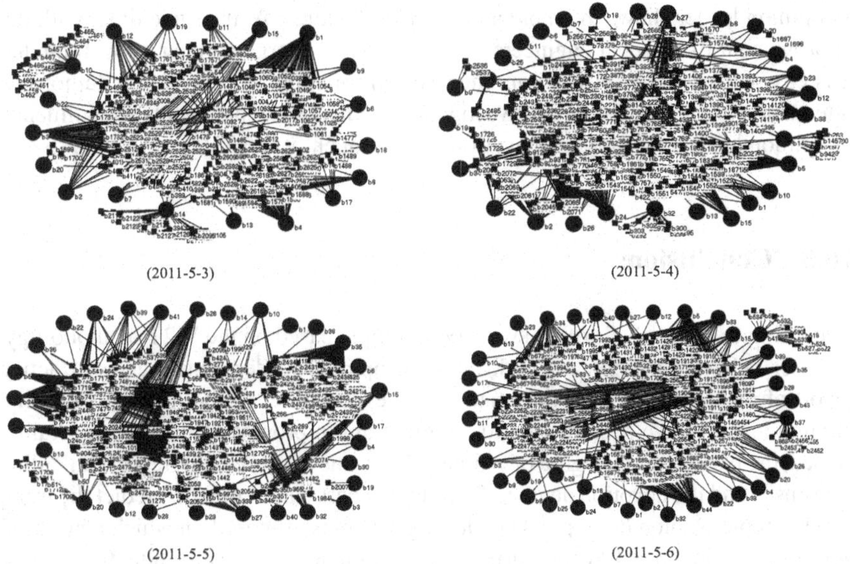

Fig. 10.14 Propagation process of the hot topic related to the news that Bin Laden is killed

killed, and the social networks in different time intervals are constructed on the basis of the interaction relationships among opinion leaders and famous bloggers. Circle nodes in the social network stand for the opinion leaders within the current time interval. Rectangle nodes stand for the famous bloggers or previous opinion leaders, and an arrow points to a responder. Those experimental results show that long-term opinion leaders are in the minority in comparison with other kinds of opinion leaders. The famous blogger in a given domain is not always an opinion leader. Opinion leaders prefer to influence other users by means of a blog post because they seldom take part in opinion interaction in other blogs. In order to analyze the influence of an opinion leader during the topic propagation, topic propagation networks within different time intervals are constructed. The information propagator who publishes the origin report and plays the role of an opinion leader in the current phase or in the previous phase is labeled in the form of a circle node, and a rectangle node stands for an information receiver in the network. The quotation of a blog post is represented as an edge between the propagator and the receiver. Figure 10.14 shows the propagation process of the topic related to the news that bin laden is killed, and the post quotation of each propagator shows a downward trend. According to the experimental results, the influence of opinion leaders during the topic propagation gradually becomes weak. Hence, opinion leaders must capture the latest information and publish sharp remarks to keep their status.

The reasons for above phenomena can be explained as follows. The real identities of bloggers are ignored so that the credibility of information is based on the reasonable explanation and the development status of the related event. Hence, the formation of an opinion leader shows the rapid and unstable features. At the same time, with the improvement of retrieval engineers and attention of a large number of Web media, it is easy for users to know comprehensive information. Moreover, the authorities often actively publish the latest investigation results on the hot event. The influence of opinion leaders on topic propagation is consequently weak.

10.5 Conclusions

According to the analysis of a news blog hot topic based on the W2T methodology, the user behavior pattern, network opinion, opinion leader, timeliness and active report of media impact on the formation and evolution of the hot topic. Especially, opinion leaders have been proven to be important in promoting the topical vitality. Hence, the participation degree of ordinary users, the development trend of an online consensus and the devotion degree of opinion leaders can be used to predict the trend of a hot topic. A blog hot topic detection algorithm is proposed, in which news blog hot topics are identified by measuring the duration, topical novelty, attention degree of users and topical growth.

Experimental results show that the proposed method is feasible and effective. However, the behavior patterns of different users in blogspace need to be further studied in future, and the theories of sociology or psychology can be adopted to understand the user behavior. At the same time, the user personality also needs to be well analyzed because the user behavior reflects his/her own need and interest. Moreover, the information is reprocessed and refined by users during the information propagation. If such information is extracted according to the human information processing mechanism, the problem solving strategy may be more effective and efficient. In future, our research will pay more attention to the latest investigation on the social contact patterns in blogspace.

Acknowledgments The study was supported by National Natural Science Foundation of China (61272345).

References

1. L. Akritidis, D. Katsaros, P. Bozanis, Identifying the productive and influential bloggers in a community. IEEE Trans. Syst. Man Cybern. **41**(5), 759–764 (2011)
2. K. Andreas, A. Henning, S. Varinder, Social activity and structural centrality in online social networks. Telematics Inform. **32**(2), 321–332 (2015)
3. E. Bakshy, B. Karrer, B.L.A. Adamic, Social influence and the diffusion of user-created content, in *Proceedings of the 2009 ACM Conference on Electronic Commerce* (2009), pp. 325–334
4. N. Bansal, F. Chiang, N. Koudas, et al., Seeking stable clusters in the blogosphere, in *Proceedings of the Thirty-Third International Conference on Very Large Data Bases* (2007), pp. 806–817

5. F. Bodendorf, C. Kaiser, Detecting opinion leaders and trends in online social networks, in *Proceedings of the Fourth International Conference on Digital Society* (2010), pp. 124–129
6. Y.Z. Cao, P.J. Shao, L.Q. Li, Topic propagation model based on diffusion threshold in blog networks, in *Proceedings of 2011 International Conference on Business Computing and Global Information* (2011), pp. 539–542
7. K.Y. Chen, L. Luesukprasert, S.C.T. Chou, Hot topic extraction based on timeline analysis and multidimensional sentence modeling. IEEE Trans. Knowl. Data Eng. **19**(8), 1016–1025 (2007)
8. C.C. Chen, Y.T. Chen, M.C. Chen, An aging theory for event life-cycle modeling. IEEE Trans. Syst. Man Cybern. **37**(2), 237–248 (2007)
9. X.Y. Dai, Q.C. Chen, X.L. Wang et al., Online topic detection and tracking of financial news based on hierarchical clustering, in *Proceedings of the Ninth International Conference on Machine Learning and Cybernetics*, vol. 6 (2010), pp. 3341–3346
10. M. Gomez-Rodriguez, J. Leskovec, A. Krause, Inferring networks of diffusion and influence, in *Proceedings of the 16th ACM SIGKDD International Conference on Knowledge Discovery and Data* (2010), pp. 1019–1028
11. H.J. Gong, *Research on Automatic Network Hot Topics Detection* (Central china normal university, Wuhan, 2008)
12. T.T. He, G.Z. Qu, S.W. Li, et al., Semi-automatic hot event detection, in *Proceedings of the Second International Conference on Advanced Data Mining and Applications* (2006), pp. 1008–1016
13. H.H. Huang, Y.H. Kuo, Cross-lingual document representation and semantic similarity measure a fuzzy set and rough set based approach. IEEE Trans. Fuzzy Syst. **18**(6), 1098–1111 (2010)
14. ICTCLAS. Home page: http://ictclas.org/
15. H. Li, J.F. Wei, Netnews bursty hot topic detection based on burtsy features, in *Proceedings of the International Conference on e-Business and e-Government* (2010), pp. 1437–1440
16. N. Li, D.D. Wu, Using text mining and sentimen analysis for online forums hotspot detection and forecast. Decis. Support Syst. **48**(2), 354–368 (2010)
17. S.H. Lim, S.W. Kim, S.J. Park, J.H. Lee, Determining content power users in a blog network: an approach and its applications. IEEE Trans. Syst. Man Cybern. **41**(5), 853–862 (2011)
18. S.A. Myers, C.G. Zhu, J. Leskovec, Information diffusion and external influence in networks, in *Proceedings of the 18th ACM SIGKDD International Conference on Knowledge Discovery and Data Mining* (2012), pp. 33–41
19. H.M. Qiu, *The Social Network Analysis of Blogosphere* (Harbin institute of technology, Harbin, 2007)
20. G. Salton, C. Buckley, Term-weighting approaches in automatic text retrieval. Inf. Process. Manage. **24**(5), 513–523 (1988)
21. Sina Blog Website. Home page: http://blog.sina.com.cn/
22. Sogou Laboratory. Home page: http://www.sogou.com/labs/dl/c.html
23. W.J. Sun, H.M. Qiu, A social network analysis on blogospheres, in *Proceedings of 2008 International Conference on Management Science and Engineering* (2008), pp. 1769–1773
24. J.H. Wang, Web-based verification on the representativeness of terms extracted from single short documents, in *Proceedings of 2011 IEEE/WIC/ACM International Conferences on Web Intelligence and Intelligent Agent Technology*, vol. 3 (2011), pp. 114–117
25. G.H. Xie, *The Research on the System of the Affect of Internet Opinion Leaders* (Central China normal university, Wuhan, 2011)
26. J.J. Yao, B. Cui, Y.X. Huang, Bursty event detection from collaborative tags. World Wide Web **15**(2), 171–195 (2012)
27. H. Yu, *Research on the Opinion Leaders of Political BBS: An Case Study on Sino-Japan BBS of Strong Nation Forum* (Huazhong university of science and technology, Wuhan, 2007)
28. Z.F. Zhang, Q.D. Li, QuestionHolic: hot topic discovery and trend analysis in community question answering sytems. Expert Syst. Appl. **38**(6), 6848–6855 (2011)
29. N. Zhong, J.H. Ma, R.H. Huang et al., Research challenges and perspectives on Wisdom Web of Things (W2T). J. Supercomput. **64**(3), 862–882 (2010)

30. N. Zhong, J.M. Bradshaw, J.M. Liu et al., Brain informatics. IEEE Intell. Syst. **26**(5), 16–21 (2011)
31. E.Z. Zhou, N. Ning, Y.F. Li, Extracting news blog hot topics based on the W2T methodology. World Wide Web (2014). doi:10.1007/s11280-013-0207-7

Part III
Wisdom Web of Things and Technologies

Chapter 11
Attention Inspired Resource Allocation for Heterogeneous Sensors in Internet of Things

Huansheng Ning, Hong Liu, Ali Li and Laurence T. Yang

Abstract Internet of things (IoT) is an attractive paradigm for intelligent interconnections among ubiquitous things through physical-cyber-social space (CPSS). During the things' cross-space interactions, heterogeneous sensors establish pervasive sensing during with the mapping from physical objects into the corresponding cyber entities in the cyber space. Such mapping depends on the available system resources, and thus resource allocation becomes challenging for resource-constrained IoT applications. In this chapter, human attention (including sustained attention, selective attention, and divided attention) is considered as limited cognitive resource to establish an attention-aware resource framework in IoT. The consideration of a heterogeneous sensors based IoT system model is built with ubiquitous attributes, and a human attention inspired resource allocation scheme is presented to facilitate the dynamic resource interaction.

11.1 Introduction

Internet of Things (IoT) as a trend of future network paradigm covers the integration of ubiquitous sensing, networking, and intelligent management technologies to enhance cyber-physical interconnections among things [1, 2]. IoT is evolving towards a big database with more human cognition and wisdom, and such complicated system confronts challenging issues that terminal components usually interact

H. Ning (✉) · A. Li
University of Science and Technology Beijing, Beijing, China
e-mail: ninghuansheng@ustb.edu.cn

H. Liu
Engineering Laboratory, Run Technologies Co., Ltd. Beijing, Beijing, China

L.T. Yang
Huazhong University of Science and Technology, Wuhan, China

L.T. Yang
St. Francis Xavier University, Antigonish, Canada

N. Zhong et al. (eds.), *Wisdom Web of Things*, Web Information Systems Engineering and Internet Technologies Book Series,
DOI 10.1007/978-3-319-44198-6_11

in resource-constrained environments. It is significant to present advanced resource strategies according to the practical application requirements.

In IoT, several novel works have been studied to address IoT issues in the perspective of imitating human and society. U2IoT (Unit IoT and Ubiquitous IoT) architecture was proposed based on manlike nervous architecture and social organization [3]. For realizing the ubiquitous intelligence, cyber-individual (Cyber-I) and brain informatics were proposed to describe the holistic wisdom considering the harmonious symbiosis of human and things [4, 5]. A social Internet of Things (SIoT) introduced social relationships among things to enhance the capability of human and devices to discover, select, and exploit things and services [6]. Towards the resource issues in IoT, existing resource solutions mainly focus on the top architecture design and traditional algorithm redesigning, referring to the online resource management [7], constrained resource allocation [8], distributed resource sharing [9], and bio-inspired resource saving [10] IoT resource research is still in its infancy, and unique insights become necessary for resource management, and human cognitive competence may be potentially available for addressing IoT resource issues. In IoT, ubiquitous resources are assigned with challenging requirements. For example, on-demand resource distribution, spontaneous resource discovery and cooperative resource sharing. In this chapter, we apply analogies from human cognition to establish an attention-aware resource framework, and present a human attention inspired resource allocation scheme for IoT applications.

11.2 Attention-Aware Resource Framework in IoT

Attention is regarded as a limited resource due to the explosions of sensing, connection, service, and intelligence in IoT, and becomes more precious during system resource allocation. In this chapter, a new challenge is identified owing to attention distribution during dynamic interactions in IoT. Figure 11.1 illustrates a familiar scenario that a person has a cup of coffee to present the main motivation. The scenario includes two steps: the persons holding a cup, and drinking coffee. During the simple human behaviors, the person may consider different aspects towards the coffee itself. Concretely, when the person has a first sight at the cup, he/she may subconsciously sense the weight of the coffee. Upon drinking the first sip, he/she may pay more attention on its taste or temperature. This scenario is a typical dynamic resource allocation process, in which multiple sense organs (e.g., hand, eyes, and tongue) are invoked to complete the action. It indicates that attention plays pivotal roles for resource allocation, and we adopt human attention and cognitive psychology to address IoT resource allocation [11].

IoT resources mainly cover the abstract attention resource and other physical-cyber-social resources. The attention resource mainly includes the sustained attention, selective attention, and divided attention. The ubiquitous things, including physical objects (e.g., sensors), cyber entities (e.g., cloud server), and the associated social attributes (e.g., ownership, and affiliation relationship), belong to the scope of the physical-cyber-social resources.

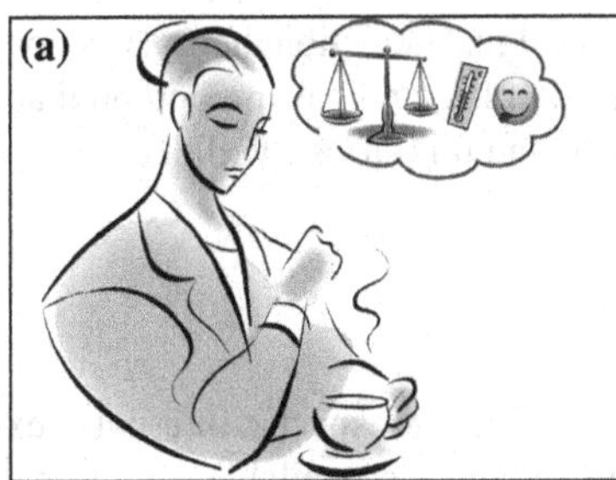

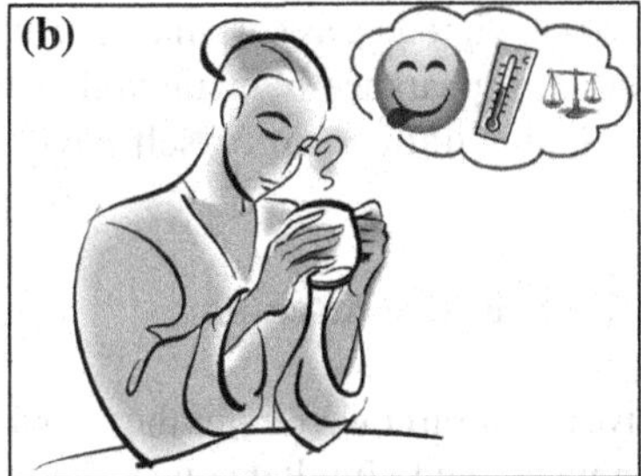

Fig. 11.1 An example of having a cup of coffee with dynamic attention. **a** Holding a cup. **b** Drinking coffee

In IoT, ubiquitous resources have several unique basic features:

- *Share ability*: Resources can be interoperated by different IoT applications to achieve enhanced resource sharing and utilization in heterogeneous networks. For instance, in cloud computing, the resources located on multiple sites are accessed by multiple resource users.
- *Power demand-supply*: In specific applications (e.g., smart grid), resources and power have subtle relationships: resources mainly consume power as an energy demand for functional operation, and resources themselves may also provide power as an energy supply.
- *Cyber-physical collaboration*: The interrelationships are established between physical resources and cyber resources, which can be jointly applied to support a particular application according to the dynamic environments.
- *Duty cycling*: Resources have the corresponding duty cycling, referring to the activity cycle and life cycle. It indicates that resources can be created, updated, released, and reloaded in practical applications.

These resources may provide various functions during interactions to achieve service accessing, discovery, and sharing.

11.2.1 Attention as Limited Cognitive Resource

11.2.1.1 Sustained Attention

Sustained attention aims to address a cognitive thing (e.g., object and activity) during a prolonged time with attention getting, holding, and releasing. It is applied to complete cognitively planned or sequenced tasks for efficient information processing, in which a distraction may arise to interrupt and consequently interfere in the attention. When a person has less sustained attention, (s)he usually presents with an accompanying inability to control the behaviors (e.g., inhibition of inappropriate behaviors, and avoidance of distraction), or to adapt to environmental requirements.

For instance, vigilance as sustained attention in signal detection theory, is an ongoing alert for the appearance of an unpredictable stimulus, and has the potential applications including traffic control, self-navigation, and military surveillance.

11.2.1.2 Selective Attention

Selective attention concentrates the resource on a specific aspect in internal or external environments, and simultaneously disregard others. An available attentional state is limited at one time, therefore it subconsciously filters out other unnecessary or unimportant issues. Cocktail party effect is a phenomenon of focusing ones auditory attention on a particular stimulus while filtering out a range of other stimuli, and a partygoer can follow a single conversation in a noisy room. Stroop effect also applies the psychological difficulty in selective attention to identify a color name (e.g., red) printed in a color not denoted by the name. Comprehensive effects realize to immediately detect sensitive information originating from the unattended stimuli, and what factors drive the attention selection? The top-down endogenous processing and bottom-up exogenous processing can jointly address the attention acquisition.

- *Endogenous goal-driven attention processing* is to steer attention towards the subjectively important stimuli themselves, for instance to read a book on a running bus, while ignoring the ongoing traffic on the road.
- *Exogenous stimulus-driven attention processing* is to notice with potentially important stimuli around the environments, and automatically activated by a sudden stimulus.

Note that it would be deleterious if attention was exclusively driven by an endogenous factor. Even when a person is concentrating on the book, the attention still needs to be susceptible to highly salient external situations (e.g., the bus arriving at the destination). Similarly, it would be also deleterious if attention was only controlled by an exogenous factor, it would be almost impossible to achieve the directed behaviors without necessarily and constantly attention distracters. The endogenous attention and exogenous attention should be interactive, and a perfect trade-off of internally and externally driven attention is crucial for an event execution.

11.2.1.3 Divided Attention

Divided attention is a capability of actively paying attention to simultaneous tasks. In the case that multiple tasks are performed in a parallel mode, attention may be divided with weaken performance, or the tasks may be proficiently performed to achieve automaticity. Examples include driving a car whilst listening to the radio, and carrying on a conversation during eating dinner. During the simultaneous task execution, attention performance on at least one of the tasks usually declines due to the limited capacity to process information. Such attention performance can be improved with practice to achieve high accuracy and low response time. It is necessary to optimize the potential resource sources, and to provide support on the relative priorities of tasks to facilitate the optimal attentional strategies.

11.2.1.4 Attention Resource Rules

The attention resource inherits the cognitive rules in cognitive psychology and satisfies the following rules.

- *Filter or bottleneck rule*: There are early selection, attenuation, and late selection models to realize the selective information processing. The environmental information and stimuli are filtered via the feature detection, extraction, and identification, in which a bottleneck is applied to filter out information not selected for data processing.
- *Central resource capacity rule*: A single undifferentiated attentional resource is assigned to all possible multiple tasks, and the available attention varies mainly depending on dynamic tasks, environmental situations, and individuals conditions (e.g., arousal level). Along with demands increasing, the supply of attention resource increases until there is no sufficient resource for compensation. During performing parallel tasks based on a single resource, it should ensure the completion of at least one task, and the enduring disposition with reasonable attention allocation.
- *Multiple resource rule*: There are multiple sources from which attention resource is allocated, and such resource is differentiated according to specific processing components (e.g., processing stages, perceptual modality, and processing codes). Performance of simultaneous multiple tasks depends on the competition for common attention resource within multiple sources.

11.3 Heterogeneous Sensors Based IoT

11.3.1 Physical-Cyber-Social Cross-Space Mapping

The ubiquitous things as the main form of resources include physical objects and cyber entities, which establish physical-cyber-social mapping in IoT. A physical object is assigned with the heterogeneous attributes, which act as feature signals to inform the sensors for sensing and identification, and the sensors resemble dendrites of a neuron for things attribute detection.The physical objects and the cyber entities have several characteristics.

- *Heterogeneous attribute matching*: Things' heterogeneous attributes and the sensors sensing capabilities should be appropriately matched, and only the adaptive sensors can obtain the appointed attributes to achieve physical object recognition.

Towards a certain thing, expandable attributes can be attached according to practical application requirements.

- *Space-time consistency*: Things can establish interconnections, and a cyber entity can interact with other cyber entities without space-time constraints. A physical object may be active and subsequently invoke the corresponding cyber entities, and a cyber entity may freely enter or leave the interactions without influencing the ongoing sessions. Note that space-time registration, synchronization, and correlation should be considered during the cross-space interconnections.
- *Pervasive connection convergence*: Things are in the contexts of pervasive networks, not only including the real communication channel networking via switches, routers, gateways, and other network components, but also including the virtual social networking via social relations based online platform. The network convergence realizes the aggregated effects on CPSS to provide the enhanced services (e.g., geographic information, cloud services, and intelligent decision support).

11.3.2 Network Framework

The IoT system model has a coupled distributed network framework. The IoT system involves sensors, actuators, network technologies and communication technologies.

The sensors and actuators are used to collect data for identifying things, gathering information, and executing tasks. Ubiquitous sensing technologies can achieve ubiquitous sensing and controlling. There are wired sensing technologies and wireless sensing technologies. The wireless sensor network is a suitable access network platform that has typical wireless sensing technologies, such as RFID, Bluetooth, Wi-Fi, and so on. The sensors are usually low-cost devices with limited energy, computation, and communication capabilities.

In IoT, network and communication technologies are pivotal for interconnection among remote things Internet and mobile communication can realize the objective. It is significant to merge fixed, mobile, and wireless communications to establish heterogeneous communications. The hybrid communication technologies should be optimized to achieve high data rate and seamless mobility. IoT accelerates the development of the next-generation Internet technology, and Internet protocol version 6 (IPv6) aims to replace the traditional Internet with its expanded address space, enables addressing, connecting, and tracking things. Meanwhile, 6LoWPAN is to realize that low-power devices with limited processing capabilities can participate in IoT.

11.4 A Human Attention Inspired Resource Allocation Scheme in IoT

Figure 11.2 shows a human attention inspired resource allocation scheme for dynamic resource interactions in IoT. The scheme refers to the physical objects (e.g., sensors, and actuators), cyber entities (e.g., online resources), and the associated social

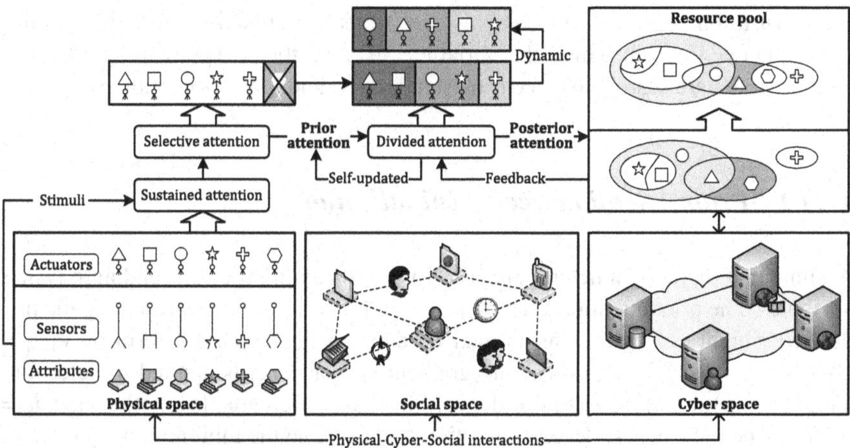

Fig. 11.2 The human attention inspired resource allocation scheme

correlation in the CPSS. The heterogeneous attributes (marked as the geometrical shapes) are attached to the things in the physical space, and the sustained, selective, and divided attention is introduced during resource allocation. Upon the sensors detecting effective stimuli triggered by things attributes, the corresponding actuators sustained attention is disarranged. The selective attention is accordingly launched to perform an adaptive selection, and some inapparent attributes may be ignored. Towards the selected attributes, divided attention dynamically varies during resource interactions. The resource pool provides common resource supports for the involved physical objects. Here, attention arrays including prior attention vector and posterior attention matrix are defined as follows.

- *Prior attention vector* considering the sustained attention, is an initial parameter obtained by the historical interactive data with self-updating capacity.
- *Posterior attention matrix* considering the selective attention and divided attention, is a multi-dimensional array with a set of time-sensitive parameters obtained by real-time data collection in an ongoing session.

In the scheme, the related parameters are listed.

- *Attention array parameters*: $\{V_{1\times n}, V'_{1\times n}\}(n \in N^{\star})$ are the initial and updated prior attention vector. $S_{T\times n}(T \in N^{\star})$ is the dynamic sensing data set. $S'_{T\times n}$ is the revised sensing data according to a criterion. $E_{1\times n}$ denotes the sensitivity on heterogeneous attributes. $M_{T\times n}$ is the posterior attention matrix.
- *Attention distribution parameters*: $\{p_{V(i)}, p_{SE(i)}\}$ are the weight percentages of $\{V_{1\times n}, M_{T\times n}\}$ at the time point T_i. $\Delta\Phi_{(i)}$ is the aggregated variation between the posterior and prior attention at T_i.
- *Normalization parameters*: $\{n_{1_{ij}}, n_{2_{ij}}\}$ are the normalized values respectively satisfying Gauss distribution and uniform distribution. $R_{T\times n}$ is the resource allocation value. $R'_{T\times n}$ is the resource allocation percentage.

- *Optimization parameters*: $f(x)$ is an objective function for determining $\min f(x) = V_{1\times n}$, in which the variable x is a vector. $\nabla f(x)$ is the gradient of $f(x)$. $\{\alpha, d\}$ are search distance (i.e., step length) and search direction of $f(x)$.

11.4.1 Prior Attention Vector Initialization

Assume that there are n heterogeneous sensors to capture the surrounding physical attributes. The prior attention vector $V_{1\times n} = [v_j](j = 1, \ldots, n)$ representing the predefined weight values of sensors, can be denoted in the variant form of $V_{1\times n} = [\frac{A_1}{A}, \frac{A_2}{A}, \ldots, \frac{A_n}{A}](\sum_{j=1}^{n} A_j = A)$. The gradient descent [12] is applied to determine $V_{1\times n}$. Let $f(x)(x \in R^n)$ be a first-order continuously differentiable function, and $d_k = -\nabla f(x_k)$ be the steepest descent direction to determine the minimum $\min f(x)$, and the iteration is performed as follows.

Step 1: Given a starting point $x_0 \in R$, and a sufficiently small value $\varepsilon > 0$, let $k := 0$;

Step 2: If $|\nabla f(x_k)| < \varepsilon$ holds, terminate the iteration to output x_k. Otherwise, continue the iteration;

Step 3: Let $d_k = -\nabla f(x_k)$, and apply the Armijo inexact line search to determine an optimal step length α_k, which satisfies Eq. (11.1). Let $x_{k+1} = x_k + \alpha_k d_k$ and $k := k + 1$, and go to Step 2.

$$f(x_k + \alpha_k d_k) = \min f(x_k + \alpha d_k) \tag{11.1}$$

In the Armijo line search [10], the global minimizer of an univariate function $\varphi(.)$ is defined as $\varphi(\alpha) = f(x_k + \alpha d_k)(\alpha > 0)$. α_k satisfies the decrease condition $(c \in (0, 0.5))$.

$$\varphi(\alpha_k) \leq \varphi(0) + c\alpha_k \varphi'(0) \tag{11.2}$$

Step 1: If $\alpha_k = 1$ satisfies (3), let $\alpha_k = 1$. Otherwise, go to Step 2;

$$f(x_k + \alpha_k d_k) \leq f(x_k) + c\alpha_k \nabla f(x_k)^T d_k \tag{11.3}$$

Step 2: Given constants $\beta > 0$ and $\varrho \in (0, 1)$, let $\alpha_k = \beta$;
Step 3: If α_k satisfies (3), output α_k. Otherwise, go to Step 4;
Step 4: Let $\alpha_k := \rho\alpha_{(k)}$, and go to Step 3.

11.4.2 Posterior Attention Matrix Assignment

During the dynamic interactions, $S_{T\times n} = [s_{ij}](i = 1, \ldots, T, j = 1, \ldots, n)$ persistently records the raw sensing data, and is further converted into $S'_{T\times n} = [s'_{ij}]$

according to a pre-defined criterion. $S'_{T\times n}$ and $E_{1\times n} = [e_j]$ are applied to define the posterior attention matrix $M_{T\times n} = [m_{ij}]$.

$$m_{ij} = p_{SE(i)} s'_{ij} e_j + p_{V(i)} v_j, \quad p_{SE(i)} + p_{V(i)} = 1$$

Assume that the initial weight percentages $\{p_{SE(0)}, p_{V(0)}\}$ are assigned with the same value at the time point T_0. Towards the adjacent time points $\{T_i, T_{i+1}\}$, the percentages performs self-adjustment according to the practical conditions.

For $\Delta\Phi_{(i+1)} \neq \Delta\Phi_{(i)}$:

$$p_{SE(i+1)} = p_{SE(i)} + \frac{\Delta\Phi_{(i+1)} - \Delta\Phi_{(i)}}{|\Delta\Phi_{(i+1)} - \Delta\Phi_{(i)}|} \times v, \quad p_{V(i+1)} = p_{V(i)} - \frac{\Delta\Phi_{(i+1)} - \Delta\Phi_{(i)}}{|\Delta\Phi_{(i+1)} - \Delta\Phi_{(i)}|} \times v$$

For $\Delta\Phi_{(i+1)} = \Delta\Phi_{(i)}$:

$$p_{SE(i+1)} = p_{SE(i)}, \quad p_{V(i+1)} = p_{V(i)}$$

Here, $\Delta\Phi_{(i)} = \sum_{j=1}^{n} |s'_{ij} e_j - v_j|$, and v is a unit variation value. Considering the posterior attentions reaction, $V_{1\times n}$ will be updated into $V'_{1\times n}$ after running a sensing session.

$$V'_{1\times n} = [v'_{1\times j}] = \left[\frac{A_j + m_{ij}}{A + \sum_{j=1}^{n} m_{ij}}\right]$$

11.4.3 Normalization and Resource Allocation

Normalization is performed to achieve a unified quality of the sensing data, and the variables $\{n_{1_{ij}}, n_{2_{ij}}\}$ are applied to normalize the elements $[m_{ij}]$. Assume that $n_{1_{ij}}$ is a major factor satisfying the Gauss distribution, and $n_{2_{ij}}$ is a cofactor satisfying the uniform distribution.

$n_{1_{ij}}$ represents the distance between m_{ij} and the arithmetic mean μ in units of the standard deviation σ. Thereinto, $\mu = \frac{1}{n}\sum_{j=1}^{n} m_{ij}$, and $\sigma = \sqrt{\frac{1}{n}\sum_{j=1}^{n}(m_{ij} - \mu)^2}$.

$$n_{1_{ij}} = \frac{1}{\sigma}(m_{ij} - \mu)$$

$n_{2_{ij}}$ is obtained by a linear function, in which the maximum value $m_i^{\max} = \max(m_{i1}, \ldots, m_{in})$ and the minimum value $m_i^{\min} = \min(m_{i1}, \ldots, m_{in})$ are used to measure m_{ij} into a non-dimensional parameter.

$$n_{2_{ij}} = \frac{m_{ij} - m_i^{\min}}{m_i^{\max} - m_i^{\min}}$$

Based on the dynamic attention, different weight coefficients are assigned to the heterogeneous attributes, which realizes that the resource allocation can be formalized in quantification. Two normalized values can be aggregated as $R_{T\times n} = [r_{ij}] = [pn_{1_{ij}} + (1-p)n_{2_{ij}}]$ ($50\,\% < p < 100\,\%$) to determine the resource allocation priority, in which $\{p, 1-p\}$ are the proportions of $\{n_{1_{ij}}, n_{2_{ij}}\}$. $R_{T\times n}$ can be transformed into the resource allocation percentage $R'_{T\times n} = [r'_{ij}]$. The attributes with larger percentage will be assigned with higher share or priority to access more resources. Note that the resource allocation is not fully unrestricted. If the pre-assigned resource for one attribute exceeds a threshold τ, the excess resource will be proportionately re-distributed to other attributes.

For $r'_{ij} \leq \tau$,

$$r'_{ij} = \frac{r_{ij} - 2\min(r_{ij})}{\sum_{j=1}^{n}(r_{ij} - 2\min(r_{ij}))}$$

For $r'_{ij} > \tau$,

$$r'_{i\eta} = \frac{r_{i\eta} - 2\min(r_{i\eta})}{\sum_{\eta=1}^{n}(r_{i\eta} - 2\min(r_{i\eta}))}(1 + \frac{(r'_{ij} - \tau)}{\sum_{j\neq\eta}^{n} r'_{ij}}), \quad (\eta \neq j)$$

$$r'_{ij} = \tau$$

Table 11.1 shows the comparisons with the heuristic resource allocation algorithms, including ant colony optimization (ACO), genetic algorithm (GA), and particle swarm optimization (PSO). It turns out that the proposed scheme is flexible and lightweight for resource-constrained IoT applications.

11.4.4 Case Study: IoT Based Environmental Monitoring

In the case study, there are four types of sensors to capture the environmental parameters: temperature (°C), relative humidity (%), UV index, and PM 2.5 value ($\mu g/m^3$). The sensors are deployed in relatively independent subsystems, associating with the corresponding actuators (i.e., thermostat, (de)humidifier, anti-ultraviolet, and purifier).

The prior attention vector $V_{1\times4} = [v_1, v_2, v_3, v_4]$ is determined by a historical prior attention vector set $V_{T\times4} = [v_{m1}, v_{m2}, \ldots, v_{m4}] (m = 1, \ldots, T)$. An objective function $f(V)$ is established to obtain $V_{1\times4} = [\frac{1}{8}, \frac{1}{4}, \frac{1}{4}, \frac{3}{8}]$.

$$f(V) = \sum_{m=1}^{T}\sum_{n=1}^{4}(v_{mn} - v_n)^2$$

Table 11.1 The comparisons with the heuristic resource allocation algorithms

	ACO	GA	PSO	Our scheme
Origin	The behavior of ants seeking a path between their colony and a source of food while laying down pheromone trails	Natural selection and genetics (e.g., inheritance, mutation, selection, and crossover)	The behavior (e.g., movement, and predator-prey behavior) of bird flocking or fish schooling	Human attention (i.e., sustained attention, selective attention, and divided attention)
Element factors	Maximum/Minimum pheromone amounts, visibility, and Tabu search	Population size, fitness function, crossover probability, and mutation probability	Inertia weight, Quasi-Newton method, and gradient descent	Prior attention vector, posterior attention matrix, and gradient descent
Feedback	Positive feedback	No feedback	No feedback	Positive feedback
Advantages	Distributed parallelism, robustness, and compatibility	Randomness, robustness, and self-adapting,	Dynamic neighborhood topology, and high accuracy	Threshold control, dynamic, and lightweight
Shortcomings	Lack of initial pheromone, slow convergence speed, and search stagnation	Blind search, low efficiency, and limited convergence speed	Premature convergence, and the local minimum	Dependence on historical experiences, and limited applicability for massive networks

$S_{T\times n}$ is obtained by continuously monitoring the 24-h sensing data during May 30–June 5, 2013 in Beijing, China. Assume that an ideal temperature and relative humidity are 22 °C and 50 %, and the UV index and PM 2.5 value are limited within 2 and 70 $\mu g/m^3$, which are defined as the criterion. Figure 11.3 illustrates the data sensing and resource allocation, in which IoT resources can be regarded as a constant, and dynamic resource proportion is distributed according to the real-time attention arrays. The scheme provides the scalability and stability properties.

- *Scalability*: The attention arrays are time-sensitive variables, and dynamic resource allocation is accordingly realized based on the real-time data sensing. A growing amount of sensing data is persistently handled during the interactions, and additional sensors can be extended to provide new functionalities at the minimal effort.
- *Stability*: The sensors are relatively independent, and an accidental breakdown of a sensor will not cause other sensors' unavailability. The associated actuators share a common IoT resource pool, and an emergency resource response can be launched to address an urgent event. Degeneratiaon may occur when the sensors or actuators persistently suffer from overload utilization or malicious abuse, and

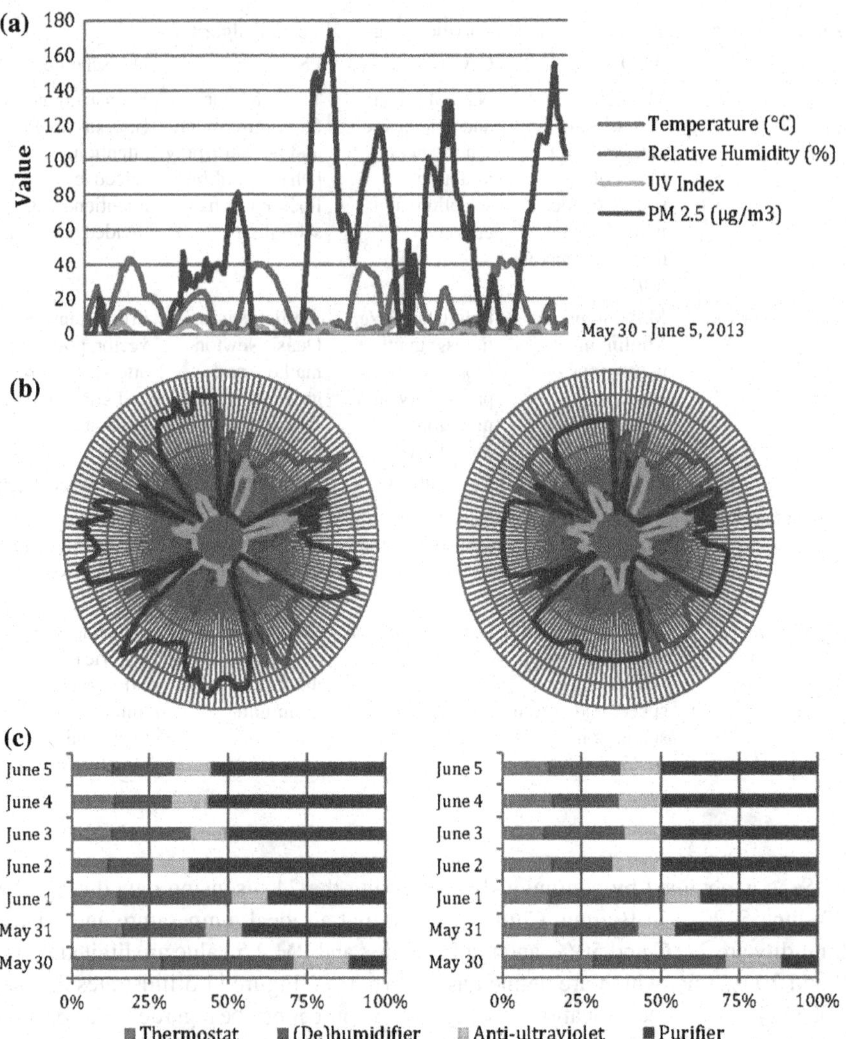

Fig. 11.3 The data sensing and resource allocation: **a** the sensing data during one week according to the defined criterion; **b** the original and revised real-time resource allocation; and **c** the original and revised daily resource allocation, in which $p = 70\,\%$, and the threshold $\tau = 50\,\%$

the threshold control mechanism ensures that an approximately corrupted system will be kept in a safe state to prevent resource exhaustion.

11.5 Conclusions

In this chapter, we identify natural correlations between human attention and resource issues, and present a heuristic resource allocation scheme for heterogeneous sensors in IoT. Considering the things physical-cyber-social cross-space mapping, the prior attention and posterior attention are jointly applied during the resource allocation to achieve dynamic resource interactions in lightweight IoT applications.

Acknowledgments We thank IEEE's authorization to use some related materials from Ref. [13].

References

1. L. Atzori, A. Iera, G. Morabito, The internet of things: a survey. Comput. Netw. **54**(15), 27872805 (2010)
2. A. Georgakopoulos, K. Tsagkaris, D. Karvounas, P. Vlacheas, P. Demestichas, Cognitive networks for future internet: status and emerging challenges. IEEE Veh. Technol. Mag. **7**(3), 4856 (2012)
3. H. Ning, Z. Wang, Future internet of things architecture: like mankind neural system or social organization framework? IEEE Commun. Lett. **15**(4), 461463 (2011)
4. J. Ma, J. Wen, R. Huang, B. Huang, Cyber-individual meets brain informatics. IEEE Intell. Syst. **26**(5), 3037 (2011)
5. N. Zhong, J. Ma, R. Huang, J. Liu, Y. Yao, Y. Zhang, J. Chen, Research challenges and perspectives on wisdom web of things (W2T). J. Supercomput. (2010). doi:10.1007/s11227-010-0518-8
6. L. Atzori, A. Iera, G. Morabito, SIoT: giving a social structure to the internet of things. IEEE Commun. Lett. **15**(11), 11931195 (2011)
7. A. Sehgal, V. Perelman, S. Kuryla, J. Schonwalder, Management of resource constrained devices in the internet of things. IEEE Commun. Mag. **50**(12), 144–149 (2012)
8. K. Zheng, F. Hu, W. Wang, W. Xiang, M. Dohler, Radio resource allocation in LTE-advanced cellular networks with M2M communications. IEEE Commun. Mag. **50**(7), 184–192 (2012)
9. P.T. Endo, A.V. de Almeida Palhares, N.M. Pereira, G.E. Goncalves, D. Sadok, J. Kelner, B. Melander, J.E. Mangs, Resource allocation for distributed cloud: concepts and research challenges. IEEE Netw. **25**(4), 42–46 (2011)
10. H. Hildmann, S. Nicolas, F. Saffre, A bio-inspired resource-saving approach to dynamic client-server association. IEEE Intell. Syst. **27**(6), 17–25 (2012)
11. R.T. Kellogg, *Cognitive Psychology*, 2nd edn (Sage Publications, 2003)
12. J. Nocedal, S.J. Wright, *Numerical Optimization* (Springer Verlag, 1999)
13. H. Ning et al., Human-attention inspired resource allocation for heterogeneous sensors in the web of things. IEEE Intell. Syst. **28**(6), 20–28 (2013)

Chapter 12
Mining Multiplex Structural Patterns from Complex Networks

Bo Yang and Jiming Liu

Abstract Wisdom Web of Things (W2T) can be modeled and studied from the perspective of complex networks. The complex network perspective aims to model and characterize complex systems that consist of multiple and interdependent components. Among the studies on complex networks, topological structure analysis is of the most fundamental importance, as it represents a natural route to understand the dynamics, as well as to synthesize or optimize the functions, of networks. A broad spectrum of network structural patterns have been respectively reported in the past decade, such as communities, multipartites, hubs, authorities, outliers, bow ties, and others. In this chapter, we show that many real-world networks demonstrate multiplex structure patterns. A multitude of known or even unknown (hidden) patterns can simultaneously exist in the same network, and moreover they may be overlapped and nested with each other to collaboratively form a heterogeneous, nested or hierarchical organization, in which different connective phenomena can be observed at different granular levels. In addition, we show that such patterns hidden in exploratory networks can be well defined as well as effectively recognized within an unified framework consisting of a set of proposed concepts, models, and algorithms. Our findings provide a strong evidence that many real-world complex systems are driven by a combination of heterogeneous mechanisms that may collaboratively shape their ubiquitous multiplex structures as we currently observe. This work also contributes a mathematical tool for analyzing different sources of networks from a new perspective of unveiling multiplex structure patterns, which will be beneficial to Wisdom Web of Things.

B. Yang
School of Computer Science and Technology, Jilin University, Changchun, China
e-mail: ybo@jlu.edu.cn

J. Liu (✉)
Hong Kong Baptist University, Kowloon Tong, Hong Kong
e-mail: jiming@comp.hkbu.edu.hk

J. Liu
International WIC Institute, Beijing University of Technology, Beijing 100124, China

N. Zhong et al. (eds.), *Wisdom Web of Things*, Web Information Systems Engineering and Internet Technologies Book Series,
DOI 10.1007/978-3-319-44198-6_12

12.1 Introduction

Wisdom Web of Things (W2T) can be modeled and studied from the perspective of complex network analysis, which provides a novel approach to examining how W2T are organized and evolving according to what basic principles, and moreover armed with such discovered principles, constructing efficient, robust as well as flexible W2T systems under different constraints. Among all studies about complex networks, structural pattern analysis is the most fundamental, and the ability to discover and visualize the underlying structural patterns of real-world networks will be greatly helpful for both topological and dynamic analysis applied to them [2]. So far, scientists have uncovered a multitude of structural patterns ubiquitously existing in social, biological, ecological or technological networks; they may be microscopic such as motifs [3], mesoscopic such as modularities [4] or macroscopic such as small world [5] and scale-free phenomena [6]. These structural patterns observed at different granular levels may collectively unveil the secrets hidden in complex networked systems. All these works have greatly triggered the common interesting as well as boosted the progress of exploring complex networks in both scientific and engineering domains.

In spite of the great efforts having been taken, the structural pattern analysis of complex networks, even restricted to the mesoscopic level, remains one of the major challenges in complex network theory mainly because most of the real-world networks are usually resulted from a combination of heterogeneous mechanisms which may collaboratively shape their non-trivial structures. More specifically one can raise the following issues.

Above all, beyond modularity the most extensively studied at the mesoscopic level [4, 7], a wide spectrum of structural patterns have been reported in the literature including bipartites or more generally multipartites [8–10], hubs, authorities and outliers [11–13], bow ties [14–16] or others. Moreover, these miscellaneous patterns may simultaneously coexist in the same networks, or they may even overlap with each other such as the overlaps between communities [17].

Figure 12.1 shows an illustrative example, in which a social network encoding the co-appearances of 77 characters in the novel "Les Miserables" is visualized in terms of both network and matrix representations. The network as shown in (a) depicts the co-appearances of 77 characters in the novel "Les Miserables (by Victor Hugo)". Nodes denote characters and links connect any pair of characters that appear in the same chapter of the novel. This data set is from "The Stanford GraphBase: A Platform for Combinatorial Computing" edited by Knuth [18]. The physical connection profiles of nodes are represented in terms of the adjacency matrix as shown in (b), in which dots denote "1" entries. In total, six blocks are detected by our method in terms of the connection profiles of nodes, as separated by solid lines, so that the nodes within the same blocks will demonstrate homogeneous connectivities. To clearly visualize the block organization, the matrix has been transformed by putting together the nodes within the same blocks which are labeled by "block 1" to "block 6" from the top down. Correspondingly, in the network as shown in (a), nodes are also

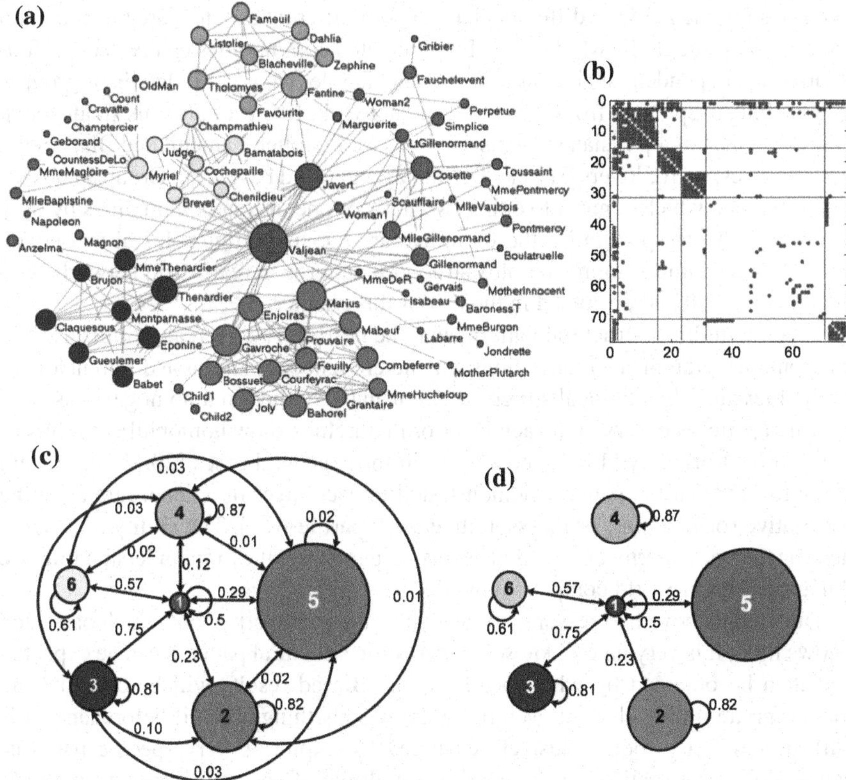

Fig. 12.1 An example of multiplex patterns consisting of hubs, outliers and communities coexisting in one social network. This figure is from [1]

colored according to their block IDs (specifically, the coloring schema is: block 1-red, block 2-green, block 3-blue, block 4-cyan, block 5-gray and block 6-yellow), and the sizes of nodes are proportional to their respective degrees. (c) shows the blocking model of the network, in which each block is colored, numbered and placed according to the nodes it contains, and the sizes of blocks are proportional to the number of nodes they contain, respectively. The weights on the arrow lines globally measure the probabilities that one node from one block will connect to another from other blocks. (d) shows the reduced blocking model by cutting the arrow lines with trivial weights. In this case, one hub pattern consisting of block 1, one outlier pattern consisting of block 5 and four community patterns consisting of blocks 2, 3, 4 and 6 will readily be recognized by referring to the probabilistic linkage among these blocks.

From the reduced blocking model, one can observe two hubs and a number of outliers coexisting with four well-formed communities. The two hubs, corresponding to *Valjean* and *Javert*, are the main characters of the novel, and their links are across all other clusters by connecting about 48 % of the overall characters. It indicates that the two roles interacting with different characters in different chapters are the two main clues going through the whole story. Four detected communities can be seen as four relatively independent social cliques. As an example, we go into details of group 4 that is almost separated from the rest of the network. Interestingly, this small social clique consists of 4 parisian students Tholomyes, Listolier, Fameuil and Blacheville with their respective lovers Fantine, Dahlia, Zephine and Favourite. Group 5 consists of 39 outliers, which connect to either two hubs or one of four communities by only a few links. Correspondingly, these outliers are the supporting roles of this novel. Besides this example, more complex structural patterns in real-world networks will be demonstrated and discussed in the rest of this chapter.

Second, multiple structural patterns may be nested. That is, real-world networks can contain hierarchical organizations with heterogeneous patterns at different levels. In the literature, hierarchical structures are usually studied in a homogeneous way, in which patterns observed in each layer of hierarchies show homophily in terms of either fractal property [19] or modularity in more general cases [20, 21]. A recent study reveals that the patterns demonstrated in each layer of a dendrogram can be assortative (or modular) or disassortative (or bipartite) [22]. The ability to observe heterogeneous patterns at different levels brings new clues for understanding the dynamics of real-world complex networks.

Due to the above two reasons, for an exploratory network about which one often knows little, it is very hard to know what specific structural patterns can be expected and then be obtained by what specific tools. Biased results will be caused if an inappropriate tool is chosen; even if we know something about it beforehand, it is still difficult for a tool exclusively designed for exploring very specific patterns, say modularity, to satisfactorily uncover a multiple of coexisting patterns possibly overlapped or even nested with each other (we call them *multiplex patterns* in this work) from networks.

To the best our knowledge, there have been little studies in the literature being able to address both of the above issues. On the other hand, human beings have the capability of modeling and simultaneously discovering multiple and significant structural patterns for various objectives. It has been believed that this kind of capability is an important form of human cognitive and intelligent functions [23].

Back to the matrix as shown in Fig. 12.1, one would observe an intuitive phenomenon: *any significant pattern contained in the underlying structures of the network can be statistically highlighted by a group of homogenous individuals with identical or quite similar connectivity profiles*. For instance, individuals from the same communities prefer to intensively interact with each other but rarely interact with the rest; hubs would prefer to connect many individuals from different parts of the whole network, whereas all outliers tend to seldom play with others by emitting only a few connections. Based on this naive observation, if one can group the majority of individuals into reasonable clusters according to their connectivity profiles, the coexisting structural patterns can be unveiled by further inferring the linkage among clusters. In this way, the first issue listed above can be promisingly solved.

The idea of grouping nodes into *equivalent* clusters in terms of their connection patterns is similar to the philosophy of the *blockmodeling* first proposed by Lorrain and White [24], in which nodes with *structural equivalence* (defined in terms of local neighborhood configurations) or more generally *regular equivalence* [25] (defined in terms of globally physical connections to all others) or more softly *stochastic equivalence* [26, 27] (defined in terms of linking probabilities between groups) will be grouped into the same blocks.

Based on the same idea, a very related study has been proposed recently by Newman and Leicht, which first (to our knowledge) shows the motivation to detect unpredefined structural patterns from exploratory networks [28]. From the perspective of machine leaning, their method can be seen as a version of naive Bayes algorithm applied to networks, whose objective is to group nodes with similar connection features into a predefined number of clusters. Although their work only shows the ability to determine whether an exploratory network is assortative or disassortative by manually analyzing the obtained clusters, it has provided one good proof supporting that the idea of grouping nodes into equivalent clusters can be an initial step of the whole process aiming to unveil multiplex patterns from networks.

In this chapter, we will introduce a novel model, by introducing the concept of granularity into stochastic connection profiles in order to properly model multiplex patterns mentioned above, and then show how the task of extracting such patterns of networks can be reduced to a simplified version of the isomorphism subgraph matching problem. To validate our ideas and strategies proposed here, different sources of networks have been analyzed. It is encouraging that our methods show a good performance, capable of uncovering multiplex patterns from the tested networks in a fully automatic way.

The rest of this chapter is organized as follows: Sect. 12.2 proposes the granular blocking model and the definitions of multiplex patterns. Based on them, Sect. 12.3 proposes the algorithms extracting multiplex patterns from networks. Section 12.4 validates the proposed models and algorithms by applying them to both real-world and synthetic networks. Finally, Sect. 12.5 concludes this chapter by highlighting our main contributions.

12.2 Modeling Multiplex Patterns

12.2.1 Granular Couplings

We will model the connection profiles of nodes in terms of probabilities instead of physical connectivity. In this way, it is expected not only to find out multiplex patterns but also to provide an explicit probabilistic interpretation for these findings within the Bayesian framework. We term such probabilities as *couplings* in that they are not just the mathematical measures subjectively defined for modeling or computing, but they do exist in many real-world systems, encoding different physical meanings such as social preferences in societies, predation habits in ecosystems, co-expression regularities in gene networks or co-occurrence likelihood of words in languages, which will be valuable to predict their situated systems.

Here the notation of *granularity* should be interpreted in terms of the resolution and precision.

On one hand, in our model we define two kinds of couplings with different resolutions, i.e., *node couplings* and *block couplings*. Formally, we define *node feedforward-coupling* matrix $P_{n\times n}$ and *node feedback-coupling* matrix $Q_{n\times n}$, where p_{ij} and q_{ij} respectively denote the probabilities that node i expects to couple with or to be coupled by node j. In the cases of indirected networks we have $P = Q$ (see Appendix for proofs). We assume nodes will independently couple with others regulated by such couplings. Nodes with similar feedforward- as well as feedback-coupling distributions will be clustered into the same blocks. In terms of matrices, homogeneous feedforward- and feedback-couplings guarantee homogeneous row and column connection profiles, respectively. Correspondingly, given the block number K, we define *block feedforward-coupling* matrix $\Phi_{K\times K}$ and *block feedback-coupling matrix* $\Psi_{K\times K}$, where ϕ_{pq} and ψ_{pq} respectively denote the probabilities that block C_p expects to couple with or to be coupled by block C_q. We will show later that block couplings can be inferred from node couplings and vice versa. Node couplings with a fine granularity are used to model networks in order to capture their local information as much as possible; while block couplings with a coarser granularity are used to define and recognize global structural patterns by intentionally neglecting trivial details.

On the other hand, in the nested patterns, node couplings and block couplings in different hierarchies will have different precisions in order to properly abstract and construct hierarchical organizations. In our model, the couplings on higher layers are the approximations of the related ones on the lower layers. Therefore, as the layers moving from the bottom (corresponding to the original networks) to the top (corresponding to the finally reduced networks) of the nested organizations, the precision of node or block couplings will gradually degenerate.

12.2.2 Defining Multiplex Patterns

The main steps of our strategies for extracting multiplex patterns from networks can be stated as follows: (1) simultaneously estimating all kinds of couplings mentioned above and clustering all nodes into nested blocks with a proposed granular blocking algorithm; and (2) in each layer of the nested blocks, recognizing and extracting structural patterns by matching predefined isomorphism subgraphs from a reduced blocking model in which trivial couplings are neglected, as illustrated in Fig. 12.1d. Multiplex patterns can be defined in terms of blocks and their couplings. Figure 12.2 shows a schematic illustration by means of some conceptual networks. By referring to them, we give following definitions.

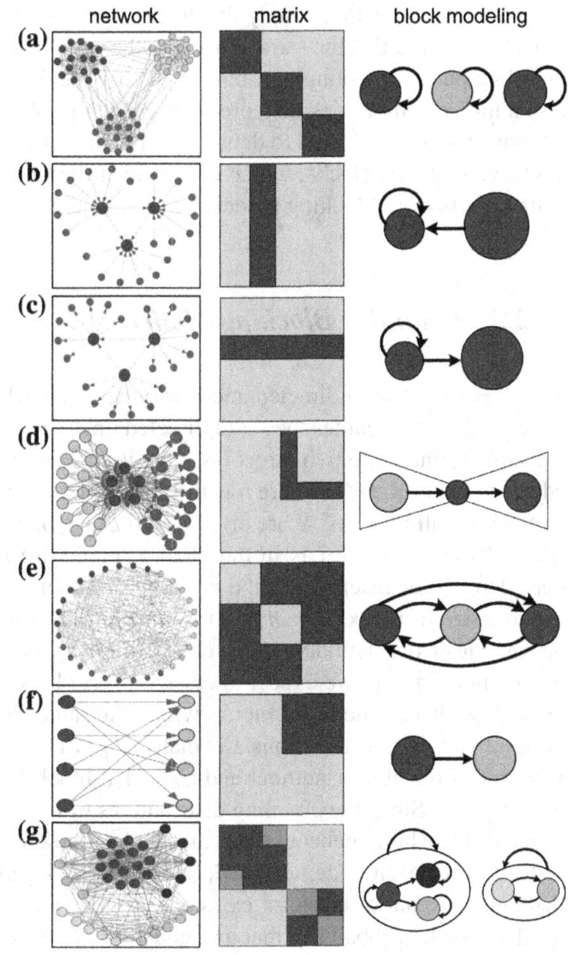

Fig. 12.2 The schematic illustrations of multiplex patterns. **a–g** shows seven structural patterns frequently observed in real-world networks, which are represented by networks, matrices and blocking models, respectively. In the matrices, *shades* represent the densities of links. In the blocking models, *circles* denote blocks and *solid arrow lines* denote block feedforward-couplings. From **a–g**, structural patterns are communities, authorities and outliers, hubs and outliers, a bow tie, a multipartite, a bipartite and a hierarchical organization, respectively. **g** shows a two-layer hierarchy; two overlapped communities (also can be seen as a hub with two communities) and one bipartite are in the first layer; two communities are in the second layer. This figure is from [1]

A *community* is a self-coupled block. An *authority* is a self-coupled block which is coupled by a number of other blocks. A *hub* is a self-coupled block which couples with a number of other blocks. An *outlier* is a block without self-coupling which is coupled by a hub or couples with an authority. *A bow-tie* is a subgraph consisting of a block b and two sets of blocks $S_l(b)$ and $S_r(b)$, which satisfy with: (1) b is coupled by and couples with the blocks of $S_l(p)$ and $S_r(p)$, respectively; (2) the intersection of $S_l(p)$ and $S_r(p)$ is empty or $\{b\}$; and 3) there are no couplings between $S_l(p)$ and $S_r(p)$; A *multipartite* is a subgraph consisting of a set of blocks without self-couplings which reciprocally couple with each other. As a special case of multipartite, a *bipartite* is a subgraph consisting of two blocks without self-loop couplings which unilaterally or bilaterally coupled with each other. A *hierarchical organization* is a set of nested blocks, in which block subgraphs in lower layers are directly or indirectly nested in the bigger blocks on higher layers.

The above definitions imply that there may exist overlaps between different patterns in the sense that the same blocks can be simultaneously involved in a multitude of subgraphs. For example, a block which is determined as a community can be also a hub, a authority or the core of one bow tie. Moreover, beyond the predefined patterns, users are allowed to define novel even more complex patterns by designing new subgraphs of blocks, which can be identified by matching their isomorphism counterparts from blocking models.

12.2.3 Granular Blocking Model

Let $N = (V, E)$ be a directed and binary network, where $V(N)$ denotes the set of nodes and $E(N)$ denotes the set of directed links. In the case of undirected network, we suppose there are two direct links between each pair of nodes. Let $A_{n\times n}$ be the adjacency matrix of N, where n is the number of nodes.

Suppose all nodes of N are divided into $L (1 \leq L \leq n)$ blocks, denotes by $B_{n\times L}$, where $b_{il} = 1$ if node i is in the block l, otherwise $b_{il} = 0$. When each block is considered to be inseparable, the *granularity* of network N can be measured by the average size of blocks $g = n/L$. As g increasing from 1 to n, the granularity of N degenerates from the finest to the coarsest. Let B_g denote the blocking model with a granularity g, and we expect to cluster all its blocks into a reasonable number of clusters so that the nodes of blocks within the same cluster will demonstrate homogeneous coupling distributions. Let matrix $Z_{L\times K} (1 \leq K \leq L)$ denote such clusters, where K is the cluster number and $z_{lk} = 1$ if block l is labeled by cluster k, otherwise $z_{lk} = 0$. Since the coupling distributions of nodes within the same clusters are expected to be homogeneous, one can characterize such distributions for each cluster instead of for each node. Given Z, define $\Theta_{K\times n}$, where θ_{kj} denotes the probability that any node out of cluster k expects to couple with node v_j; define $\Delta_{K\times n}$, where δ_{kj} denotes the probability that any node out of cluster k expects to be coupled by node v_j; define $\Omega = (\omega_1, \cdots, \omega_K)^T$, where ω_k denotes the prior probability that a randomly selected node will belong to the cluster C_k. It is easy to show $P = B_g Z\Theta$ and $Q = B_g Z\Delta$ (see Proposition 1 in Appendix).

Let $X = (K, Z, \Theta, \Delta, \Omega)$ be a model with respect to N and B_g. We expect to select an optimal X from its hypothesis space to properly fit as well as to precisely predict the behaviors of N under B_g in terms of node couplings characterized by it. According to the MAP principle (maximum a posteriori), the optimal X for a given network N under B_g will be the one with the maximum posterior probability. Moreover, we have: $P(X|N, B_g) \propto P(N|X, B_g)P(X|B_g)$, where $P(X|N, B_g)$, $P(N|X, B_g)$ and $P(X|B_g)$ denote the posteriori of X given N and B_g, the likelihood of N given X and B_g and the priori of X given B_g, respectively.

12.3 Extracting Multiplex Patterns

12.3.1 Likelihood Maximization

We first consider the simplest case by assuming all the prioris of X given B_g are equal. In this case, we have: $P(X|N, B_g) \propto P(N|X, B_g)$. Let $L(N|X, B_g) = \ln P(N|X, B_g)$, we have (see Proposition 2 in Appendix):

$$L(N|X, B_g) = \sum_{l=1}^{L} \sum_{b_{il} \neq 0} \ln \sum_{k=1}^{K} \Pi_{j=1}^{n} f(\theta_{kj}, a_{ij}) f(\delta_{kj}, a_{ji}) \omega_k \tag{12.1}$$

where $f(x, y) = x^y (1 - x)^{1-y}$.

Let $L(N, Z|X, B_g)$ be the log-likelihood of the joint distribution of N and Z given X and B_g, we have (see Proposition 3 in Appendix):

$$L(N, Z|X, B_g) = \sum_{l=1}^{L} \sum_{b_{il} \neq 0} \sum_{k=1}^{K} z_{lk} (\sum_{j=1}^{n} (\ln f(\theta_{kj}, a_{ij}) + \ln f(\delta_{kj}, a_{ji})) + \ln \omega_k) \tag{12.2}$$

Considering the expectation of $L(N, Z|X, B_g)$ on Z, we have:

$$E[L(N, Z|X, B_g)] = \sum_{l=1}^{L} \sum_{b_{il} \neq 0} \sum_{k=1}^{K} \gamma_{lk} (\sum_{j=1}^{n} (\ln f(\theta_{kj}, a_{ij}) + \ln f(\delta_{kj}, a_{ji})) + \ln \omega_k) \tag{12.3}$$

where $E[z_{lk}] = \gamma_{lk} = P(y = k|b = l, X, B_g)$, i.e., the probability that block l will be labeled as cluster k given X and B_g.

Let $J = E[L(N, Z|X, B_g)] + \lambda(\sum_{k=1}^{K} \omega_k - 1)$ be a Lagrangian function constructed for maximizing $E[L(N, Z|X, B_g)]$ with a constraint $\sum_{k=1}^{K} \omega_k = 1$, we have:

$$\begin{cases} \frac{\partial J}{\partial \theta_{kj}} = 0 \\ \frac{\partial J}{\partial \delta_{kj}} = 0 \\ \frac{\partial J}{\partial \omega_k} = 0 \\ \frac{\partial J}{\partial \lambda} = 0 \end{cases} \Rightarrow \begin{cases} \theta_{kj} = \frac{\sum_{l=1}^{L} \sum_{b_{il} \neq 0} a_{ij} \gamma_{lk}}{\sum_{l=1}^{L} \sum_{b_{il} \neq 0} \gamma_{lk}} \\ \delta_{kj} = \frac{\sum_{l=1}^{L} \sum_{b_{il} \neq 0} a_{ji} \gamma_{lk}}{\sum_{l=1}^{L} \sum_{b_{il} \neq 0} \gamma_{lk}} \\ \omega_k = \frac{\sum_{l=1}^{L} \sum_{b_{il} \neq 0} \gamma_{bk}}{n} \end{cases} \tag{12.4}$$

According to the Bayesian theorem,we have (see Proposition 4 in Appendix):

$$\gamma_{lk} = \frac{1}{\sum_{i=1}^{n} b_{il}} \sum_{b_{il} \neq 0} \frac{\Pi_{j=1}^{n} f(\theta_{kj}, a_{ij}) f(\delta_{kj}, a_{ji}) \omega_k}{\sum_{k=1}^{K} \Pi_{j=1}^{n} f(\theta_{kj}, a_{ij}) f(\delta_{kj}, a_{ji}) \omega_k} \tag{12.5}$$

Using the similar treatment as proposed by Dempster and Laird [29], we can prove that a local optimum of Eq. 12.1 will be guaranteed by recursively calculating Eqs. 12.4 and 12.5 (see Theorem 1 in Appendix). The time complexity of this iterative computing process is $O(In^2K)$, where I is the iterations required for convergence, which is usually quite small. An approximate but much faster version with a time $O(ILnK)$ is given in the Appendix.

12.3.2 Priori Approximation

Without considering the priori of the model, the above-proposed likelihood maximization algorithm will be cursed by the overfitting problem. That is, $L(N|X, B_g)$ will monotonically increase as K approaching to L. In this section, we will discuss how to approximately estimate the prior $P(X|B_g)$ by means of the information theory.

Note that $1 \leq K \leq L = n/g$, which implies that the coarser granularity the smaller K. It will be shown in the following that a smaller K will indicate a less complexity of X. So, we have: a coarser granularity prefer simpler models, which can be mathematically written as $P(X|B_g) = \eta(X)^g$, where the function $\eta(X)$ measures the complexity of X in terms of its parameters. In this work, we set $\eta(X) = P(X|B_1) = P(X)$, where $P(X)$ is the priori of X in the hypothesis space in which K can be freely valued from 1 to n. According to Shannon and Weaver [30], $\ln(1/P(X))$ is the minimum description length of X with a prior $P(X)$ in its model space. Let $OC(X)$ denote the optimal coding schema for X, and let $L_{OC}(X)$ be the minimum description length of X under this schema. We have: $-\ln P(X|B_g) = -g \ln P(X) = gL_{OC}(X)$. Now, to estimate the prior $P(X|B_g)$ is to design a good coding (or compressing) schema as close to OC as possible.

In terms of the parameter of X, i.e.,Θ, Δ, Z and Ω, we have (see Proposition 5 in Appendix):

$$\Phi = \Theta B_g Z D^{-1}, \quad \Psi = \Delta B_g Z D^{-1} \tag{12.6}$$

where $D = diag(n\Omega)$.

Note that matrices Z and B_g can be compressed into a map y, where $y(i) = k$ if the entry (i, k) of $B_g Z$ is equal to one. Given y, Φ and Ψ, node couplings p_{ij} and q_{ij} can be measured by:

$$p_{ij} = \phi_{y(i),y(j)}, \quad q_{ij} = \psi_{y(i),y(j)} \tag{12.7}$$

Equation 12.7 says that, all node couplings can be approximately characterized by y, Φ and Ψ. In other word, the compressing schema close to $OC(X)$ we have found out is:

$$\widehat{OC}(X) = (K, \Phi_{K\times K}, \Psi_{K\times K}, y_{n\times 2}) \tag{12.8}$$

Now, we have,

$$L_{\widehat{OC}}(X) = 1 \times (-\ln \tfrac{1}{1}) + 2K^2(-\ln \tfrac{1}{K^2}) + 2n(-\ln \tfrac{1}{2n})$$
$$= 2K^2 \ln K^2 + 2n \ln 2n$$

Moreover, we have:

$$\begin{aligned}
&\arg\max_X P(X|N, B_g) \\
&= \arg\min_X(-\ln P(N|X, B_g) - \ln P(X|B_g)) \\
&= \arg\min_X(-\ln P(N|X, B_g) + gL_{\widehat{OC}}(X)) \\
&= \arg\min_X(-L(N|X, B_g) + g(2K^2 \ln K^2 + 2n \ln 2n)) \\
&= \arg\min_X(-L(N|X, B_g) + 2gK^2 \ln K^2)
\end{aligned} \tag{12.9}$$

Equation 12.9 tries to seek a good tradeoff between the accuracy of model (or the precision of fitting observed data) measured by the likelihood of a network, and the complexity of a model (or the generalization ability to predict new data) measured by its optimal coding length.

12.3.3 Optimum Searching

For a given K, the penalty term is a constant, and thus to maximize $P(X|N, B_g)$ is to maximize $L(N|X, B_g)$. In our algorithm, K will be systematically checked from 1 to L, and the model with the minimum sum of negative likelihood and penalty will be returned as the optimal one. In the landscape of K and $P(X|N, B_g)$, a well-like curve will be shaped during the whole search process (see Fig. 12.6b for an example). So, in practice, rather than mechanically checking K for exact L times, an ongoing searching can be stopped after it has safely passed the well bottom. By means of this greedy strategy, the efficiency of our algorithm would be greatly improved. The complete algorithm is given as follows.

Algorithm 1 *Searching optimal X given N and* B_g

```
X=GBM(N,B_g)
    K = 1;
    X^(0) = LM(N, K, B_g);
    L^(0) = -ln(N|X^(0), B_g);
    for K=2:n
        X^(1) = LM(N, K, B_g);
        L^(1) = -ln(N|X^(1), B_g) + 2gK^2 ln K^2;
        if L^(1) < L^(0) then
            X^(0) = X^(1); L^(0) = L^(1);
```

endif
if $L^{(1)}$ *keeps increasing for predefined steps*
return $X^{(0)}$;
endif
endfor
return $X^{(0)}$;

Algorithm 2 *Searching optimal* X *given* N, K *and* B_g

X=*LM*(N,K,B_g)
randomly initialing $\Gamma^{(0)} = (\gamma_{lk})_{L\times K}$
$s \leftarrow 1$;
repeat until convergence:
compute $\Theta^{(s)}$, $\Delta^{(s)}$ *and* $\Omega^{(s)}$;
compute $\Gamma^{(s)}$;
$s \leftarrow s + 1$;
compute Z *from* $\Gamma^{(s)}$ *according to Bayesian rule;*

12.3.4 Hierarchy Construction

Assume we have constructed h layers, in which the i-th layer corresponds to a blocking model characterized by B_{g_i}. Now, we want to construct the $(h+1)$-th layer by selecting an X with a maximum posterior given a set of blocking models on different layers. We have shown that (see Proposition 6 in Appendix): $P(X|N, B_{g_1}, \cdots, B_{g_h}) \propto P(N|X, B_{g_h})P(X|B_{g_h}) \propto P(N|X, B_{g_h})P(X)^{g_h}$. This Markov-like process indicates that the new model to be selected for layer h is only based on the information of the layer $h-1$. So, for a given network, its hierarchical organization can be incrementally constructed as follows.

Firstly, we construct the first layer by taking each node as one block, and cluster it into K_1 clusters by selecting an model with a maximum $P(X|N, B_1)$. Next, we form B_{n/K_1} by capsuling each cluster on the first layer as one block, and cluster these blocks into K_2 clusters by selecting an new model with a maximum $P(X|N, B_{n/K_1})$, which forms the second layer. We repeat the same procedure until it converges (the cluster number obtained keeps fixed). In this way, the number of layers of a hierarchical organization will be automatically determined. The above procedure can be seen as a semi-supervised learning process; in the cases that the granularity is more than one, we have already known a priori that which nodes will be definitely within the same clusters. As the layer in the constructed hierarchy increases, the homogeneity of the nodes within the same cluster in terms of their connection profiles keeps degenerating, and correspondingly more global patterns are allowed to be observed by tolerating such increasing diversities.

12.3.5 Isomorphism Subgraph Matching

Based on the obtained blocks in the level $h + 1$ of the hierarchy, all potential patterns hidden in the level h can be revealed through an isomorphism subgraph matching procedure, whose input is the block feedforward-coupling matrix Φ. First we construct a reduced blocking model by taking each block as one node, and for each pair of blocks p and q we insert a link from p to q if ϕ_{pq} is above a threshold computed based on Φ (see below algorithm). Then for each block, we pick up the matched isomorphism subgraphs it will be involved in, and put them into categorized reservoirs labeled by different patterns. During this procedure, the subgraph to be put into a reservoir will be discarded if it is a subgraph of an existing one, as illustrated by Fig. 12.4d.

Algorithm 3 *Computing the threshold of a blocking model based on* Φ
01. sort all entries of Φ *into a non-increasing sequence* S*;*
02. cluster all entries of Φ *by the remarkable gaps of* S*;*
03. return the biggest entry of the cluster with the minimum mean as the threshold;

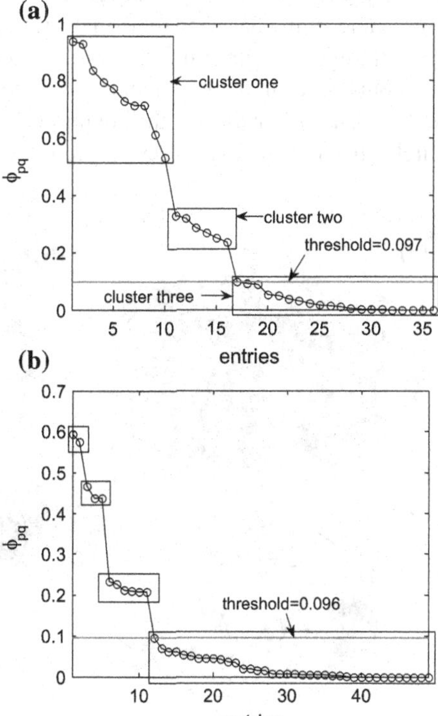

Fig. 12.3 The illustrations of calculating thresholds for reducing blocking models. **a** calculating the threshold for the blocking model of the first layer of the world trade net. **b** calculating the threshold for the blocking model of the first layer of the co-purchased political book network. In both figures, the x denotes the sorted entries and the y denotes the values of block couplings in terms of Φ. These couplings are clustered into three or four groups, as separated by *rectangles*, by remarkable gaps. The calculated thresholds are the maximum entries of the clusters with minimum means pointed out by *red solid lines*, respectively

As examples, Fig. 12.3 illustrates, by means of the above algorithm, how to choose reasonable thresholds for reducing blocking models of the world trade net and the co-purchased political book network to be discussed in the next section.

12.4 Experimentation and Validation

12.4.1 Exploring the Cash Flow Patterns of the World Trade System

The discovered multiplex patterns as well as their granular couplings can be used to understand some dynamics of networks. Here we give one example to show how cash possibly flow through a world trade net. Figure 12.4a shows a directed network encoding the trade relationship among eighty countries in the world in 1994, which was originally constructed by Nooy [31] based on the commodity trade statistics published by the United Nations. Nodes denote countries, and each arc $i \rightarrow j$ denotes the country i imported high technology products or heavy manufactures from the country j. Analogous to the "structural world system positions" initially suggested by Smith and White based on their analysis of the international trade from 1965 to 1980 [32], the eight countries in 1994 were categorized into three classes according to their economic roles in the world: core, semi-periphery and periphery [31]. Accordingly, in the visualized network, the countries labeled by them are distributed along three circles from inside to outside, respectively.

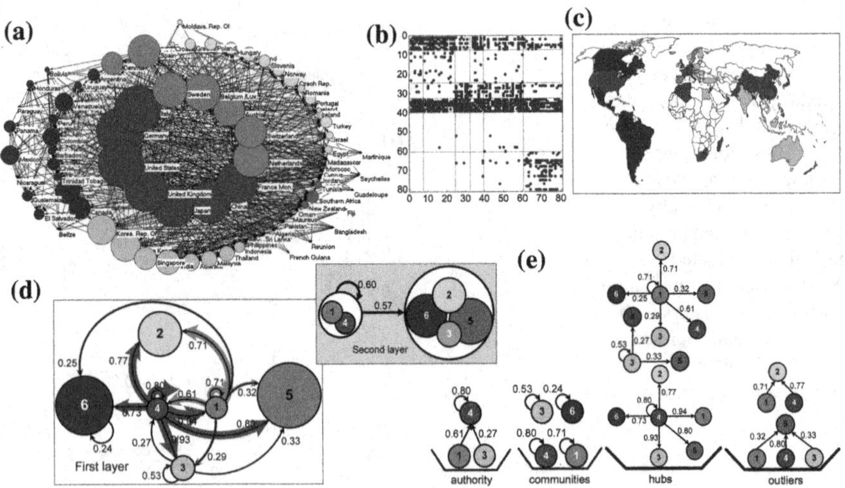

Fig. 12.4 Detecting the nested core-periphery organization and the cash flow patterns from a world trade net. This figure is from [1]. **b** Matrix. **c** Colored map. **d** Nested block modeling. **e** Patterns

Specifically, in Fig. 12.4, the network as shown in (a) encodes the trade relationship among 80 countries. Nodes denote countries and arcs denote countries imported commodities from others. The physical connection profiles of nodes are represented in terms of its adjacency matrix as shown in (b), in which dots denote "1" entries. In total, six blocks are detected as separated by solid lines so that the nodes within the same blocks will demonstrate homogeneous row- and column- connection distributions. As before, the matrix has been transformed by putting together the nodes within the same blocks which labeled by "block 1" to "block 6" from the top down. Correspondingly, in the network shown in (a), nodes are colored according to their block IDs (specifically, block 1-green, block 2-yellow, block 3-cyan, block 4-red, block 5-gray and block 6-blue), and the sizes of nodes are proportional to their respective out-degrees. (c) shows the world map in which 80 countries are colored by the same coloring schema defined above. (d) shows the detected two-layer hierarchical organization, in which each block is colored by the same coloring schema defined above and the sizes of blocks are proportional to the number of nodes they contain, respectively. In the first layer, a reduced blocking model is given by neglecting the trivial block couplings. By referring the matrix of the network as presented in Fig. 12.4b, one can observe that the nodes within the same blocks demonstrate homogeneous row as well as column connection profiles. The arrow lines with weights denote the cash flows from the countries within one block to others. The cash flows from two hubs (blocks 4 and 1) are highlighted by thicker arrow lines, of which the thickness is proportional to their strength measured by respective block couplings. These highlighted cash flows would outline the backbone of the cash circulation in the world trade system. A macroscopic hub-outlier pattern on the second layer is detected; together with the microscopic hub-outlier patterns on the first layer, the whole trade system would demonstrate a nested core-periphery organization. (e) shows the multiplex patterns discovered from the reduced blocking model on the first layer by a procedure of matching isomorphism subgraphs as defined before. Specifically, ten isomorphism subgraphs of the patterns as defined in Fig. 12.2 are recognized, which, respectively, are one authority, four communities, three hubs and two outliers.

Quite a few interesting things can be read from these uncovered multiplex patterns. Globally, the countries near center tend to have larger out-degrees, while those far from center have smaller even zero out-degrees. Specifically, (1) according to the coupling strength from strong to weak, three detected hubs can be ranked into the sequence of blocks 4, 1 and 3. The first two hubs consist of the "core" of the trade system except for Spain and Denmark; (2) the countries from blocks 3, 2 and 6 consist of the backbone of the "semi-periphery"; (3) more than a half of "periphery" countries (10 of 17) have zero out-degrees; (4) interestingly, the detected blocks are also geography-related, as illustrated in Fig. 12.4c. Most countries of hubs 4 and 1 are from western Europe expect America, China and Japan; most of hub 3 are from southeastern Asia; most of the community block 6 are from north or south America; most of the outlier block 2 are from eastern Europe; most of the outlier block 5 are from Africa or some areas of Asia.

In the second layer, a macroscopic hub-outlier pattern with strong couplings is recognized. Hub blocks 4 and 1 in the first layer collectively form a more global hub of the whole network as the core of the entire trade system; other blocks form a more global outlier of the network corresponding to the semi-periphery and periphery of the trade system. This nested hub-outlier patterns perhaps give us an evidence about how cash flowed through the world in different levels in 1994. Note that arc $i \rightarrow j$ denotes that country i imported commodities from country j, which also indicates that the spent cash has flowed from i to j. In this way, one can image cash flows along these arcs from one country to another. According to the global pattern in the second layer, the dominant cash flux will flow from the core countries to themselves with a probability 0.6, and to the rest with a probability 0.57. Locally, the blocking model in the first layer shows the backbone of the cash flow through the entire world with their respective strength in terms of block couplings, as illustrated in Fig. 12.4d.

12.4.2 Mining Granular Association Rules from Networks

When a network encodes the co-occurrence of events, its underlying node- or block-coupling matrices would imply the probabilistic associations among these events in different granular levels, respectively. Formally, we have: *node association rule (NAR)*: $i \rightarrow j \langle p_{ij} \rangle$, and *block association rule (BAR)*: $B_p \rightarrow B_q \langle \phi_{pq} \rangle$. A *NAR* means that event j would happen with a probability p_{ij} given event i happens. A *BAR* means that any event of block q would happen with a probability ϕ_{pq} given any event of block p happens. Such association rules with different granularities can be used in making prediction in a wide range of applications, such as online recommender systems. We will demonstrate this idea with a political book co-purchasing network compiled by V. Krebs, as given in Fig. 12.5a, where nodes represent books about US politics sold by the online bookseller Amazon.com, and edges connects pairs of books that are frequently co-purchased, as indicated by the "customers who bought this book also bought these other books" feature on Amazon. Moreover, these books have been labeled as "liberal", "neutral" or "conservative" according to their stated or apparent political alignments based on the descriptions and reviews of the books posted on Amazon.com [33].

Specifically, in Fig. 12.5, the network in (a) encodes the co-purchased relationship among 105 books, in which the nodes with large, median and small sizes are labeled by "liberal", "conservative" and "neutral(including one unlabeled)", respectively.

A two-layer hierarchical organization is detected. In the first layer, seven blocks are detected as shown in Fig. 12.5b. As before, the matrix as shown in (b) has been transformed by putting together the nodes within the same blocks which labeled by "block 1" to "block 7" from the top down. Correspondingly, in the network shown in (a), nodes are colored according to their block IDs (specifically, block 1-blue, block 2-red, block 3-gray, block 4-brown, block 5-green, block 6-cyan and block 7-yellow). In the blocking model as shown in (b), each block is colored by the same coloring schema defined above, the sizes of blocks are proportional to the number of nodes they contain, respectively; the arrow lines to be reserved in its reduced blocking model are highlighted by thicker arrow lines. By matching isomorphism subgraphs

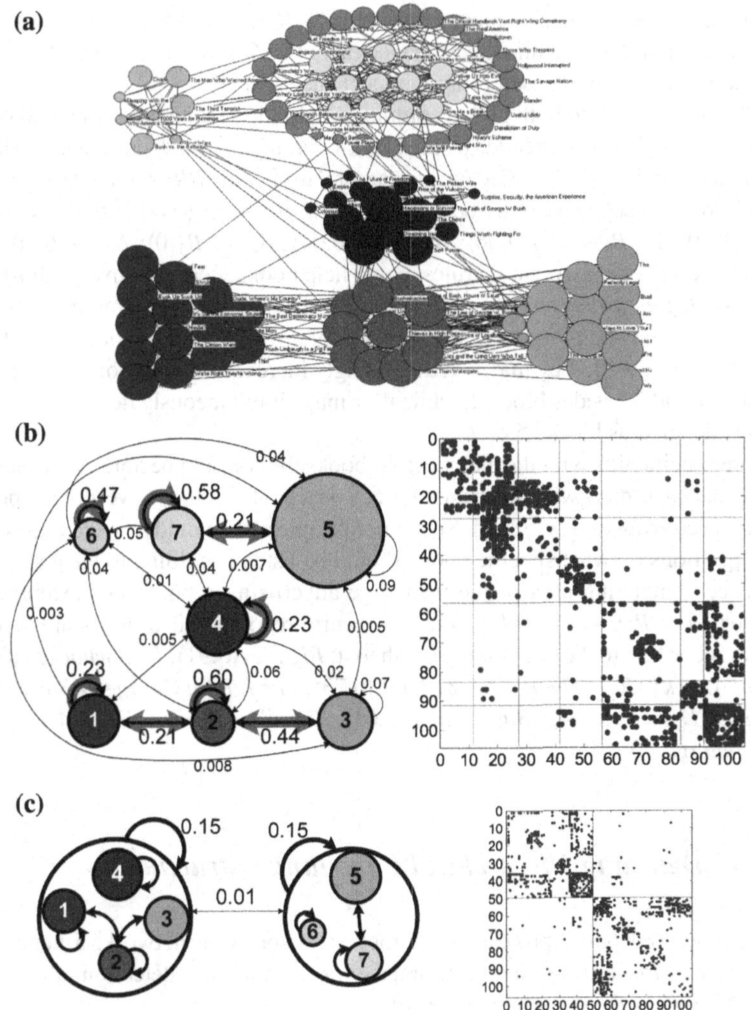

Fig. 12.5 Mining granular association rules from a co-occurrence net. This figure is from [1]. **a** Ground layer (g = 1). **b** First layer (g = 15). **c** Second layer (g = 52.5)

in its reduced blocking model, nine patterns are recognized, which respectively are five communities (blocks 1,2,4,6,7), two cores (blocks 2 and 7), two outliers (blocks 3 and 5) and a bow tie (blocks 1,2,3). Note that, in indirected networks, the core of a bow tie (block 2 in this case) can be seen as the overlapping part of its two wings (blocks 1 and 3 in this case) by neglecting the direction of links.

The blocking model and its corresponding matrix of the second layer are shows in (c). In the second layer, a macroscopic community structure is recognized. Interestingly, the left and right communities can be globally labeled as "left-wing" and "right-wing" according to the types of the books they contain respectively. Such a global pattern can be seen as one macroscopic *BAR*: the books with common labels would be co-purchased with a great chance (about 15 %); while, those with different labels are rarely co-purchased (only with a chance of 1 %).

When zooming in to both global communities in the second layer, one will obtain 7×7 mesoscopic *BAR*s encoded by the block-coupling matrix Φ, as illustrated by the weighted arrow lines Fig. 12.5b. As an example, we list the *BRA*s related to the block 2 in a decreasing sequence of association strength: $B_2 \rightarrow B_2\langle 0.60\rangle$; $B_2 \rightarrow B_3\langle 0.44\rangle$; $B_2 \rightarrow B_1\langle 0.21\rangle$; $B_2 \rightarrow B_4\langle 0.06\rangle$; $B_2 \rightarrow B_6\langle 0.04\rangle$; $B_2 \rightarrow B_5\langle 0\rangle$; $B_2 \rightarrow B_7\langle 0\rangle$.

Such mesoscopic association rules would help booksellers adaptively adjust their selling strategies to determine what kinds of stocks they should increase or decrease based on the statistics of past sales. For example, if they find the books labeled as block 2 are sold well, they may correspondingly increase the order of books labeled as blocks 1 and 3 besides block 2, while they may simultaneously decrease the order of books labeled as blocks 5 or 7.

More specifically, with the aid of *NAR*s, booksellers would be able to estimate the chance that customers will spend their money on a book j if they have already bought book i by referring to $i \rightarrow j\langle p_{ij}\rangle$. Such microscopic rules would provide booksellers the suggestions on what specific books should be listed according to what sequence in the recommending area of the web page advertising a book. For example, for the book *"The Price of Loyalty"*, the most worth recommended books are listed as follows according to the coupling strength to it: *Big Lies*$\langle 0.91\rangle$; *Bushwhacked*$\langle 0.73\rangle$; *Plan of Attack*$\langle 0.73\rangle$; *The Politics of Truth*$\langle 0.73\rangle$; *The Lies of George W.Bush*$\langle 0.73\rangle$; *American Dynasty*$\langle 0.64\rangle$; *Bushwomen*$\langle 0.64\rangle$; *The Great Unraveling*$\langle 0.64\rangle$; *Worse Than Watergate*$\langle 0.64\rangle$.

12.4.3 Detecting Hierarchical Community Structure

We have applied our approach to the football association network, a benchmark widely used for testing the performance of community detection algorithms. Figure 12.6 gives the experimental results.

Our approach automatically find out 10 clusters or communities from this network. Figure 12.6a shows the clustered network, and Fig. 12.6c1, shows the clustered matrix, in which dots denote the non-zero entries, and the rows and column corresponding to the same cluster will be put together and be separated by the solid lines. Figure 12.6b shows the searching process, in which the cost in terms of $-L(N|X, B_1) + L_{\overline{OC}}(X)$ firstly drops down quickly, and then goes up sharply after a local minimum corresponding to $K = 10$. This iterative searching process shapes a well-like landscape by penalizing both small likelihood and big coding complexity or smaller priori, and a good compromise between them is what we expect. Notice that, this estimated community number is a little bit smaller than the real one, in total 12 real associations, among which the teams from two small independent associations prefer to play matches with outside teams. (c)–(e) show the nested blocking models of this network. A hierarchical organization with three layers have been constructed.

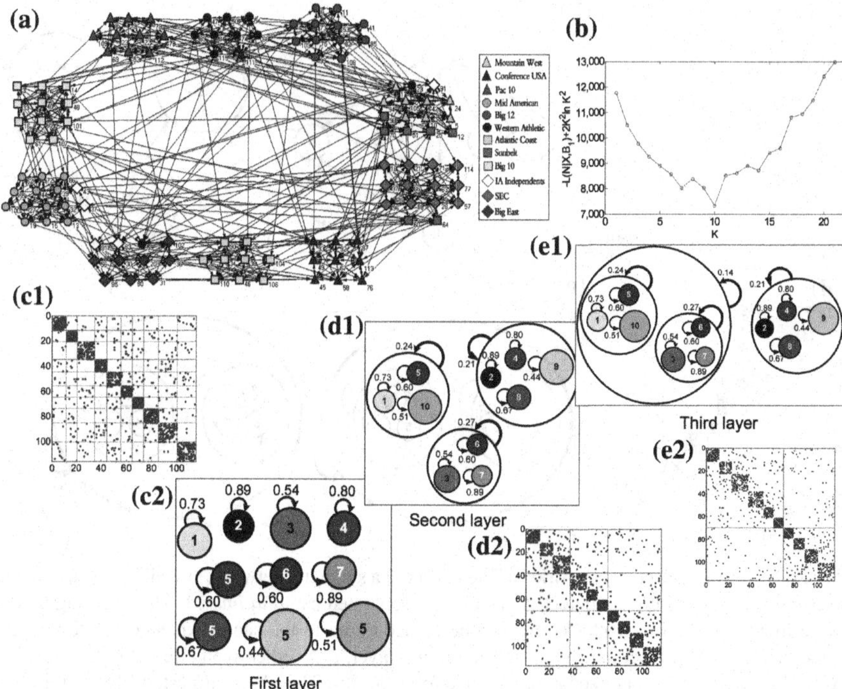

Fig. 12.6 Detecting the hierarchical community structure of the football association network. **a** The discovered football associations; **b** The iterative searching landscape. **c1–c2** The matrix and blocking model of the first layer. **d1–d2** The matrix and blocking model of the second layer. **e1–e2** The matrix and blocking model of the third layer. The coloring schemes used in **a** and **c2**, **d1** and **e1** are same

12.4.4 Testing Against Synthetic Networks

We have tested our approach against several synthetic networks, and here we give two examples. Figure 12.7a gives one synthetic network, in which a 2-community pattern and two bipartite patterns coexist together. A two-layer nested organization is found out. In the first layer, six clusters with homogeneous row as well as column connection distributions are detected; in the second layer, such detected clusters are grouped in pairs according to the node couplings with coarser granularity. This time, a 2-community pattern, a reciprocal bipartite pattern and an unilateral bipartite pattern are emerged. Figure 12.7d give another synthetic network, in which 12 communities are organized in a 3-layer hierarchical structure according to the density of connections. Correspondingly, a three-layer nested blocking model is constructed as given in Fig. 12.7e.

The script defining the stochastic block model of two-layer multiplex patterns as shown by Fig. 12.7a is given as follows.

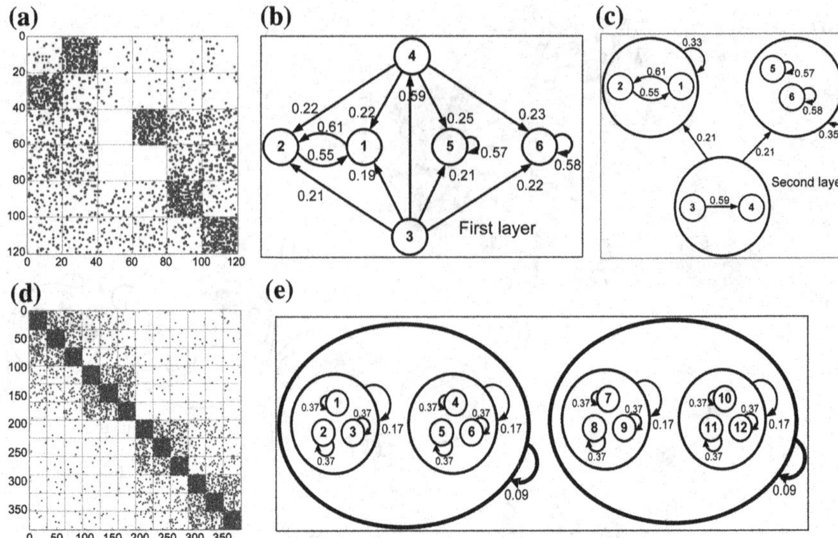

Fig. 12.7 Testing synthetic networks. **a** The matrix of a synthetic network, in which *dots* denote the non-zero entries, and the six detected clusters are separated by *solid lines*; **b** The blocking model in the first layer, in which blocks are numbered according to the same sequence of the clusters in the matrix. **c** The blocking model in the second layer. **d** Another synthetic network, in which twelve detected clusters are separated by the *solid lines*. **e** The obtained nested blocking model corresponding to the hierarchical organization with three layers, in which blocks are numbered according to the same sequence of the clusters in the matrix

Algorithm 4 *The script of defining a hierarchical stochastic block model*

layers = 2;
[define the first layer]
blocks = 6;
block_size = [20 20 20 20 20 20];
block_couplings = [1 2 0.61; 2 1 0.55; 3 4 0.59; 5 5 0.57; 6 6 0.58];
newlayer;
[define the second layer]
blocks = 3;
[define the nested relations]
nested_relation = [1 2; 3 4; 5 6;];
block_couplings = [1 1 0.33; 2 2 0.35; 3 1 0.21; 3 2 0.21];

The algorithm that sampling a random synthetic network from a SBM defined by an input script is given as follows.

Algorithm 5 *Sampling a random network from a SBM script*
A = ***Sampling(script_file_name)***

1. *A = zeros(n,n);*
2. *for i=1:layers*
   a. *r = rows(block_couplings);*
   b. *for j=1:r*
      i. *block1 = block_couplings(j,1);*
      ii. *block2 = block_couplings(j,2);*
      iii. *p = block_coplings(j,3);*
      iv. *let B be the submatrix of A determined by block1 and block2;*
      v. *old_ones = the number of "1" of B;*
      vi. *new_ones = p×rows(B)×cols(B) - old_ones;*
      vii. *randomly put new_ones "1" into the unoccupied areas of B;*
      viii. *label B as "occupied";*
      endfor

   endfor
3. *return A.*

12.5 Conclusions

In this chapter, we have shown through examples that the structural patterns coexisting in the same real-world complex network can be miscellaneous, overlapped or nested, which collaboratively shape a heterogeneous hierarchical organization. We have proposed an approach based on the concept of granular couplings and the proposed granular blocking model to model and uncover such multiplex structure patterns of networks. From the output of patterns, hierarchies and granular couplings generated by our approach, one can analyze or even predict some dynamics of networks, which are helpful for both theoretical studies and practical applications.

Moreover, based on the rationale behind this work, we suggest that the evolution of a real-world network may be driven by the co-evolution of its structural patterns and its underlying couplings. On one hand, statistically significant patterns would be gradually highlighted and emergently shaped by the aggregations of homogeneous individuals in terms of their couplings. On the other hand, individuals would adaptively adjust their respective couplings according to the currently evolved structural patterns.

Acknowledgments This chapter is based on the authors' work published in [1], with further extended materials on detailed theoretical analysis as well as additional experimental results.
This work was supported in part by National Natural Science Foundation of China under grants 61373053 and 61572226, Program for New Century Excellent Talents in University under grant NCET-11-0204, Jilin Province Natural Science Foundation under grants 20150101052JC, and Hong Kong Research Grants Council under grant RGC/HKBU211212 and HKBU12202415.

Appendix

Proposition 1 *For an indirected network, its feedforward-coupling matrix is equal to its feedback-coupling matrix, i.e., we have:* $P = Q$.

Proof $p_{ij} = P(i \rightarrow j|y = k)$
$= \sum_{k=1}^{K} m_{ik} P(i \rightarrow j|y = k)$
$= \sum_{k=1}^{K} (\sum_{l=1}^{L} b_{il} z_{lk}) P(i \rightarrow j|y = k)$
$= \sum_{l=1}^{L} \sum_{k=1}^{K} b_{il} z_{lk} \theta_{kj}$
where $i \rightarrow j$ denote the event that node v_i couples with v_j, and $y = k$ denote the event that v_i is labeled by cluster k; $m_{ik} = 1$ if v_i is labeled by cluster k, otherwise $m_{ik} = 0$. So we have:

$$P = B_g Z \Theta.$$

$q_{ij} = P(i \dashleftarrow j|y = k)$
$= \sum_{k=1}^{K} m_{ik} P(i \dashleftarrow j|y = k)$
$= \sum_{k=1}^{K} (\sum_{l=1}^{L} b_{il} z_{lk}) P(i \dashleftarrow j|y = k)$
$= \sum_{l=1}^{L} \sum_{k=1}^{K} b_{il} z_{lk} \delta_{kj}$
where $i \dashleftarrow j$ denote the event that node v_i except to be coupled by v_j. So we have:

$$Q = B_g Z \Delta.$$

If A is symmetry, from the Eq. 12.4 in the chapter, we have

$$\theta_{kj} = \frac{\sum_{l=1}^{L} \sum_{b_{il} \neq 0} a_{ij} \gamma_{lk}}{\sum_{l=1}^{L} \sum_{b_{il} \neq 0} \gamma_{lk}} = \frac{\sum_{l=1}^{L} \sum_{b_{il} \neq 0} a_{ji} \gamma_{lk}}{\sum_{l=1}^{L} \sum_{b_{il} \neq 0} \gamma_{lk}} = \delta_{kj}.$$

So we have $P = Q$. □

Proposition 2

$$L(N|X, B_g) = \sum_{l=1}^{L} \sum_{b_{il} \neq 0} \ln \sum_{k=1}^{K} \Pi_{j=1}^{n} f(\theta_{kj}, a_{ij}) f(\delta_{kj}, a_{ji}) \omega_k \qquad (12.10)$$

where $f(x, y) = x^y (1 - x)^{1-y}$.

Proof Let $v = i$ denote the event that a node with linkage structure $< a_{i1}, \cdots, a_{in}, a_{1i}, \cdots, a_{ni} >$ will be observed in network N. Let $y = k$ denote the event that the cluster label assigned to a node is equal to k. Let $i \rightarrow_{a_{ij}} j$ denote the event that node v_i link to node v_j or not depending on a_{ij}. Let $i \leftarrow_{a_{ji}} j$ denote the event that node v_i will be linked by node v_j or not depending on a_{ji}. We have:
$L(N|X, B_g) = \ln \Pi_{i=1}^{n} P(v = i) = \sum_{i=1}^{n} \ln P(v = i)$
$= \sum_{i=1}^{n} \ln P((v = i) \cap (\cup_{k=1}^{K} y = k))$
$= \sum_{i=1}^{n} \ln \sum_{k=1}^{K} P(v = i, y = k)$
$= \sum_{i=1}^{n} \ln \sum_{k=1}^{K} (P(v = i|y = k) P(y = k))$
$= \sum_{i=1}^{n} \ln \sum_{k=1}^{K} (P(< a_{i1}, \cdots, a_{in}, a_{1i}, \cdots, a_{ni} > |y = k) P(y = k))$
$= \sum_{i=1}^{n} \ln \sum_{k=1}^{K} (\Pi_{j=1}^{n} P(i \rightarrow_{a_{ij}} j|y = k) P(i \leftarrow_{a_{ji}} j|y = k) P(y = k))$
$= \sum_{i=1}^{n} \ln \sum_{k=1}^{K} (\Pi_{j=1}^{n} (\theta_{kj}^{a_{ij}} (1 - \theta_{kj})^{1-a_{ij}}) (\delta_{kj}^{a_{ji}} (1 - \delta_{kj})^{1-a_{ji}}) \omega_k)$

$= \sum_{i=1}^{n} \ln \sum_{k=1}^{K} (\Pi_{j=1}^{n} f(\theta_{kj}, a_{ij}) f(\delta_{kj}, a_{ji}) \omega_k)$
$= \sum_{l=1}^{L} \sum_{b_{il} \neq 0} \ln \sum_{k=1}^{K} (\Pi_{j=1}^{n} f(\theta_{kj}, a_{ij}) f(\delta_{kj}, a_{ji}) \omega_k)$ □

Proposition 3

$$L(N, Z|X, B_g) = \sum_{l=1}^{L} \sum_{b_{il} \neq 0} \sum_{k=1}^{K} z_{lk} (\sum_{j=1}^{n} (\ln f(\theta_{kj}, a_{ij}) + \ln f(\delta_{kj}, a_{ji})) + \ln \omega_k) \quad (12.11)$$

Proof Let $y(i)$ denote the cluster label assigned to node i under the given partition Z, we have:
$L(N, Z|X, B_g)$
$= \ln \Pi_{i=1}^{n} P(v = i, y = y(i))$
$= \sum_{i=1}^{n} \ln \sum_{k=1}^{K} m_{ik} P(v = i, y = k)$
$= \sum_{i=1}^{n} \ln \sum_{k=1}^{K} m_{ik} P(v = i | y = k) P(y = k)$
$= \sum_{i=1}^{n} \sum_{k=1}^{K} \ln(P(v = i | y = k) P(y = k))^{m_{ik}}$
$= \sum_{i=1}^{n} \sum_{k=1}^{K} m_{ik} \ln(P(v = i | y = k) P(y = k))$
$= \sum_{i=1}^{n} \sum_{k=1}^{K} m_{ik} \ln(\Pi_{j=1}^{n} (\theta_{kj}^{a_{ij}} (1 - \theta_{kj}^{1-a_{ij}}) \delta_{kj}^{a_{ji}} (1 - \delta_{kj}^{1-a_{ji}})) \omega_k$
$= \sum_{i=1}^{n} \sum_{k=1}^{K} m_{ik} (\sum_{j=1}^{n} (\ln f(\theta_{kj}, a_{ij}) + \ln f(\delta_{kj}, a_{ji})) + \ln \omega_k)$
$= \sum_{b_{i1} \neq 0} \sum_{k=1}^{K} z_{1k} (\sum_{j=1}^{n} (\ln f(\theta_{kj}, a_{ij}) + \ln f(\delta_{kj}, a_{ji})) + \ln \omega_k) + \cdots$
$+ \sum_{b_{iL} \neq 0} \sum_{k=1}^{K} z_{Lk} (\sum_{j=1}^{n} (\ln f(\theta_{kj}, a_{ij}) + \ln f(\delta_{kj}, a_{ji})) + \ln \omega_k)$
$= \sum_{l=1}^{L} \sum_{b_{il} \neq 0} \sum_{k=1}^{K} z_{lk} (\sum_{j=1}^{n} (\ln f(\theta_{kj}, a_{ij}) + \ln f(\delta_{kj}, a_{ji})) + \ln \omega_k)$. □

Notice that, in the proofs of Propositions 2–3, all probabilities such as $P(y = k | v = i)$ and $P(y = k)$ are discussed under the conditions of X and B_g. To simplify the equations, we omit them without losing correctness.

Proposition 4

$$\gamma_{lk} = \frac{1}{\sum_{i=1}^{n} b_{il}} \sum_{b_{il} \neq 0} \frac{\Pi_{j=1}^{n} f(\theta_{kj}, a_{ij}) f(\delta_{kj}, a_{ji}) \omega_k}{\sum_{k=1}^{K} \Pi_{j=1}^{n} f(\theta_{kj}, a_{ij}) f(\delta_{kj}, a_{ji}) \omega_k} \quad (12.12)$$

Proof let $P(y = k | v = i)$ be the probability that node i belongs to cluster k given X and B_g. We have:
$\gamma_{lk} = P(y = k | b = l, X, B_g)$
$= \sum_{b_{il} \neq 0} \frac{1}{\sum_{i=1}^{n} b_{il}} P(y = k | v = i)$
where $\frac{1}{\sum_{i=1}^{n} b_{il}}$ is the probability of selecting node i from block l.
According to the Bayesian theorem, we have:
$$P(y = k | v = i) = \frac{P(y=k) P(v=i | y=k)}{\sum_{k=1}^{K} P(y=k) P(v=i | y=k)}.$$
Based on the proof of Proposition 1, we have:
$$P(y = k) P(v = i | y = k) = \Pi_{j=1}^{n} f(\theta_{kj}, a_{ij}) f(\delta_{kj}, a_{ji}) \omega_k.$$
So, we have Eq. 12.12. □

As an approximate version of Eq. 12.12, we have:

$$\begin{aligned}\gamma_{lk} &= P(y=k|b=l) = P(y=k|v=i, b_{il} \neq 0) \\ &= \frac{P(y=k)P(v=i, b_{il} \neq 0|y=k)}{\sum_{k=1}^{K} P(y=k)P(v=i, b_{il} \neq 0|y=k)} \\ &= \frac{\exists_{b_{il} \neq 0} \Pi_{j=1}^{n} f(\theta_{kj}, a_{ij}) f(\delta_{kj}, a_{ji}) \omega_k}{\sum_{k=1}^{K} \exists_{b_{il} \neq 0} \Pi_{j=1}^{n} f(\theta_{kj}, a_{ij}) f(\delta_{kj}, a_{ji}) \omega_k}\end{aligned} \tag{12.13}$$

where $\exists_{b_{il} \neq 0}$ denotes that randomly selecting a node from block l.

That is, instead of averaging all nodes in the block l, the real value of γ_{lk} can be approximately estimated by a randomly selected node from block l.

Correspondingly, an approximate version of the log-likelihood of Eq. 12.10 is given by:

$$\begin{aligned}L(N|X, B_g) = \sum_{l=1}^{L} N_l (\exists_{b_{il} \neq 0} \ln \sum_{k=1}^{K} \Pi_{j=1}^{n} f(\theta_{kj}, a_{ij}) \\ f(\delta_{kj}, a_{ji}) \omega_k)\end{aligned} \tag{12.14}$$

where N_l denotes the size of block l.

The time calculating Eqs. 12.12 and 12.10 will be bounded by $O(n^2 K)$. While, the time calculating Eqs. 12.13 and 12.14 will be bounded by $O(LnK)$. This will be much efficient for constructing the hierarchical organizations of networks.

Theorem 1 *A local optimum of Eq. 12.10 will be guaranteed by recursively calculating Eqs. 12.4 and 12.5 in the chapter.*

Proof From the Proposition 1, we have:
$L(N|X, B_g)$
$= \sum_{i=1}^{n} \ln P(v=i|X, B_g)$
$= \sum_{i=1}^{n} \ln \sum_{k=1}^{K} P(v=i, y=k|X, B_g)$
$= \sum_{i=1}^{n} \ln \sum_{k=1}^{K} P(y=k|v=i, X^{(s)}, B_g)$
$\frac{P(v=i,y=k|X,B_g)}{P(y=k|v=i,X^{(s)},B_g)}$
(by Jensen's inequality)
$\geq \sum_{i=1}^{n} \sum_{k=1}^{K} P(y=k|v=i, X^{(s)}, B_g) \ln \frac{P(v=i,y=k|X,B_g)}{P(y=k|v=i,X^{(s)},B_g)}$
$\equiv G(X, X^{(s)})$.

Furthermore, we have:
$G(X^{(s)}, X^{(s)})$
$= \sum_{i=1}^{n} \sum_{k=1}^{K} P(y=k|v=i, X^{(s)}, B_g) \ln \frac{P(v=i,y=k|X^{(s)},B_g)}{P(y=k|v=i,X^{(s)},B_g)}$
$= \sum_{i=1}^{n} \sum_{k=1}^{K} P(y=k|v=i, X^{(s)}, B_g) \ln P(v=i|X^{(s)}, B_g)$
$= \sum_{i=1}^{n} \ln P(v=i|X^{(s)}, B_g) \sum_{k=1}^{K} P(y=k|v=i, X^{(s)}, B_g)$
$= \sum_{i=1}^{n} \ln P(v=i|X^{(s)}, B_g)$

$= L(N|X^{(s)}, B_g)$.

Let $P(y = k|b = l, X^{(s)}, B_g) = \gamma_{ik}^{(s)}$, we have:

$G(X, X^{(s)})$

$= \sum_{l=1}^{L} \sum_{b_{il}\neq 0} \sum_{k=1}^{K} \gamma_{lk}^{(s)} \ln P(v = i, y = k|X, B_g) - \sum_{l=1}^{L} \sum_{b_{il}\neq 0} \sum_{k=1}^{K} \gamma_{ik}^{(s)} \ln P(y = k|v = i, X^{(s)}, B_g)$.

So, we have:

$\arg\max G(X, X^{(s)})$

$= \arg\max(\sum_{l=1}^{L} \sum_{b_{il}\neq 0} \sum_{k=1}^{K} \gamma_{lk}^{(s)} \ln P(v = i, y = k|X, B_g) - \sum_{l=1}^{L} \sum_{b_{il}\neq 0} \sum_{k=1}^{K} \gamma_{ik}^{(s)} \ln P(y = k|v = i, X^{(s)}, B_g))$

$= \arg\max(\sum_{l=1}^{L} \sum_{b_{il}\neq 0} \sum_{k=1}^{K} (\gamma_{ik}^{(s)} \ln P(v = i, y = k|X, B_g)))$

$= \arg\max E[L(N, Z^{(s)}|X, B_g)]$

$= X^{(s+1)}$.

Recall that, the $\Theta^{(s+1)}$, $\Delta^{(s+1)}$ and $\Omega^{(s+1)}$ of $X^{(s+1)}$ can be computed in terms of $\gamma_{lk}^{(s)}$ by Eq. 12.4 in the chapter. So, we have:

$$G(X^{(s+1)}, X^{(s)}) \geq G(X^{(s)}, X^{(s)}) = L(N|X^{(s)}, B_g).$$

Recall that $L(N|X, B_g) \geq G(X, X^{(s)})$, we have:

$L(N|X^{(s+1)}, B_g) \geq G(X^{(s+1)}, X^{(s)}) \geq G(X^{(s)}, X^{(s)}) = L(N|X^{(s)}, B_g)$.

That is to say, the $X^{(s+1)}$ obtained in the current iteration will be not worse than $X^{(s)}$ obtained in last iteration. So, we have the theorem. □

Proposition 5 *In terms of the parameter of* X, Θ, Δ, Z *and* Ω, *we have:*

$$\Phi = \Theta B_g Z D^{-1}, \quad \Psi = \Delta B_g Z D^{-1} \tag{12.15}$$

where $D = diag(n\Omega)$.

Proof We have

$$\phi_{pq} = \sum_{i\in C_q} \frac{1}{N_q} \theta_{pi}$$

where $i \in C_q$ denotes node i is in the cluster q with a size N_q, and $\frac{1}{N_q}$ is the probability of selecting node i from cluster q. Furthermore, we have:

$$\phi_{pq} = \frac{1}{n\omega_q} \sum_{i=1}^{n} \theta_{pi} (B_g Z)_{iq}.$$

Similarly, we have:

$$\psi_{pq} = \frac{1}{n\omega_q} \sum_{i=1}^{n} \delta_{pi} (B_g Z)_{iq}.$$

So, we have

$$\Phi = \Theta B_g Z D^{-1}, \quad \Psi = \Delta B_g Z D^{-1}.$$

□

Proposition 6 *Let* B_{g_i} *denotes the blocking model on the* $i-th$ *layer of the hierarchical organization of network* N, *we have:*

$P(X|N, B_{g_1}, \cdots, B_{g_h}) \propto P(N|X, B_{g_h}) P(X)^{g_h}$

Proof $P(X|N, B_{g_1}, \cdots, B_{g_h})$

$= \frac{P(X,N,B_{g_1},\cdots,B_{g_h})}{P(N,B_{g_1},\cdots,B_{g_h})}$

$\propto P(X, N, B_{g_1}, \cdots, B_{g_h})$

$$= P(N|X, B_{g_1}, \cdots, B_{g_h})P(X, B_{g_1}, \cdots, B_{g_h})$$
$$= P(N|X, B_{g_1}, \cdots, B_{g_h})P(X|B_{g_1}, \cdots, B_{g_h})$$
$$P(B_{g_h}|B_{g_1}, \cdots, B_{g_{h-1}}) \cdots P(B_{g_2}|B_{g_1})P(B_{g_1})$$
$$\propto P(N|X, B_{g_1}, \cdots, B_{g_h})P(X|B_{g_1}, \cdots, B_{g_h})$$

Since two nodes from the same block of $B_{g_{i-1}}$ will also be in the same block of B_{g_i}, we have:

$$P(X|N, B_{g_1}, \cdots, B_{g_h}) \propto P(N|X, B_{g_h})P(X|B_{g_h}) = P(N|X, B_{g_h})P(X)^{g_h} \qquad \square$$

References

1. B. Yang, J. Liu, D. Liu, Characterizing and extracting multiplex patterns in complex networks. IEEE Trans. Syst. Man Cybernet. (Part B—Cybernetics) **42**(2), 469–481 (2012)
2. S. Boccaletti, V. Latora, Y. Moreno, M. Chavez, D.U. Hwang, Complex networks: structure and dynamics. Phys. Rep. **424**, 175–308 (2006)
3. R. Milo, S.S. Orr, S. Itzkovitz, N. Kashtan, D. Chklovskii, U. Alon, Network motifs: simple building blocks of complex networks. Science **298**, 824–827 (2002)
4. M. Girvan, M.E.J. Newman, Community structure in social and biological networks. Proc. Natl. Acad. Sci. USA **99**(12), 7821–7826 (2002)
5. D.J. Watts, S.H. Strogatz, Collective dynamics of small-world networks. Nature **393**, 440–442 (1998)
6. A.L. Barabasi, R. Albert, Emergence of scaling in random networks. Science **286**, 509–512 (1999)
7. S. Fortunato, Community detection in graphs. Phys. Rep. **486**, 75–174 (2010)
8. P. Holme, F. Liljeros, C.R. Edling, B.J. Kim, Network bipartivity. Phys. Rev. E. **68**, 056107 (2003)
9. J.L. Guillaume, M. Latapy, Bipartite structure of all complex networks. Inform. Process. Lett. **90**, 215–221 (2004)
10. A. Brady, K. Maxwell, N. Daniels, L.J. Cowen, Fault tolerance in protein interaction networks: stable bipartite subgraphs and redundant pathways. PLoS ONE **4**, e5364 (2009)
11. J.M. Kleinberg, Authoritative sources in a hyperlinked environment. J. ACM **46**, 604–632 (1999)
12. R. Albert, H. Jeong, A.L. Barabasi, The internet's achilles heel: error and attack tolerance of complex netowrks. Nature **406**, 378–382 (2000)
13. O. Sporns, C. Honey, R. Kotter, Identification and classification of hubs in brain networks. PLoS ONE **2**(10), e1049 (2007)
14. A. Broder, R. Kumar, F. Maghoul, P. Raghavan, S. Rajagopalan, R. Stata, A. Tomkins, J. Wiener, Graph structure in the web. Comput. Netw. **33**, 309–320 (1999)
15. News Feature, The web is a bow tie. Nature **405**, 113 (2000)
16. H.W. Ma, A.P. Zeng, The connectivity structure, giant strong component and centrality of metabolic networks. Bioinformatics **19**, 1423–1430 (2003)
17. G. Palla, I. Derenyi, I. Farkas, T. Vicsek, Uncovering the overlapping community structures of complex networks in nature and society. Nature **435**, 814–818 (2005)
18. D.E. Knuth, *The Stanford GraphBase: A Platform for Combinatorial Computing* (Addison-Wesley press, Reading, MA, 1993)
19. E. Ravasz, A.L. Somera, D.A. Mongru, Z.N. Oltvai, A.L. Barabasi, Hierarchical organization of modularity in metabolic networks. Science **297**, 1551–1555 (2004)
20. C. Zhou, L. Zemanova, G. Zamora, C.C. Hilgetag, J. Kurths, Hierarchical organization unveiled by functional connectivity in complex brain networks. Phys. Rev. Lett. **97**, 238103 (2006)
21. M.S. Pardo, R. Guimera, A.A. Moreira, L.A.N. Amaral, Extracting the hierarchical organization of complex systems. Proc. Natl. Acad. Sci. USA **104**, 7821–7826 (2007)

22. A. Clauset, C. Moore, M.E.J. Newman, Hierarchical structure and the prediction of missing links in networks. Nature **453**, 98–101 (2008)
23. C. Kemp, J.B. Tenenbaum, The discovery of structural form. Proc. Natl. Acad. Sci. USA **105**, 10687–10692 (2008)
24. F. Lorrain, H.C. White, Structural equivalence of individuals in social networks. J. Math. Sociol. **1**, 49–80 (1971)
25. D.R. White, K.P. Reitz, Graph and semigroup homomorphism on networks of relations. Soc. Netw. **5**, 193–235 (1983)
26. S.E. Fienberg, S. Wasserman, Categorical data analysis of single sociometric relations. Sociol. Methodol. **12**, 156–192 (1983)
27. P.W. Holland, K.B. Laskey, S. Leinhardt, Stochastic blockmodels: some first steps. Soc. Netw. **5**, 109–137 (1983)
28. M.E.J. Newman, E.A. Leicht, Mixture models and exploratory analysis in networks. Proc. Natl. Acad. Sci. USA **104**, 9564–9569 (2007)
29. A.P. Dempster, N.M. Laird, D.B. Rubin, Maximum likelihood from incomplete data via the EM algorithm. J. R. Stat. Soc. B. **39**, 185–197 (1977)
30. C.E. Shannon, W. Weaver, *The Mathematical Theory of Communication* (University of Illinois Press, Urbana, 1949)
31. W.D. Nooy, A. Mirvar, V. Batagelj, *Exploratory Social Network Analysis with Pajeck* (Cambridge University Press, 2004)
32. D.A. Smith, D.R. White, Structure and dynamics of the global economy—network analysis of international-trade 1965–1980. Soc. Forces **70**, 857–893 (1992)
33. M.E.J. Newman, Finding community structure in networks using the eigenvectors of matrices. Phys. Rev. E. **74**, 036104 (2006)

Chapter 13
Suitable Route Recommendation Inspired by Cognition

Hui Wang, Jiajin Huang, Erzhong Zhou, Zhisheng Huang and Ning Zhong

Abstract With the increasing popularity of mobile phones, large amounts of real and reliable mobile phone data are being generated every day. These mobile phone data represent the practical travel routes of users and imply the intelligence of them in selecting a suitable route. Usually, an experienced user knows which route is congested in a specified period of time but unblocked in another period of time. Moreover, a route used frequently and recently by a user is usually the suitable one to satisfy the user's needs. ACT-R (Adaptive Control of Thought-Rational) is a computational cognitive architecture, which provides a good framework to understand the principles and mechanisms of information organization, retrieval and selection in human memory. In this chapter, we employ ACT-R to model the process of selecting a suitable route of users. We propose a cognition-inspired route recommendation method to mine the intelligence of users in selecting a suitable route, evaluate the suitability of the routes, and recommend an ordered list of routes for subscribers. Experiments show that it is effective and feasible to recommend the suitable routes inspired by cognition.

H. Wang · J. Huang · E. Zhou · Z. Huang
International WIC Institute, Beijing University of Technology, Beijing, China

J. Huang
e-mail: hjj@emails.bjut.edu.cn

N. Zhong (✉)
Beijing Advanced Innovation Center for Future Internet Technology, The International WIC Institute, Beijing University of Technology, Beijing, China
e-mail: zhongn@bjut.edu.cn; zhong@maebashi-it.ac.jp

N. Zhong
Department of Life Science and Informatics, Maebashi Institute of Technology, Maebashi, Japan

Z. Huang
Department of Computer Science, Vrije University of Amsterdam, Amsterdam, The Netherlands
e-mail: z.huang@vu.nl; huang@cs.vu.nl; huang.zhisheng.nl@gmail.com

N. Zhong et al. (eds.), *Wisdom Web of Things*, Web Information Systems Engineering and Internet Technologies Book Series,
DOI 10.1007/978-3-319-44198-6_13

13.1 Introduction

Routing service is an important application in our daily life. Suitable routing can not only benefit subscribers on their daily journeys but also improve the traffic condition of the city. Although many routing services like Baidu and Google Maps have been emerging, existing routing services generally search the routes between the origin and destination, calculate the travel time of each route (usually based on the distance and speed constraint), and recommend the routes ordered by time. In these routing services, the real traffic condition is not often taken into account and the recommended order of the routes is static. Another observation is that a route may heavily be congested in the morning and evening but unblocked in other periods of time. We can see that it is necessary to evaluate the routes according to the real traffic condition and recommend them in a suitable order in different periods of time.

Nowadays, mobile phones are often used as 'monitors' of users' travel routes due to the fact that the users tend to carry mobile phones with them all days. And with the increasing popularity of mobile phones, large amounts of real and reliable mobile phone data are being generated every day. In the real world, an experienced user knows which route is congested in a specified period of time but unblocked in another period of time. And the user can select a suitable route according to his/her experience and cognition in real traffic condition. These mobile phone data represent the practical travel routes of users and imply the intelligence of them in selecting a suitable route. Hence we can learn the intelligence from these mobile phone data and evaluate the suitability of the routes for subscribers.

Adaptive control of thought-rational (ACT-R) is a computational cognitive architecture, which provides a good framework to understand the principles and mechanisms of information organization, retrieval and selection in human memory [1, 2]. ACT-R deems that human memory is composed of many units of information and each unit of information can be viewed as a chunk. ACT-R uses an activation equation to model the process of information retrieval based on these chunks.

Inspired by ACT-R, we present an application of the activation equation in ACT-R to mine the intelligence of users in selecting a suitable route and evaluate the suitability of the routes for subscribers, which is based on the architecture of three-level granularity of information organization by using a large number of real mobile phone data.

In order to reach this goal, we need to face the following three challenges:

- In order to evaluate the suitability of the routes, we need to discover the routes which users deem suitable. In general, a user's mobile phone data between the origin and destination of a trip can represent a suitable route for the user. However, the mobile phone data of a user may contain many trips. The first challenge for us is how to detect the origins and destinations exactly and extract the suitable routes from the mobile phone data of a user.
- After detecting the origins and destinations from these mobile phone data, many suitable routes will be extracted. As a route to be evaluated may be starting from any origin and ending at any destination, there would be no extracted suitable

route passing the route to be evaluated. In other words, we cannot directly match the route to be evaluated with the extracted suitable routes. How to model these extracted suitable routes that can tackle the problem above is another challenge for us.

- After modeling these extracted suitable routes properly, any route to be evaluated will be matched directly. Although ACT-R provides a good framework to understand the process of information retrieval in human memory, how to employ ACT-R correctly to simulate the process of selecting a suitable route in human memory still is a big challenge, which concerns whether we can evaluate the routes accurately.

The remainder of this chapter is organized as follows: We give the preliminary to our work and briefly review the related work in Sect. 13.2. Then the problem is stated in Sect. 13.3. In Sect. 13.4, we describe the proposed method, in detail. The empirical evaluation for performance study is made in Sect. 13.5. Finally, we conclude our work in Sect. 13.6.

13.2 Foundation and State of the Art

In this section, we give the foundation about mobile phone data obtained from the GSM (Global Systems for Mobile Communications) network, and review the related work.

13.2.1 Foundation

To begin with, we clarify the concepts of location area and cell briefly. In a GSM network, the service coverage area is divided into smaller areas of hexagonal shape, referred to as cells (as shown in Fig. 13.1). In each cell, a base station (namely, an antenna) is installed. And within each cell, mobile phones can communicate with a certain base station. In other words, a cell is served by a base station. A location area consists of a set of cells that are grouped together to optimize signaling, which is identified distinctively by a location area identifier (LAI) in the GSM network. A cell is also identified uniquely by a cell identity (CI) in a location area. That is to say, a cell in a GSM network is identified by a LAI and a CI. For convenience, we use CID to indicate a cell uniquely in a GSM network instead of a LAI and a CI. In urban areas, cells are close to each other and small in area whose diameter can be down to one hundred meters, while in rural areas the diameter of a cell can reach kilometers.

When a mobile phone corresponds with the GSM network, the signal sent by the mobile phone contains the location information (in the form of a CID) of the mobile phone. In order to provide service for mobile phones effectively, the location information will be stored by the GSM network. That the mobile phone sends a signal to the GSM network is triggered by one of the following events:

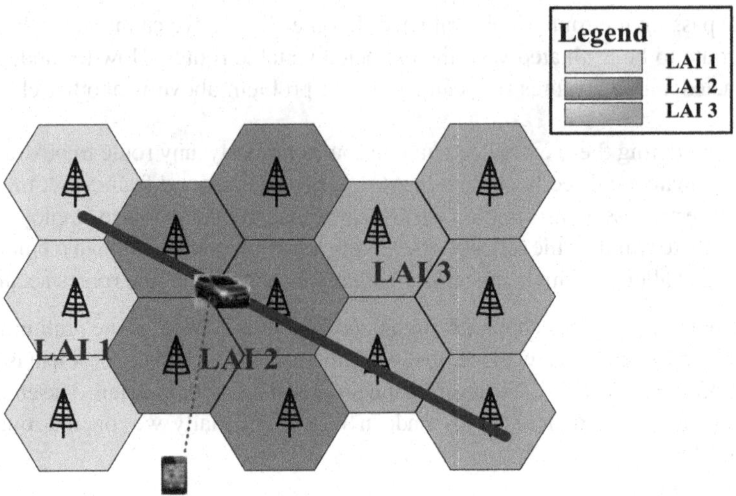

Fig. 13.1 The concepts of location area and cell

- The mobile phone is switched on or switched off.
- The mobile phone receives or sends a short message.
- The mobile phone places or receives a call (both at the beginning and end of the call).
- The mobile phone connects the Internet (for example, browsing the web).
- The mobile phone moves into a cell belonging to a new location area, which is called Normal Location Updating.
- The mobile phone during a call is entering into a new cell, which is called Handover.
- The timer set by the network comes to an end when there is no any event mentioned above that happened to the mobile phone, which is called Periodical Location Updating.

13.2.2 State of the Art

Mobile Phone Data Mining.
Many studies have been conducted on mobile phone data for urban computing. Caceres and Calabrese exploited mobile phone data to acquire high-quality origin-destination information for traffic planning and management respectively [3, 4]. Calabrese developed a real-time urban monitoring system to sense city dynamics which range from traffic conditions to the movements of pedestrians throughout the city, using mobile phones [5]. Ying mined the similarity of users by using their mobile phone data [6]. Ying and Lu predicted the next location of the user with mobile phone data respectively [7, 8]. Liu studied the annotation of mobile phone data with activity purposes, which can be used to understand the travel behavior of users [9]. Our work

aims to mine the intelligence of users in selecting a suitable route and recommend the routes to subscribers, which is totally different from the work above.

Route Recommendation Systems.
In recent years, some researches have been performed for route recommendation based on large amounts of trajectories. Yuan et al. developed a smart driving direction system that analyzed the trajectories of GPS-equipped taxis [10]. The system aimed to leverage the intelligence of experienced taxi drivers in choosing driving directions and provide a subscriber with the fastest route. Wei presented a route inference framework to construct the popular routes from uncertain trajectories [11]. Explicitly, given a location sequence, the route inference framework was able to construct the top-k routes which sequentially passed through the locations within the specified time span, by aggregating such uncertain trajectories in a mutual reinforcement way. Chen investigated the problem of discovering the most popular route between two locations by using a huge collection of historical truck trajectories generated by GPS-enabled devices [12]. The discovery of the most popular route between two locations is the most similar one to our work. However, we are also different in the following aspects. (1) The data we use are mobile phone data which are totally different from GPS trajectories. The mobile phone data are a sequence of cells, each of which covers an area rather than being a GPS point. And the sampling frequencies between mobile phone data and GPS trajectories are different. (2) Our aim is to evaluate a given route rather than discover a popular route. (3) We use a cognition-inspired method which is more consistent with the thinking pattern of human.

13.3 Problem Statement

In this section, we define some terms used in this chapter and give the representation of our problem.

Definition 1 (Mobile Phone Record Set and Mobile Phone Trajectory). *A mobile phone record set is a sequence of records R*: $r_1 \rightarrow r_2, ..., \rightarrow r_n$, *each of which* r_i $(1 \leq i \leq n)$ *contains a LAI*(r_i.LAI), a CI(r_i.*CI*), *a timestamp*(r_i.T), *an event*(r_i.E), *and an antenna*(r_i.*A*) *with the constraint* $(r_i.T \leq r_{i+1}.T\ \forall 1 \leq i \leq n-1)$, *representing that an event* $r_i.E$ *happens in cell* $r_i.CI$ *belonging to location area* $r_i.LAI$ *at time* $r_i.T$ *and the antenna* $r_i.A$ *(whose latitude and longitude can be obtained) is located in cell* $r_i.CI$.

As shown in the left part of Fig. 13.2, r_1, r_2, ..., r_{12} constitute a mobile phone record set. We can connect these cells within r_i $(1 \leq i \leq 12)$ into a mobile phone trajectory according to their time serials, as shown in the right part of Fig. 13.2.

Definition 2 (Stay Area). *A stay area stands for a geographic region where a user stayed over a certain time interval. A stay area carries a particular semantic meaning, such as a place we work/live in, a business district we walk around for shopping, or*

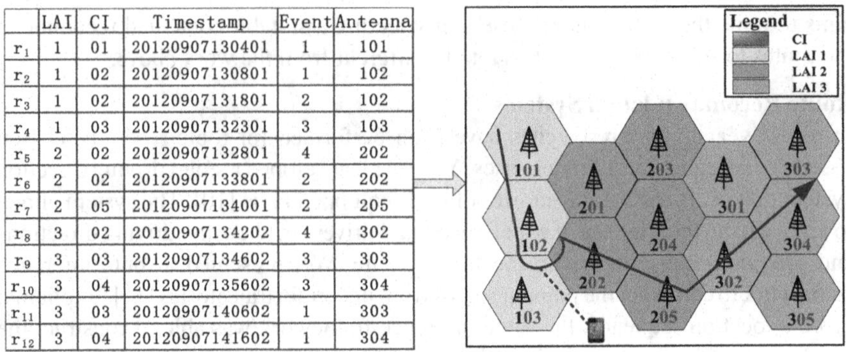

	LAI	CI	Timestamp	Event	Antenna
r_1	1	01	20120907130401	1	101
r_2	1	02	20120907130801	1	102
r_3	1	02	20120907131801	2	102
r_4	1	03	20120907132301	3	103
r_5	2	02	20120907132801	4	202
r_6	2	02	20120907133801	2	202
r_7	2	05	20120907134001	2	205
r_8	3	02	20120907134202	4	302
r_9	3	03	20120907134602	3	303
r_{10}	3	04	20120907135602	3	304
r_{11}	3	03	20120907140602	1	303
r_{12}	3	04	20120907141602	1	304

Fig. 13.2 The example of a mobile phone record and a mobile phone trajectory

a spot we wander in for sightseeing. Owing to the fact that the user cannot be located accurately, a stay area can be regarded as a cell or a group of consecutive cells. The detection of a stay area depends on two scale parameters, a time threshold θ_t representing the minimum stay time interval, and a distance threshold θ_d representing the maximum distance between any two antennas in the stay area. Given a mobile phone record set R: $r_1 \rightarrow r_2, ..., \rightarrow r_n$, if there exists a sub-sequence R': $r_{i'} \rightarrow r_{i'+1}, ..., \rightarrow r_{j'}$, where $r_{j'}.T - r_{i'}.T \geq \theta_t$ and $\forall i' \leq i \leq j \leq j'$, Distance($r_i.CID, r_j.CID$) $\leq \theta_d$, a stay area can be defined as s=$\{r_{i'}$.CID, $r_{i'+1}$.CID, ..., $r_{j'}$.CID$\}$. The function Distance(r_i.CID, r_j.CID) indicates the Euclidean distance between the antenna $r_i.A$ and the antenna $r_j.A$.

Definition 3 (Landmark Cell). *If a cell is traversed frequently by users, we call this cell a landmark cell. Generally speaking, the more frequently the place is traversed, the more important the place is. In the real route planning, we often use a sequence of important places to represent our routes (e.g., from Beijing University of Technology to Dawanglu Station to The Imperial Palace). In order to match with the natural thinking pattern of human, we can represent a route with a sequence of landmark cells which are some important places.*

Definition 4 (Suitable Route). *Given a user's mobile phone record set R: $r_1 \rightarrow r_2$, ..., $\rightarrow r_n$, if there exists a sub-sequence R': $r_{i'} \rightarrow r_{i'+1}, ..., \rightarrow r_{j'}$, which can represent a trip of the user completely (namely, the sub-sequence R' starts from the origin of the trip and ends at the destination of the trip), we call this sub-sequence R' a suitable route. To avoid ambiguity, we use R^s: $r^s_1 \rightarrow r^s_2, ..., \rightarrow r^s_m$ (m = $j' - i' + 1$) to indicate the suitable route.*

Definition 5 (Transition). *Given a set of suitable routes, two cells u, v, we say e_{uv} is a transition (or a edge) if it holds the two following conditions: (1) Cell u and cell v are two landmark cells. (2) There exists a sub-sequence $R^{s'}$: $r^s_{i'} \rightarrow r^s_{i'+1}, ..., \rightarrow r^s_{j'}$, cell $r^s_{i'}$.CID and cell $r^s_{j'}$.CID are two landmark cells and $\forall i' < k < j'$, cell r^s_k.CID is not a landmark cell.*

Definition 6 (Transition Network). *A transition network $G = (V,E)$ is a directed graph that consists of a set of landmark cells V and a set of transitions E.*

Problem Representation. With the definitions above, the main problem we are addressing in this chapter is formulated as follow: Given some routes queried by a subscriber and represented as a set of cell sequences, our goal is to develop a system to evaluate the suitability of the queried routes. In other words, we mine the intelligence of users in selecting a suitable route from their mobile phone data and employ the intelligence to evaluate the suitability of the queried routes for a subscriber.

13.4 Proposed Method

In this section, we describe our system design and discuss three important issues in the process of evaluating the routes inspired by cognition: detection of the stay areas, construction of the transition network, and route evaluation inspired by cognition.

13.4.1 System Framework

Figure 13.3 gives an overview of our system, which realizes a data cycle in the physical world, the cyber world, and the social world [13].

Mobile phones are used to probe the traffic behavior of users in the physical world, which will generate large amounts of mobile phone data. In the cyber world, a

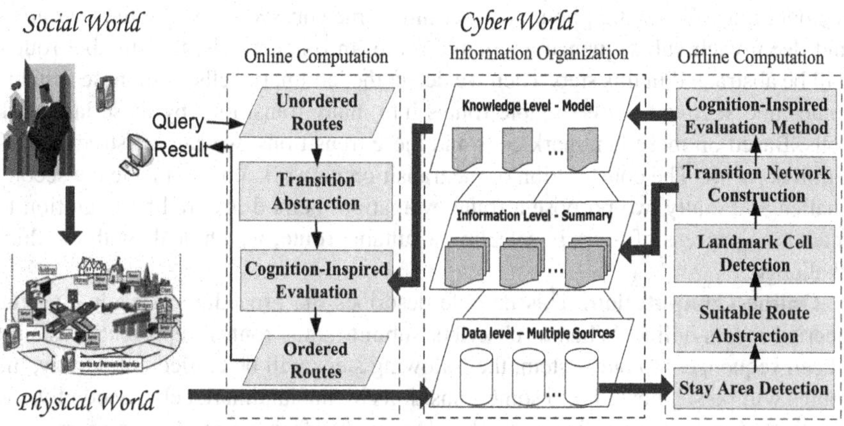

Fig. 13.3 Architecture of our system

cognition-inspired route evaluation method is implemented to mine the intelligence of users in selecting a suitable route from these mobile phone data. The system provides route evaluation service to the subscribers and the subscribers can share their experiences of the real traffic condition in the social world. In turn, the subscribers/users travel again in the physical world.

In the cyber world, our system consists of an information organization module, an offline computation module and an online computation module.

Information Organization: This module aims to organize our information using the principles and mechanisms of information organization in human memory.

As mentioned in Sect. 13.1, human memory is composed of many chunks and each chunk can be viewed as a granule. In other words, we can decompose the information in human memory into many granules. Moreover, granules can be grouped into multiple levels to form a hierarchical granular structure. The theory above inspires us to employ a conceptual architecture of three-level of granularity to represent our information organization: the data level, the information level, and the knowledge level. The data level is used to store the original data (e.g., the mobile phone data). The information level is used to store the information (e.g., the transition network G) summarized from the data level. The knowledge level is used to store the used models (e.g., the route evaluation method). The information of each level is decomposed into many granules.

It is convenient to switch among the three levels according to different needs, which is based on the architecture of three-level granularity for information organization.

Offline Computation: The offline computation module aims to prepare the needed information for the module of information organization and lighten the burden on online computation. Firstly, we detect the stay areas from a user's mobile phone data set. Generally speaking, a stay area indicates the origin or destination of a trip. The detection of the stay areas is to handle the first challenge. Secondly, we segment a user's mobile phone data set into some sub-sequences by the stay areas and deem each sub-sequence a suitable route. In other words, the suitable routes will be abstracted in this step. Then we detect the landmark cells from these suitable routes and segment these suitable routes into many transitions by these landmark cells. Based on these landmark cells and these transitions, we can construct a transition network. The construction of the transition network aims to tackle the second challenge. Finally, we propose a route evaluation method inspired by cognition to model the process of users in selecting a suitable route, which deals with the third challenge.

Online Computation: This module describes the procedure of evaluating the queried routes online. When a subscriber submits some routes (represented as a set of cell sequences) to our system, the following steps will be carried out. Firstly, the routes will be segmented into some transitions by the landmark cells. Secondly, the cognition-inspired evaluation method will be invoked from the module of information organization and make some evaluations to these routes represented by these transitions. Finally, the routes ordered by the evaluation method will be returned to the subscriber.

In the process of evaluating the routes, detection of the stay area concerns whether suitable routes can be extracted exactly, construction of the transition network concerns whether any queried route can be matched directly, and cognition-inspired evaluation method concerns whether routes can be evaluated accurately. We will pay more attention to these three important issues in this chapter.

13.4.2 Detection of the Stay Areas

As mentioned earlier, the stay area plays an important role in understanding the traffic routes of a user. The general method for detecting the stay areas is made up of two steps: (1) Deriving the stay time interval in a cell by calculating the difference between the times of the first event and the last event in this cell. (2) Setting a time threshold and judging a cell as a stay area when the stay time interval in this cell is greater than the time threshold.

However, it is complicated in the real physical world and the general method cannot deal with the two following situations effectively.

One is that the user is located in the overlapped signal coverage area of several adjacent antennas, where the signal drift may exist (namely the user can be served by any of these adjacent antennas according to their signal quality). As depicted in the right part of Fig. 13.2, the user may be located in the intersection of cell 303, cell 304 and be static. Although the user is static, the corresponding mobile phone record set may be generated as depicted in the left part of Fig. 13.2 ranging from r_9 to r_{12}, which means the user is moving.

The other situation is that the user may be wandering in a business district or a spot, where several antennas may be situated. As shown in the right part of Fig. 13.2, cell 102, cell 103, and cell 202 may be situated in a business district and the user is randomly wandering among them for shopping. The mobile phone record set may be generated as shown in the left part of Fig. 13.2 ranging from r_2 to r_6.

Assuming that we take the general method to deal with these two situations, the stay interval time in cell 102, cell 103, cell 202, cell 303, and cell 304 will be 10 min, 0, 10 min, 0, and 0 respectively. Then we set the time threshold as 30 min and no cell will be judged as a stay area. In fact, the user is staying 30 min in the intersection of cell 303 and cell 304 or the user is wandering 30 min among cell 102, cell 103, and cell 202.

Algorithm 3 shows the procedure of detecting the stay areas for the general and particular situations.

Algorithm 3 StayAreaDetection(R, θ_t, θ_d)

Require:
A mobile phone record set R: $r_1 \rightarrow r_2$, ..., $\rightarrow r_n$, a time interval threshold θ_t and a distance threshold θ_d

Ensure:
A set of stay areas S={s}

1: i'=1, j'=i';
2: **while** ($i' < n - 1$) and ($j' < n$) **do**
3: k=i';
4: **while** $k \leq j'$ **do**
5: **if** $Distance(r_k.CID, r_{j'+1}.CID)$>$\theta_d$ **then**
6: break;
7: **end if**
8: k++;
9: **end while**
10: **if** $k > j'$ **then**
11: j'++;
12: **else**
13: Δt=$r_{j'}.T$-$r_{i'}.T$;
14: **if** $\Delta t > \theta_t$ **then**
15: $s \leftarrow \{r_{i'}.CID, r_{i'+1}.CID, ..., r_{j'}.CID\}$;
16: S.Insert(s);
17: i'=j'+1;
18: **else**
19: i'=k+1;
20: **end if**
21: j'=i';
22: **end if**
23: **end while**
24: **return** S;

In Algorithm 3, the input data are a mobile phone record set of a user, a time interval, and a distance threshold. The output data are a set of stay areas of the user. The variables i' and j' in line 1 indicate that there exists a sub-sequence R': $r_{i'} \rightarrow r_{i'+1}$, ..., $\rightarrow r_{j'}$ satisfying the constraint $\forall i' \leq i \leq j \leq j'$, Distance$(r_i.CID, r_j.CID) \leq \theta_d$. Lines 4–9 checks whether the distance constraint between cell $r_k.CID$ and cell $r_{j'+1}.CID$ is also satisfied. If the distance constraint is not be satisfied and the time interval between $r_{j'}.T$ and $r_{i'}.T$ is greater than the time threshold, these cells contained in the sub-sequence r' are judged as a stay area s and are inserted into the set S (lines 13–16). The main idea of this algorithm is to try and detect the stay area continuously and the time complexity of this algorithm is O(n^2).

13.4.3 Construction of the Transition Network

After stay areas are detected, these stay areas can be used to segment a user's mobile phone data set into many suitable routes. From these suitable routes of all users, some landmark cells can be detected. Furthermore, these suitable routes can be segmented into many transitions. These landmark cells and these transitions constitute a transition network. In order to evaluate the suitability of a route, the suitability of these transitions in the transition network need to be evaluated first.

As traffic condition is changing all day, a route may be suitable in a period of time but congested in another period of time. For reflecting this feature, a two-level granularity of suitability measurement for these transitions is constructed, namely the base-suitability (BS) level and the context-suitability (CS) level. According to the idea that granulation involves "decomposition of whole into parts", a day can be segmented into a set of consecutive periods of time [14]. The suitability of a transition in a day and in a period of time is deemed to be a coarse granule and a fine granule respectively. The BS level indicates the suitability of each transition in a day while the CS level indicates the suitability of each transition in each period of time.

The suitability of a transition e_{uv} in the BS level can be evaluated by

$$\oint_1 (e_{uv}) = \frac{e_{uv}.support}{\sum_x e_{ux}.support} \tag{13.1}$$

where u and v are two landmark cells, e_{ux} is a transition which starts from the landmark cell u and ends in the landmark cell x, $e_{uv}.support$ is the total traverse frequency of the transition e_{uv} in a day, and $e_{ux}.support$ is the total traverse frequency of the transition e_{ux} in a day.

Equation (13.1) focuses on the condition that these transitions from the same origin are all related to the destination of a trip. However, this condition often doesn't exist in the real physical world. As shown in Fig. 13.4, cell 101, cell 202, cell 203, cell 302 and cell 303 are all landmark cells. A user starts from cell 202 and ends in cell 303. For computing the suitability of the transition $e_{(202)(302)}$, all adjacent transitions that start from cell 202 need to be enumerated according to Eq. (13.1). In fact, the transition $e_{(202)(101)}$ is not related to the destination (cell 303). In this condition, Eq. (13.2) is used to reflect whether the transition is correlative to the destination (cell d).

$$correlate(e_{uv}, d) = \begin{cases} 1, & if \quad Distance(u, d) > Distance(v, d) \\ 0, & if \quad Distance(u, d) \le Distance(v, d) \end{cases} \tag{13.2}$$

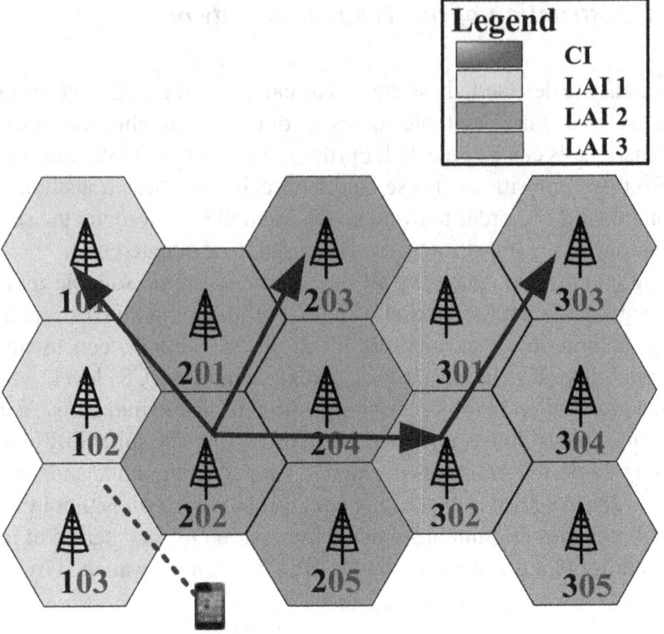

Fig. 13.4 The example of a transition network

Based on Eq. (13.2), the suitability of a transition e_{uv} in the BS level can be evaluated by

$$\oint_2 (e_{uv}) = \frac{e_{uv}.support}{\sum_x correlate(e_{ux}, d) \quad e_{ux}.support} \tag{13.3}$$

In the CS level, Eq. (13.3) can be changed into Eq. (13.4) to evaluate the suitability of a transition e_{uv}.

$$\oint_3 (e_{uv}) = \frac{e_{uv}.support^p}{\sum_x correlate(e_{ux}, d) \quad e_{ux}.support^p} \tag{13.4}$$

where $e_{uv}.support^p$ is the traverse frequency of the transition e_{uv} in any period of time p, and $e_{ux}.support$ is the traverse frequency of the transition e_{ux} in any period of time p.

According to the suitability measurements above for these transitions in the transition network, the procedure of constructing the transition network is depicted in Algorithm 4. In Algorithm 4, the input data are a set of suitable routes, the number of the landmark cells, and a set of periods of time. The number of the landmark cells can be set according to the real traffic condition. Firstly, each cell's traverse frequency from all suitable routes is calculated (lines 1–5). Secondly, the top l cells are selected as landmark cells (line 6). Furthermore, the traverse frequency of each transition $e_{uv}.support^p$ in any period of time p and the total traverse time of each transition $e_{uv}.totalT^p$ in any period of time p are computed (lines 7–27). And the total traverse frequency of each transition $e_{uv}.support$ in a day is also computed (lines 7–27). Finally, the average traverse time of each transition $e_{uv}.averageT^p$ in any period of time p is calculated (lines 28–32). And the time complexity of this algorithm is $O(n^2)$.

Algorithm 4 TansitionNetworkConstruction($\Re$, l, P)

Require:
A set of suitable routes $\Re=\{R^s\}$, the number of the landmark cells l, a set of periods of time $P=\{p\}$

Ensure:
The transition network G.

1: **for** each $R^s \in \Re$ **do**
2: **for** each r_k^s in R^s **do**
3: Count[$r_k^s.CID$]++; //$r_k^s.CID$ is counted only once in Count[]
4: **end for**
5: **end for**
6: select top l cells from *Count*[] as a set of landmark cells V
7: **for** each $R^s \in \Re$ **do**
8: k=1, $m=|R^s|$; //u and v are not two landmark cells initially.
9: **while** $k < m$ **do**
10: **if** $r_k^s.CID$ is a landmark cell **then**
11: **if** u is a landmark cell **then**
12: $v=r_k^s.CID$;
13: j=k;
14: compute the period of time p which $r_i^s.T$ is belonging to;
15: **if** $e_{uv} \notin E$ **then**
16: E.Insert(e_{uv});
17: **end if**
18: $e_{uv}.support^p$++;
19: $e_{uv}.totalT^p += r_j^s.T - r_i^s.T$;
20: $e_{uv}.support$++;
21: **end if**
22: $u=r_k^s.CID$;
23: i=k;
24: **end if**
25: k++;
26: **end while**
27: **end for**
28: **for** each p in P **do**
29: **for** each $e_{uv} \in E$ **do**
30: $e_{uv}.averageT^p = e_{uv}.totalT^p \div e_{uv}.support^p$;
31: **end for**
32: **end for**
33: $G \leftarrow (V, E)$
34: **return** G;

13.4.4 Route Evaluation Inspired by Cognition

After constructing the transition network, a method inspired by ACT-R can be used to evaluate a route. ACT-R uses the rational analysis methodology to represent the process of information retrieval in human memory. The process assumes that, selections are often made once they are good enough instead of searching for the optimal one. In order to represent the procedure of information retrieval above, a spreading activation model in ACT-R is implemented. Spreading activation model uses chunks to represent information. In a common formula of the spreading activation model, the activation of a chunk is a sum of a base-level activation, reflecting its general usefulness in the past, and an associative activation, reflecting its relevance to the current context. The activation A_i of a chunk i is defined as

$$A_i = B_i + \sum_j W_j S_{ji} \tag{13.5}$$

where B_i is the base-level activation of the chunk i, the W_js reflect the attentional weighting of the elements that are part of the current goal, and the S_{ji}s are the strengths of association from the elements j to chunk i.

ACT-R also considers that the frequently and recently used selections in human memory are often good enough to satisfy the needs of human. As we know, the route used frequently and recently is often the suitable one in our real life, which is consistent with the process of information retrieval in human memory. From this point of view, ACT-R provides a good model to understand the intelligence of users in selecting a suitable route and we can employ ACT-R to model the process of retrieving a suitable route in human memory.

In our study, a transition is regarded as a chunk. The base-level activation of a transition (chunk) e_{uv} can be indicated by $\oint_2(e_{uv})$. And the associative activation of the transition e_{uv} can be indicated by $\oint_3(e_{uv})$, which represents the associative context (namely, the suitability of the transition in the period of time p).

As a route consists of some transitions, we can see a route as chunks. The retrieval of a route can be seen as the retrieval of chunks in human memory. The base level activation B_i of a route (chunks) i can be defined as follow:

$$B_i = \frac{1}{n_i} \sum \oint_2 (e_{uv}) \tag{13.6}$$

where n_i is the total number of the transitions contained in the route i and $\sum$ indicates the sum of the suitability of each transition e_{uv} contained in the route i.

The activation A_i of a route (chunks) i can be represented by

$$A_i = \frac{1}{n_i} \sum \oint_2 (e_{uv}) + \frac{1}{n_i} \sum_j W_j \oint_3 (e_{uv}) \tag{13.7}$$

Meanwhile, we set W_j as 1.

The period of time p which each transition e_{uv} belongs to can be obtained due to the following two aspects: (1) When a subscriber submits a route to be evaluated, the subscriber must submit a start time. (2) In Algorithm 4, we can estimate the needed traverse time of each transition in different periods of time.

According to our real experience, the more transitions a route contains, the more intersections the route contains. If a route contains more intersections, it may be not suitable to the subscriber. A penalty can be set if a route contains more intersections and we modify A_i by

$$A_i' = \frac{n_a}{n_i} A_i \tag{13.8}$$

where n_a is the average number of the transitions in route i.

After completing these steps above, we can compute an activation A_i for the route i. According to the ACT-R, the higher the activation A_i is, the more easily the route (chunks) is retrieved. We can order the queried routes by their activation and recommend them to the subscriber.

As $\oint_2(e_{uv})$ and $\oint_3(e_{uv})$ are employed to measure the suitability of each transition in the BS level and in the CS level respectively, the use of the activation equation in ACT-R can be seen as a combination between the granules of the BS level and the CS level.

As mentioned in Sect. 13.1, a chunk in ACT-R could be a granule. Because a route is made up of many chunks (transitions) and the activation equation in ACT-R is based on these chunks, the application of the activation equation in evaluating the suitability of a route is a process that makes use of granules.

13.5 Experiments

In this section, we conduct a series of experiments to evaluate the performance for the proposed cognition-inspired route evaluation method, using the real mobile phone data. We present the representation for the experimental data and introduce the evaluation methodology. We also give our experimental results followed by discussions. All the experiments are implemented in Java on an Intel Core Quad CPU Q9550 2.83 GHz machine with 4 GB of memory running Windows 7.

13.5.1 Dataset

The dataset is a mobile phone data set which recorded the mobile phone trajectories of about 100,000 users from 7 September, 2010 to 13 September, 2010 in Beijing. The data are shown in the left part of Fig. 13.2 and all the phone numbers are anonymous for protecting the privacy of users. As there exist are missing data in the dataset, we must preprocess the data. In addition, the dataset contains some mobile phone trajectories of taxies. The mobile phone trajectories of the taxies must be deleted from the dataset owing to the fact that the taxies are moving always and we cannot get their origin-destinations precisely. The rules of preprocessing data are as follows:

- If the distance between any two consecutive antennas in a mobile phone data set is more than a threshold, this mobile phone data set will be segmented into two mobile phone data sets from these two antennas.
- If the number of different antennas contained in a mobile phone data set of a user for a whole day is less than a threshold, we delete this mobile phone data set from the dataset. Otherwise, we consider this user an experienced user and use this user's mobile phone data set.
- If the number of different antennas contained in a mobile phone data set of a user for a whole day is more than a threshold, we think that this mobile phone data set comes from a taxi and delete it from the dataset.

13.5.2 Evaluation Methodology

Existing route recommendation systems generally provide some fast routes for subscribers, which consists of two main stages: (1) When a subscriber submits his/her origin and destination to the route recommendation systems, the systems search some routes which connect the origin and destination. (2) The route recommendation systems estimate the travel time on each route and order the routes by time, then recommend them to the subscriber. As our route evaluation system mainly focuses on evaluating whether the routes are suitable to the subscribers, we can employ the routes provided by other route recommendation systems and evaluate them by the proposed method.

In order to evaluate our method, there are three issues needed to be solved.

Ground Truth: We invited 9 subjects who often traveled in Beijing to take part in our experiments and used Baidu Map service as the basic route recommendation system for providing the routes between the origins and destinations. Firstly, each subject submitted his/her origin and destination to the route recommendation system and obtained some routes (each subject may do this many times). Secondly, each subject evaluated every recommended route with the criterion (as shown in Table 13.1) according to their real experiences. Finally, we aggregated all subjects' ratings as our ground truth.

Baseline and Methods: As many recommendation systems often recommend the most popular things to subscribers, we can use this idea in our experiments [15]. Equation (13.6) reflects the travel frequency of a route, which can be used as our baseline (called *M0* for short). And we use Eq. (13.7) as our original method (called *M1* for short) and Eq. (13.8) as our improved method (called *M2* for short).

Table 13.1 Rating criteria for routes

Ratings	Explanations
4	In this period of time, I would like to use this route preferentially
3	In this period of time, I would like to use this route
2	In this period of time, I would use this route if I have no other alternatives
1	In this period of time, I would not use this route if I have no other alternatives

Evaluation Criterion: As our evaluation system is based on ordering the routes, we employ the normalized discounted cumulative gain (*nDCG*) to measure the list of ordered routes [16]. *nDCG* is commonly used in information retrieval to measure the search engine's performance. A higher *nDCG* value to a list of search results means that the highly relevant items have appeared earlier (with higher scores) in the result list. For each list of ordered routes by our method, we can obtain a score list where scores are provided by ground truth. Such a list is called relevance vector, denoted as G (e.g., G=⟨4, 1, 2, 2, 2⟩). The discounted cumulative gain of G is computed as follows (in our experiments, b=2):

$$DCG[i] = \begin{cases} G[i], & if \quad i = 1 \\ DCG[i-1] + G[i], & if \quad i < b \\ DCG[i-1] + \dfrac{G[i]}{\log_b i}, & if \quad i \geq b \end{cases} \tag{13.9}$$

In particular, nDCG[i] or referred as nDCG@i, measures the relevance of top i results as shown in the following equation:

$$nDCG[i] = \frac{DCG[i]}{IDCG[i]} \tag{13.10}$$

where *IDCG*[i] is the *DCG*[i] value of ideal ordered list.

13.5.3 Experimental Results and Discussions

Figure 13.5 presents nDCG@3 and nDCG@5 of the original method, the improved method and the baseline changing over the time threshold θ_t defined in Algorithm 3. In Fig. 13.5, let the distance threshold θ_d in Algorithm 3 be 700 meters.

Figure 13.6 presents nDCG@3 and nDCG@5 of the original method, the improved method and the baseline changing over the distance θ_d defined in Algorithm 3. In Fig. 13.6, let the time interval threshold θ_t in Algorithm 3 be 40 min.

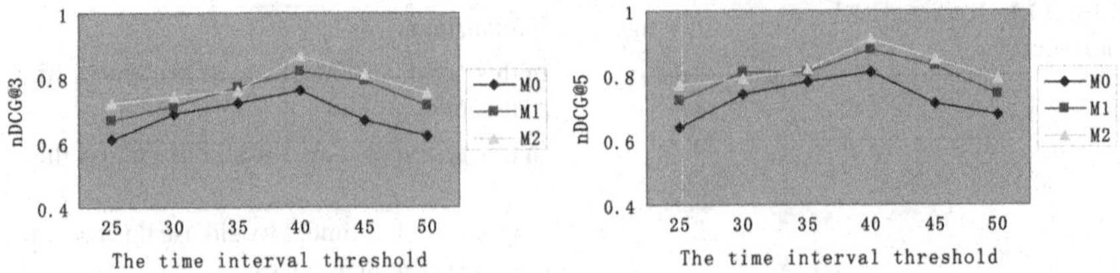

Fig. 13.5 nDCG@3 and nDCG@5 changing over the time interval threshold

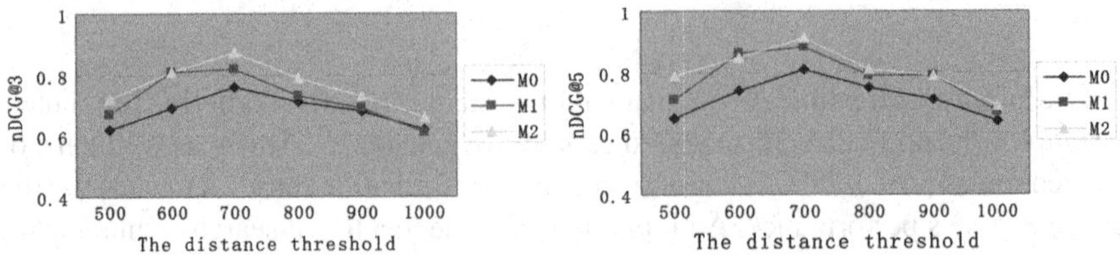

Fig. 13.6 nDCG@3 and nDCG@5 changing over the distance threshold

Figures 13.5 and 13.6 also present that the original method and the improved method show clear advantages over the baseline. In other words, the method inspired by cognition is effective in tackling the real problems. The reason is that the activation equation not only takes into account the suitability of a route in the general condition but also consider the associative context (namely, the real traffic condition in different periods of time). In addition, the experimental results present that the performance of the improved method is better than the original method. That is to say, the fewer transitions the route contains, the more suitable the route is.

In Figs. 13.5 and 13.6, we also observe that in the beginning the performance of these three methods is improved as the parameters θ_t and θ_d increase respectively. When the parameters θ_t and θ_d increase to some certain values, the performance of these three methods reaches their summits. Then, the performance of these three methods declines as the parameters θ_t and θ_d continue increasing. These observations indicate that the performance of these methods depends on the parameters θ_t and θ_d, which are employed to detect the stay areas of a user. These observations can be explained as follows: (1) As a route between the origin and destination is a suitable one for a trip and a stay area is generally the origin or destination for a trip, the stay areas of a user are used to abstract these suitable routes from the mobile phone data of the user. (2) The abstractions of the landmark cells and the transitions are based on these suitable routes of all users while the transition network is made up of these landmark cells and these transitions. Hence, the detection of a stay area plays an important role in evaluating the suitability of a route exactly. However, the parameters θ_t and θ_d are related to the distribution of the antennas in a city. In order to detect the stay areas exactly, we need to try different values for the parameters θ_t and θ_d repeatedly according to the mobile reality dataset in a city.

13.6 Conclusions

Mobile phone data of users imply their experiences in selecting a suitable route. In this chapter, we propose a cognition-inspired route recommendation method to mine the intelligence of experienced users in selecting a suitable route, using the mobile reality dataset in Beijing. The major contributions of this chapter are as follows:

- We proposed a new stay area detection method, which can deal with what the general methods cannot tackle.
- We constructed a transition network which allows for a route from any origin and any destination to be evaluated, and defined a function to measure the suitability of a transition.
- We proposed a cognition-inspired evaluation method, which is more consistent to the thinking pattern of human.

Experimental results show that the proposed method is feasible and effective. However, the representation of data, information and knowledge in the proposed architecture of three-level granularity for information organization is not discussed deeply, which is a challenge for us. Semantic technology uses Resource Description Framework to integrate and represent multi-source data, which provides a good way for tackling the challenge above [17]. In addition, the selection of a route may be related to the preferences of subscribers, which are also not taken into account. Hence, based on semantic technology, we intend to provide more personalized route evaluation services for subscribers by using the cognition-inspired methods in the future.

Acknowledgments This work is partially supported by the National Science Foundation of China (No. 61272345), the International Science & Technology Cooperation Program of China (2013DFA32180), and the CAS/SAFEA International Partnership Program for Creative Research Teams.

References

1. J.R. Anderson, D. Bothell, M.D. Byrne, S. Douglass, C. Lebiere, Y.L. Qin, An integrated theory of the mind. Psychol. Rev. **111**(4), 1036–1060 (2004)
2. W.-T. Fu, P. Pirolli, A cognitive model of user navigation on the World Wide Web. Human-Comput. Interact. **22**(4), 355–412 (2007)
3. N. Caceres, J.P. Wideberg, F.G. Benitez, Deriving origin destination data from a mobile phone network. IET Intell. Transp. Syst. **1**(1), 15–26 (2007)
4. F. Calabrese, G.D. Lorenzo, L. Liu, C. Ratti, Estimating origin-destination flows using mobile phone location data. IEEE Pervas. Comput. **10**(4), 36–44 (2011)
5. F. Calabrese, M. Colonna, P. Lovisolo, D. Parata, C. Ratti, Real-time urban monitoring using cell phones: a case study in Rome. IEEE Trans. Intell. Transp. Syst. **12**(1), 141–151 (2011)
6. J.J.-C. Ying, E.H.-C. Lu, W.-C. Lee, Mining user similarity from semantic trajectories, in *Proceedings of the 2nd ACM SIGSPATIAL International Workshop on Location Based Social Networks* (ACM, 2010), pp. 19–26

7. J.J.-C. Ying, W.-C. Lee, T.-C. Weng, Semantic trajectory mining for location prediction, in *Proceedings of the 19th ACM SIGSPATIAL International Conference on Advances in Geographic Information Systems* (ACM, 2011), pp. 34–43
8. E.H.-C. Lu, V.S. Tseng, P.S. Yu, Mining cluster-based temporal mobile sequential patterns in location-based service environments. IEEE Trans. Knowl. Data Eng. **23**(6), 914–927 (2011)
9. F. Liu, D. Janssens, G. Wets, M. Cools, Annotating mobile phone location data with activity purposes using machine learning algorithms. Expert Syst. Appl. **40**(8), 3299–3311 (2013)
10. J. Yuan, Y. Zheng, X. Xie, G.Z. Sun, T-Drive: enhancing driving directions with taxi drivers' intelligence. IEEE Trans. Knowl. Data Eng. **25**(1), 220–232 (2011)
11. L.-Y. Wei, Y. Zheng, W.-C. Peng, Constructing popular routes from uncertain trajectories, in *Proceedings of the 18th ACM SIGKDD International Conference on Knowledge Discovery and Data Mining* (ACM, 2012), pp. 195–203
12. Z.B. Chen, H.T. Shen, X.F. Zhou, Discovering popular routes from trajectories, in *Proceedings of the 2011 IEEE 27th International Conference on Data Engineering* (IEEE Computer Society, 2011), pp. 900–911
13. N. Zhong, J.H. Ma, J.H. Huang, J.M. Liu, Y.Y. Yao, Y.X. Zhang, J.H. Chen, Research challenges and perspectives on Wisdom Web of Things (W2T). J. Supercomput. **64**(3), 862–882 (2013)
14. L.A. Zadeh, Toward a theory of fuzzy information granulation and its centrality in human reasoning and fuzzy logic. Fuzzy Sets Syst. **90**(2), 111–127 (1997)
15. A. Rajaraman, J. Ullman, *Ming of Masssive Datasets* (Cambridge University Press, Cambridge, England, 2011), pp. 305–338
16. D. Manning, P. Raghavan, H. Schtze, *Introduction to Information Retrieval* (Cambridge University Press, Cambridge, England, 2008), pp. 158–164
17. G. Antoniou, F. von Harmelen, *A Semantic Web Primer* (The MIT Press, Cambridge, Massachusetts London, 2003), pp. 63–111

Chapter 14
A Monitoring System for the Safety of Building Structure Based on W2T Methodology

Haiyuan Wang, Zhisheng Huang, Ning Zhong, Jiajin Huang, Yuzhong Han and Feng Zhang

Abstract With the development of the Internet of things, monitoring systems for the safety of building structure (SBS) provide people with the important data about the main supporting points in the buildings. More and more data give the engineers an overload work problem, which can be solved by a systematic method making these monitoring systems more reliable, efficient and intelligent. Under the framework of the Wisdom Web of Things (W2T), we design a monitoring system for the SBS, by using the semantic technology. This system establishes a data cycle among the physical world (buildings), the social world (humans) and the cyber world (computers), and provides various services in the monitoring process to alleviate the engineers' workload. In this system, the sensors which are connected via cable or wireless way, are used to monitor the different parameters of building structure. The semantic data can be obtained and represented by RDF to describe the meanings of sensor data,

H. Wang (✉) · Z. Huang · J. Huang
International WIC Institute, Beijing University of Technology,
Beijing 100124, China
e-mail: wang_hai_yuan@163.com

Z. Huang
e-mail: huang.zhisheng.nl@gmail.com; z.huang@vu.nl; huang@cs.vu.nl

J. Huang
e-mail: hjj@emails.bjut.edu.cn

N. Zhong
Beijing Advanced Innovation Center for Future Internet Technology,
The International WIC Institute, Beijing University of Technology,
Beijing, China
e-mail: zhong@maebashi-it.ac.jp; zhongn@bjut.edu.cn

N. Zhong
Department of Life Science and Informatics, Maebashi Institute of Technology,
460-1 Kamisadori-Cho, Maebashi 371-0816, Japan

Z. Huang
Department of Computer Science, Vrije University Amsterdam,
Amsterdam, The Netherlands

Y. Han · F. Zhang
China Academy of Building Research, Beijing 100013, China

N. Zhong et al. (eds.), *Wisdom Web of Things*, Web Information Systems Engineering and Internet Technologies Book Series,
DOI 10.1007/978-3-319-44198-6_14

and can provide the application background for users. LarKC, a platform for scalable semantic data processing, is used for semantic querying about the data. Based on this uniform representation of data and semantic processing, intelligent services can be provided by the effective data analysis. This provides the possibility to integrate all of the monitoring systems for the safety of building structure in urban computing.

14.1 Introduction

With the development of information technology, Internet can be accessed almost anywhere through Ethernet, Wi-Fi, GPRS, or 3G. It becomes more and more convenient for the embedded devices to access the internet, and some new application technologies and new services are emerging based on the internet of things (IoT). The Wisdom Web of Things (W2T) is an extension of the Wisdom Web in the IoT age. The "Wisdom" means that each of things in the Web of things can be aware of both itself and others to provide the right service for the right object at a right time and context [1, 2]. Under the W2T framework, a monitoring system for the safety of building structure (SBS) is developed, which contains a variety of techniques and knowledge, such as sensor technology, semantic technology, communications technology, signal analysis and processing, structural mechanics and building materials. The monitoring system aims to find the potential danger timely and fix its position accurately, when the potential danger is about to happen. So the assessment of the SBS and the calculation of the broken structure lifetime can be done, according to the data collected by this monitoring system. This is important to make the building maintenance plan, improve the efficiency of maintenance, and avoid structural accident. Meanwhile, many experience and knowledge about the SBS can be formed based on the analysis of these data.

14.2 Semantic Sensor Web and LarKC Platform

W2T is not a simple combination of humans, things and computers. It contains a data cycle. The basic data of things are collected by sensors. All the data are transmitted through the internet and stored in the server of data center. In the data server, the data analysis is done by the professionals, and intelligent services can be provided to those people who focus on the data collected from the sensors. People can perform some operations that influence the things such as reinforcing structure, and the results will be reflected in the data server again. Then the data cycle is formed, and the physical world (things) and the social world (people) are connected [3].

When the data of things explodes, the data expression and the data management become problems, and it is needed to integrate these big heterogeneous data by using an effective way. Semantic Web is a solution to these problems, so Semantic Sensor Web (SSW) comes out, in which sensor data is annotated with semantic metadata to increase interoperability as well as provide contextual information essential for situational knowledge [4, 5]. The SSW can be considered as a sub web of W2T, which can analyzes the semantic data from sensors using semantic tools. Through semantic model of things, the meaning of the data and the relation among the data are obvious.

The scalable semantic data from SSW can be retrieved and reasoned by the Large Knowledge Collider (LarKC) platform. LarKC (Large Knowledge Collider) is a semantic platform for scalable semantic data processing and reasoning.[1] LarKC was developed by the European Unions Seventh Framework Program, aiming to remove the scalability barriers of currently existing reasoning systems for the Semantic Web. The main features of the LarKC platform are:

- *Configurability*: LarKC provides a flexible and modular environment where users and developers are able to build their own workflows and plug-ins respectively in an easy and straightforward manner. This platform has a pluggable architecture in which it is possible to exploit techniques and heuristics from diverse areas such as databases, machine learning, cognitive science, Semantic Web, and others [6].
- *Scalability*: In LarKC, massive, distributed and necessarily incomplete reasoning is performed over web-scale knowledge sources. Massive inference is achieved by distributing problems across heterogeneous computing resources and coordinated by the LarKC platform [7].
- *Parallelism*: LarKC supports for parallel reasoning and processing by using cloud computing and cluster computing techniques, and is engineered to be ultimately scalable to very large distributed computational resources [8].

With the urbanization development, many landmark buildings have been designed and built, which have novel appearance, unique structure. New building technologies, new building materials are also used in them. The traditional way of ensuring the SBS is making the testing schedule executed by man. According to the testing result, the maintenance and repairment can be arranged. However, the testing done by man will cause some problems: (1) because of different personnel experience between engineers, the differences exist in testing results; (2) continuous testing data cannot be obtained, and real-time warning cannot be realized; (3) the cost of manpower will grow higher as time goes by. The monitoring system within the frame of W2T is suitable for big data and long-time testing, and it also has advantages in sensor and data management, and can ensure the SBS timely.

14.3 Prototype Monitoring System for SBS

14.3.1 System Composition

The monitoring system architecture for the SBS under the W2T framework [9] is shown in Fig. 14.1. The physical world is the world that surrounds us and should be

[1] https://gate.ac.uk/projects/larkc/.

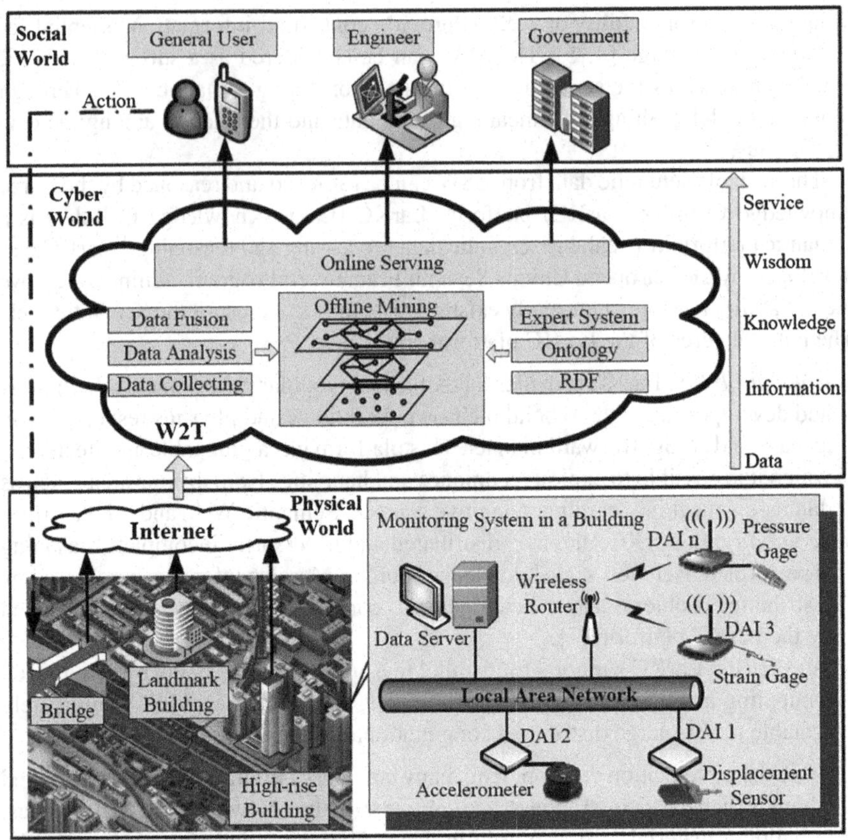

Fig. 14.1 System composition of the monitoring system

sensed. The social world is the world that humans act and think. The cyber world is the world in computers, and it is a bridge between the other two worlds. More specifically, in the cyber world the services can be derived from the data collected by the sensors in the physical world and the knowledge created by the humans in the social world. The humans can act and affect the building according to these services, so the social world, the physical world and the cyber world are connected together through data, service and action, and the effective data cycle is formed.

14.3.2 The Physical World

Within the scope of a building, the monitoring system we developed is mainly composed of three parts: (1) data server in monitoring center; (2) sensors in monitoring

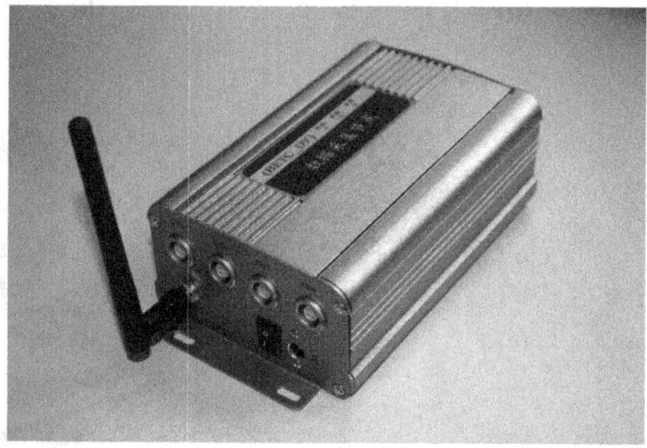

Fig. 14.2 Data acquisition instrument with four channels

points; (3) data acquisition instruments (DAIs). The DAIs are the keys that make these sensors in this system work harmonically.

These DAIs must have the following characteristics: (1) access the internet via a wired or wireless way; (2) accept commands from data server to start or stop data acquisition; (3) convert sensor data format to standard format [10]. In the area with network cables, a wired transmission can be chosen, but in some special points of the structure, where have no proper condition for laying cables, Wi-Fi is used to connect the DAIs and the data server [11]. The wireless DAI is shown in Fig. 14.2.

Sensors are used for measuring the parameters that can reflect the change of building structure. Generally, there are two types of sensor output signal: analog and digital, so the DAI can convert different signal format into standard format.

The building structure is a complex mechanical structure which is influenced by various loads and a variety of materials together, so its mechanical features cannot be reflected by only one type sensor. Different parameters need to be measured by different sensors, Fig. 14.3 shows the sensors often used in building monitoring (A: accelerometer B: inclinometer C: thermohygrometer D: vibrating wire strain sensor). The environment where sensors are installed is harsh, and the change of parameters about the building structure is tiny. So the sensor used for building monitoring should have the following characteristics: high sensitivity, convenient installation, low power consumption, and high reliability [12, 13].

14.3.3 The Cyber World

The cyber world not only plays a role in controlling the data sampling according to the monitoring plan, but also under the W2T framework it is a key part to form the data cycle, which contains a variety of techniques and knowledge. Semantic Web uses RDF to represent sensor data that can be shared and reused across the disparate information systems, and RDF has been widely acknowledged in many domains,

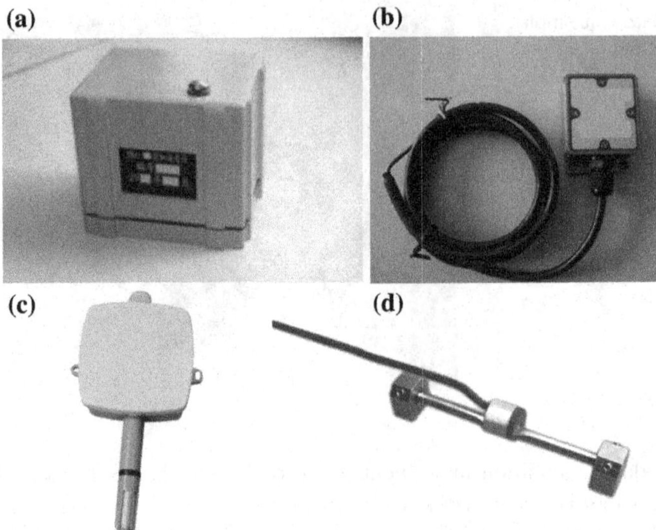

Fig. 14.3 Sensors often used in Monitoring System for the SBS

e.g. life science, information integration. The World Wide Web Consortium (W3C) has formulated a series of standards about semantic data description language (such as RDF and OWL) [14]. The semantic description and the query language provide common basis for a unified data description format, for the interoperability of data. It is not possible to provide intelligent services without the support of corresponding background knowledge. According to the characteristics of the building structure monitored, the mathematical model is established. The weak points of the building where sensors are placed are found out, and the threshold value of each point is calculated and is bound up with the corresponding sensor.

The software block diagram of data server is shown as Fig. 14.4, which is consisted of the following parts: LarKC platform, jetty web server and tcp server. The LarKC provides the wanted results by using Sparql semantic query. The Sparql proposed by RDF Data Access Working Group in 2004, has become a W3C recommendation. Sparql query language can be used to get information from RDF. It provides facilities to extract information in the form of URIs, blank nodes, plain and typed literals, to construct new RDF based on information in the queried graphs [12].

Semantic rules are created according to the relationship and the threshold value of each measuring point. After loading the semantic data, the LarKC can response the request submitted by Jetty. Jetty submits the Sparql statements, which are formed according to the user's query, to LarKC platform. When the results are returned from the LarKC, Jetty displays these results in user's web page. The DAIs will connect the data server automatically, according to its internal settings of target IP. Tcp server will establish a socket connection for each DAI, and save the sensor data from the DAIs.

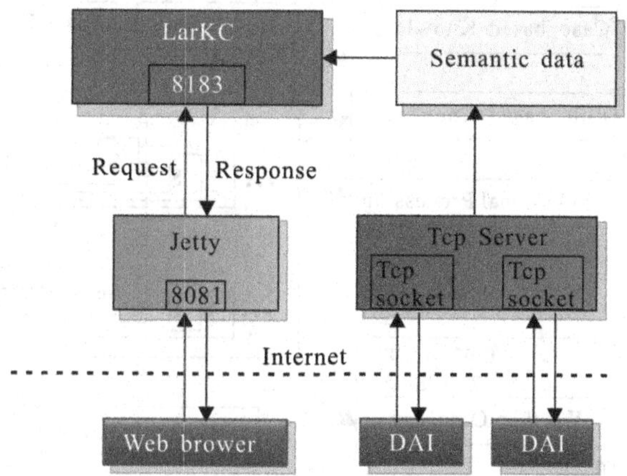

Fig. 14.4 Software block diagram of data server

Users can access the monitoring center server using a web browser, and Jetty provides web services, such as the sensor data tables, the status of SBS, and the results of queries. To identify the current status of the structural safety is the key task, by analyzing the semantic sensor data and extracting feature parameters [15, 16].

As shown in Fig. 14.5, the multi-source knowledge gained through study or investigation combines facts, truths, or principles together, which can form case-based or rule-based knowledge. Aiming at the different application cases the mechanics models are set up, and the professional analysis methods are also applied to the system. There is no perfect way to model these knowledge, ontology is one of the feasible method, which is a formal explicit description of the concept in a domain of knowledge and can standardize the representation of these knowledge. The main elements of an ontology are class, property, individual, and restriction. Class in ontology is a classification of the individuals into the group which share the same characteristics. Object property is used to associate with each class. Individual is the instance of the class, and realizes the combination between the knowledge and the application case [17]. The ontologies used in this system are divided into two categories: the commonsense ontologies and the domain ontologies. The domain ontology is the standard expression of the domain knowledge and the related concept including sensor technology, building standards, and design models, which are professional and should be maintained by the engineers in this project. There may be other type of ontologies which are developed and employed for other domain knowledge. The commonsense ontologies quoted here are these ontologies which contain the commonsense concepts of daily life [18], and have been created and maintained by other engineers.

When the sensed data is delivered into this system and the semantic information is created correspondingly by the semantic annotation, the sensed data is connected with the existed knowledge resources. The sensed data is directly related to an individual of the sensor ontology, which contains the measuring point's link. With the measuring point, the building ontology can be integrated with the real-time sensed data. Through

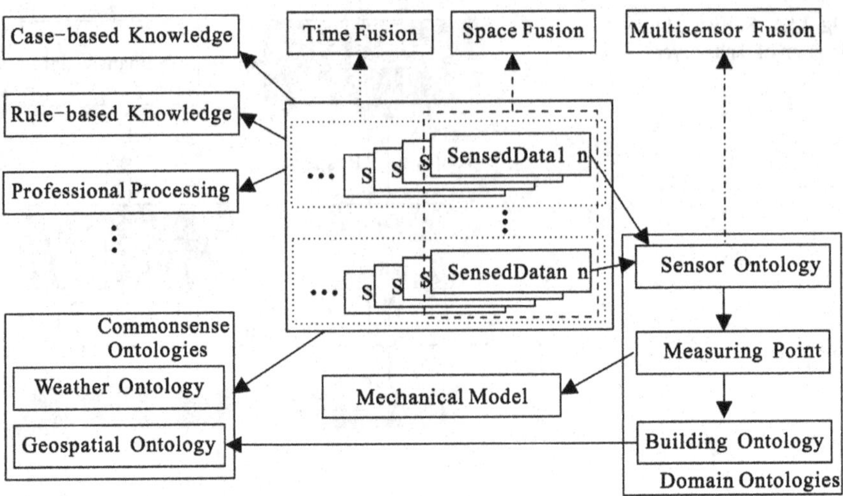

Fig. 14.5 The multi-source knowledge organization

the sampling time of the sensed data and the geographic information of the building, the commonsense ontologies such as the weather ontology and geographic ontology, can be used. So the real-time sensed data drops into a knowledge net, a series of results can be reasoned or concluded based on these knowledge.

14.3.4 The Social World

All the instruments in the physical world and all the data in the cyber world aim to serve the people in the social world. The social world here is the knowledge supplier, the service demander and the physical world's influencer, is not the cyber world's intervenor. The knowledge in the social world is effectively extracted and summarized, represented in the form of ontologies. When the knowledge and the sensed data are combined, the service becomes an interface between the social world and the cyber world. Providing the right service for the right people at a right time and context is an important question, so the personalized service model can be created for the different users [19]. For most structural engineers, they don't care how this system works and what the characteristics of the DAIs are. The things they really want to know are what the data is and when and where the data was collected, and the final goal is to know how the health status is and what kind of action should be taken. The general users maybe only care about some safety tips, and the Government requires to provide more macroscopical suggestions.

In a word, this system can collect a large number of data about the SBS in the physical world, fuse with the existing knowledge in the cyber world and serve people in the social world who will react to the physical world again. So the humans, the computers and the things will work in a dynamic state. The basis of all these services is the data and their relationships. The data organization is the key effective pre-processing before the data mining.

14.4 Data About the SBS

14.4.1 Data Query

When a large amount of data saves in the data server, there are the following questions that need to be solved:

1. How to get the background information about these data?
2. How to retrieve a series of data wanted from the vast data?
3. How to get the specific data value?
4. How to intelligentize the system and ease engineers' burden?

In this case, we design the SPARQL queries to achieve the above goals. The LarKC platform with built-in query workflow uses port 8183 to receive http request about SPARQL queries from the remote computers.

Figure 14.6 shows the SPARQL queries submitted to the LarKC platform. The code in Fig. 14.7 shows a fragment of the results returned, the details of the measuring point can be got from the results.

Strain and acceleration are most commonly parameters used for building structure monitoring, and some analysis of SBS can be done based on data about these parameters [20].

```
select distinct ?sampleTime ?tempValue ?sensor ?pointInfo ?building ?city
where {
?dataRecord rdf:type              ss:SensedData.
?dataRecord ss:TimeStamp           ?sampleTime.
?dataRecord ss:SensedValue         ?tempValue.

?dataRecord ss:FromSensor          ?sensor.
?testPoint  rdf:type              ss:ObservationPoint.
?testPoint  ss:HasTemputreSensor  ?sensor.
?testPoint  ss:Description         ?pointInfo.
?testPoint  ss:atBuilding         ?building.
?building   ss:inCity             ?city
}
```

Fig. 14.6 The SPARQL statements about the measuring points

```
<result>
 <binding name="sampleTime">
  <literal datatype="http://www.w3.org/2001/XMLSchema#dateTime">2013-12-16T18:41:20.069</literal>
 </binding>
 <binding name="tempValue">
  <literal datatype="http://www.w3.org/2001/XMLSchema#double">-23.9</literal>
 </binding>
 <binding name="sensor">
  <uri>http://www.w2t-waas.com/WHY#2013B1sensor4</uri>
 </binding>
 <binding name="pointInfo">
  <literal>at the middle of the second pile</literal>
 </binding>
 <binding name="building">
  <uri>http://www.w2t-waas.com/WHY#2013BJbuilding1</uri>
 </binding>
 <binding name="city">
  <literal>Beijing</literal>
 </binding>
</result>
```


Fig. 14.7 A fragment of the results about the measuring point

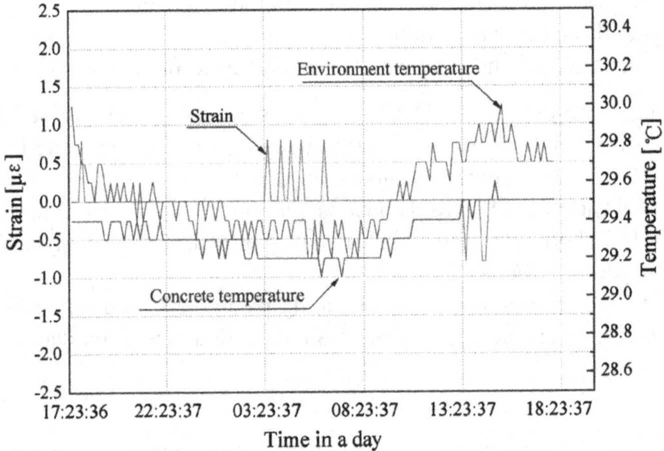

Fig. 14.8 Strain curve of a concrete block during a day

14.4.2 Strain Data

Figure 14.8 shows the testing data of a concrete block in a building during a day, and an arc weldable strain gage is used in this example. Not only the strain of the concrete is measured, the concrete temperature are obtained too. The engineer firstly establishes the mechanical model about the testing concrete block, and then analyzes the strain data with the environment condition. The status of the concrete block can be estimated, further more the change trend of strain can be predicted.

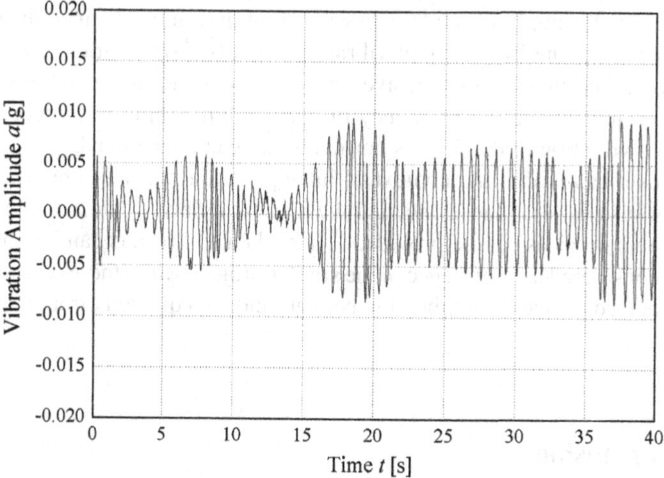

Fig. 14.9 Vibration curve of a floor

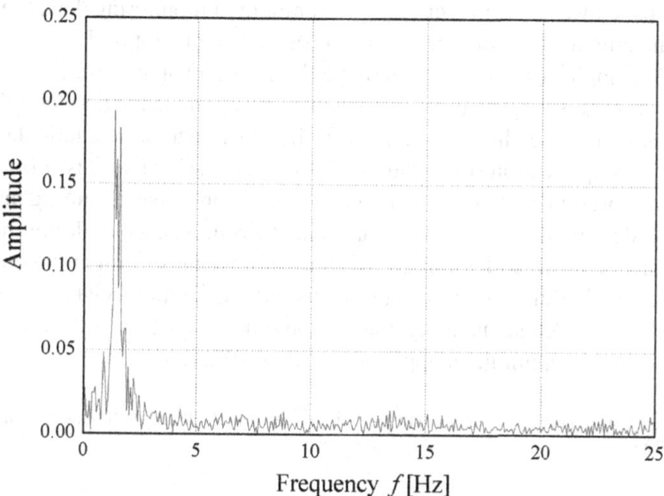

Fig. 14.10 Frequency curve of a floor vibration

14.4.3 Acceleration Data

Before the dynamic parameters of the building structure are monitored, the dynamic model of the building should be analyzed, and the natural frequency should be calculated. If it is possible, a short time testing should be done, and natural frequency can be got from this testing [21]. After the installation of monitoring system, the intensity and the law of vibration at different locations are recorded. Figure 14.9 shows a segment of data about the vibration of a floor in a residential building in Beijing.

In this case, the amplitude and the law of vibration can be obtained through time domain data. Then the frequency of vibration is got by Fourier transform as shown in Fig. 14.10. Through comprehensive analysis about the inherent frequency, the measured frequency and the frequency of surrounding vibration source, the result whether this vibration of the floor is normal or not can be obtained.

The above data within the context of its application plays an important role in monitoring system. With these data and the results engineers can estimate the SBS, and intelligent services can be provided. These data and results can be understood, reused, or considered as a reference in the similar project, while these data and results are semanticized, added the application background, and queried through the LarKC platform.

14.5 Conclusions

In recent years, the monitoring system for SBS plays an important role in intelligent building area. However, with increasing the amount of monitoring data, the relationship and the effectiveness of data become problems, and a lot of data, which has no context of its application, become garbage data. This chapter describes a monitoring system for the safety of building structure based on semantic technology. The system uses semantic technology to convert the sensor data to semantic data, so that the data has its application background, and semantic sensor web is formed. Based on uniform representation of the data and semantic processing, intelligent services can be provided by the effective data analysis. Currently, each building monitoring system is independent, and a unified building monitoring system in the city has not formed yet. The building monitoring systems with different format and networking can be unified through semantic technology and these systems will develop to be a branch of urban computing, an application case of W2T.

Acknowledgments The study was supported by National Natural Science Foundation of China (61272345).

References

1. N. Zhong, J.M. Liu, Y.Y. Yao, Envisioning intelligent information technologies through the prism of web intelligence. Commun. ACM **50**(3), 89–94 (2007)
2. N. Zhong, J.H. Ma, R.H. Huang et al., Research challenges and perspectives on Wisdom Web of Things (W2T). J. Supercomput. **64**(3), 862–882 (2013)
3. N. Zhong, J.M. Liu, Y.Y. Yao, Advances in web intelligence, in *Chinese Web Intelligence and Web Science book series*, vol. 1 (Higher Education Press, Beijing, 2011), pp. 4–10
4. S. Amit, H. Cory, Semantic sensor web. IEEE Internet Comput. 78–83 (2008)
5. K. Shyamaladevi, T.T. Mirnalinee, Integration of semantics, sensors and services on the ubiquitous web, in *International Conference on Recent Trends in Information Technology* (2012), pp. 168–173

6. D. Fensel, F. Van Harmelen, B. Andersson, P. Brennan, H. Cunningham, E.D. Valle, et al., Towards LarKC: a platform for web-scale reasoning, in *2008 IEEE International Conference on Semantic Computing* (2008), pp. 524–529
7. Z.S. Huang, N. Zhong, Scalable semantic data processing: platform, technology and applications, in *Chinese Web Intelligence and Web Science book series*, vol. 2 (Higher Education Press, Beijing, 2012), pp. 5–12
8. E.D. Valle, I. Celino, D. Dell'Aglio, R. Grothmann, F. Steinke, V. Tresp, Semantic traffic-aware routing using the larkc platform. Internet Comput. IEEE **15**(6), 15–23 (2012)
9. H.Y. Wang, Z.S. Huang, N. Zhong, J.J. Huang, Y.Z. Han, F. Zhang, An intelligent monitoring system for the safety of building structure under the w2t framework. Int. J. Distrib. Sens. Netw. **1**, 2015 (2015)
10. H.Y. Wang, Y.Z. Han, J.M. Li, Design and implementation of dynamic data acquisition system used in the construction area, in *2010 International Conference on Engineering Computation* (2010), pp. 149–152
11. A. Giuseppe, WSNs for structural health monitoring of historical buildings, in *The 2nd International Conference on Human System Interaction* (2009), pp. 574–579
12. A. Grigoris, V.H. Frank, *A Semantic Web Primer* (The MIT Press, London, 2008), pp. 65–94
13. T. Tom, Low power wireless sensor network for building monitoring. IEEE Sens. J. **13**(3), 909–915 (2009)
14. C. Michael, The SSN ontology of the W3C semantic sensor network incubator group. Web Semant. Sci. Serv. Agents World Wide Web **17**, 25–32 (2012)
15. F. Florian. Towards semantics-based monitoring of large-scale industrial system, in *2006 The International Conference on Computational Intelligence for Modelling Control and Automation,and International Conference on Intelligent Agents* (2006), pp. 261–266
16. A. Stefan, A proposal for ontology-based integration of heterogeneous decision support systems for structural health monitoring, in *2010 The 12th International Conference on Information Integration and Web-based Applications and Services* (2010), pp. 168–175
17. P. Křemen, Z. Kouba, Ontology-driven information system design. IEEE Trans. Syst. Man Cybern. Part C Appl. Rev. **42**(3), 334–344 (2012)
18. L.J. Zang, C. Cao, Y.N. Cao, Y.M. Wu, C.G. Cao, A survey of commonsense knowledge acquisition. J. Comput. Sci. Technol. **28**(4), 689–719 (2013)
19. J. Chen, J. Ma, N. Zhong, Y. Yao, J. Liu, R. Huang et al., Waas: wisdom as a service. Intell. Syst. IEEE **29**(6), 40–47 (2014)
20. H.Y. Wang, Z.S. Huang, N. Zhong, Y.Z. Han, A monitoring system for the safety of building structure based on semantic technology, in *2013 Fourth International Conference on Intelligent Systems Design and Engineering Applications* (IEEE, 2013), pp. 15–18
21. D.P. Theodor, M. Mariane, Blind Source separation of traffic-induced vibrations in building monitoring, in *2007 IEEE International Conference on Control and Automation* (2007), pp. 2101–2106

Part IV
Future Vision of W2T

Chapter 15
Brain Big Data in Wisdom Web of Things

Ning Zhong, Stephen S. Yau, Jianhua Ma, Shinsuke Shimojo, Marcel Just, Bin Hu, Guoyin Wang, Kazuhiro Oiwa and Yuichiro Anzai

Abstract The chapter summarizes main aspects of brain informatics based big data interacting with a social-cyber-physical space of Wisdom Web of Things (W2T). It describes how to realize human-level collective intelligence as a big data sharing mind—a harmonized collectivity of consciousness on the W2T by developing brain inspired intelligent technologies to provide wisdom services, and it proposes five

N. Zhong (✉)
Department of Life Science and Informatics, Maebashi Institute of Technology, 460-1 Kamisadori-Cho, Maebashi 371-0816, Japan
e-mail: zhong@maebashi-it.ac.jp; zhongn@bjut.edu.cn

N. Zhong
Beijing Advanced Innovation Center for Future Internet Technology, The International WIC Institute, Beijing University of Technology, Beijing 100124, China

S.S. Yau
Arizona State University, Tempe, USA

J. Ma
Faculty of Computer and Information Science, Hosei University, Tokyo 84-8584, Japan
e-mail: jianhua@hosei.ac.jp

S. Shimojo
California Institute of Technology, Pasadena, USA

M. Just
Carnegie Mellon University, Pittsburgh, USA

B. Hu
School of Information Science and Engineering, Lanzhou University, Lanzhou 730000, China
e-mail: bh@lzu.edu.cn

G. Wang
Chongqing University of Posts and Telecommunications, Chongqing, China

K. Oiwa
National Institute of Information and Communication Technology, Koganei, Japan

Y. Anzai
Japan Society for the Promotion of Science, Tokyo, Japan

N. Zhong et al. (eds.), *Wisdom Web of Things*, Web Information Systems Engineering and Internet Technologies Book Series,
DOI 10.1007/978-3-319-44198-6_15

guiding principles to deeper understand the nature of the vigorous interaction and interdependence of brain-body-environment.

15.1 Introduction

Wisdom Web of Things (W2T) provides a social-cyber-physical space for all human communications and activities, in which big data are used as a bridge to connect relevant aspects of humans, computers, and things [1]. It is a trend to integrate brain big data and human behavior big data in the social-cyber-physical space for realizing the harmonious symbiosis of humans, computers and things. Brain informatics provides the key technique to implement such an attempt by offering informatics-enabled brain studies and applications in the social-cyber-physical space, which can be regarded as a brain big data cycle [2]. This brain big data cycle is implemented by various processing, interpreting, and integrating multiple forms of brain big data obtained from molecular level to neuronal circuitry level. The implementation would involve the use of advanced neuroimaging technologies, including functional Magnetic Resonance Imaging (fMRI), Magnetoencephalography (MEG), Electroencephalography (EEG), functional Near-Infrared Spectroscopy (fNIRS), Positron Emission Tomography (PET), as well as other sources like eye-tracking and wearable, portable, micro and nano devices. Such brain big data will not only help scientists improve their understanding of human thinking, learning, decision-making, emotion, memory, and social behavior, but also help cure diseases, serve mental health-care and well-being, as well as develop brain inspired intelligent technologies to provide wisdom services in the social-cyber-physical space.

15.2 Developing a Big Data Sharing Mind on the W2T

Currently, various Internet of Things/Web of Things (IoT/WoT), and cloud computing based applications accelerate the amalgamation among the social, cyber and physical worlds (namely a social-cyber-physical space). As shown in Fig. 15.1, the wisdom Web of Things (W2T) has been developing as an extension of the wisdom Web in the social-cyber-physical space with big data [1]. The wisdom means that each of things in the IoT/WoT can be aware of both itself and others to provide the right service for the right object at a right time and context. Furthermore, WaaS (Wisdom as a Service) has been proposed as a content architecture of the big data cycle and a perspective of W2T in services for the large-scale converging of big data applications on the W2T [3]. In other words, WaaS is an open and interoperable intelligence service architecture for contents of IT applications, i.e., data, information, knowledge, and wisdom (DIKW). The social-cyber-physical space with its big data cycle would serve this purpose. Because of the fusion of humans, computers, and things in the social-cyber-physical space, today we live within a huge network of

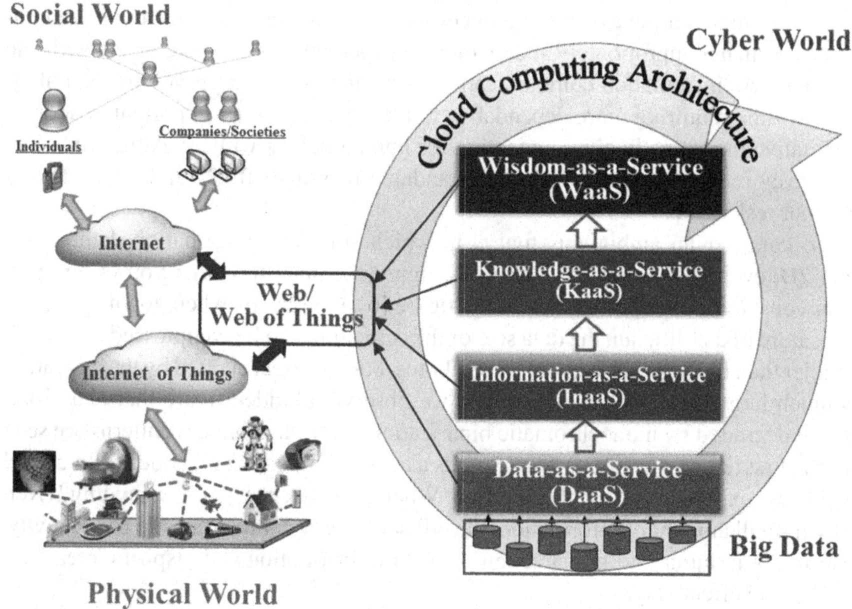

Fig. 15.1 The framework of wisdom Web of Things (W2T) in the social-cyber-physical space

numerous computing devices, measuring devices, and u-things, where real physical objects are attached, embedded, or blended with computers, networks, or some other devices such as sensors. Adapting and utilizing this kind of new human-machine relationship and developing human-level collective intelligence become a tangible goal of the DIKW related research. Realizing it will depend on a holistic intelligence research with two ways. On one hand, human brain needs to be investigated in depth as information processing system with big data for understanding the nature of intelligence and limits of human brain [4]; on the other hand, brain big data are collected in the social-cyber-physical space and integrated with human behavior big data and worldwide knowledge bases to realize human level collective intelligence as a big data sharing mind a harmonized collectivity of consciousness [5].

If we could apply this concept to the Shannon-Weaver model of communication in the social-cyber-physical space, the information in the senders mind would be converted into data, and in this process the sender would take what is necessary and discard what is not. The sender's data would be transferred through channels and received by the receiver. The receiver would decode the data and interpret the meaning of the data and generate new information in his/her mind. Thus, there is no direct relation between the information of the sender and that of the receiver. When we assume that the productivities of the society, community and persons are proportional to the amount of information transferred, we can introduce the factor of efficiency that can be expressed as a percentage of what ideally could be expected. In machine to machine communication, the efficiency should be 100 %, but in human to human communication, the efficiency varies from minus infinity to plus infinity.

The ultimate purpose of communication between humans is "a meaning communicated which is appropriately understood while people cooperate creatively with one another". As information communication more high-speed, high-volume and ubiquitous while requiring more dependability, it has become more important to address qualitative problems in communication for human beings while making it possible to convey real, meaningful and understandable messages freely and appropriately without restriction.

To consider an ambiguous figure, in which some 3D information deteriorates into 2D, even if you and I see the same figure, I cannot tell what you bring up in your consciousness or how you see the figure [6]. Contrarily, when you may draw a caricature of a politician, the data size of the caricature can be compressed into much smaller than his/her high-density (HD) photos, but the effect elicited by the caricature is much larger than HD photos. When we observe a hidden figure that is a visual image degraded by monochromatic binarization, only meaningless patterns are seen for the first time while after some seconds a meaningful object is suddenly perceived [6]. These experiences raise the question: What is the essence of understanding? Even with a small amount of information, the efficiency may compensate the productivity. Especially in human-to-human communication, inspiration and inspiring creativity work quite effectively.

While considering such circumstances, heart-to-heart science (HHS) conducts research and development to assist people to understand the meaning of words and recognize the content of information by scientifically analyzing the higher-level brain functions related to "understanding of meaning", "recognition" and "affect", which are the core of communication. When an ambiguous and/or incomplete information is presented, a computer cannot understand the meaning. On the other hand, if you see such information, you can guess the meaning of the information by inspiration. The inspiration of awareness is a key for improvement of the efficiency of information transfer. For information communication technology (ICT), especially for communication between humans in the social-cyber-physical space, it is crucial to improve the efficiency. Brain informatics should provide opportunities for this improvement by understanding and applying how the brain identifies the "heart" of the information, as well as developing the brain inspired W2T technology for communicating only the true information, namely sending what we need to send, and receiving only what we need to receive.

15.3 Network Based Big Data in the Social-Cyber-Physical Space

In the relation between the neuroscience and big-data, there are several interactions. Brain function measurements generate big data, which could be used by the information networks. Sensor networks generate human behavior data, which is also big data. Both types of data offer the stimulus set for brain researches. Network science provides analysis of network for such network based big data in the social-cyber-physical space. The analysis methods will be applicable to brain network analysis [7, 8]. When we found the new topologies, brain research gives new concept of the network.

Due to the emergence of the popularity of using smartphones, ICT has impacted by many IC cards and passes with IC tags. Furthermore, wearable sensors attached to a person continuously send information of his/her health conditions, such as heart rates, blood pressure, blood glucose levels and so on, to hospitals or doctors. These technologies have accurately recorded daily lives and social behavior of individuals as digital data logs. These types of data are all big data and would be utilized for various analyses and studies. From the ethics point of view, establishing rules for utilizing big data while taking into account of privacy protection are required.

Since big data implicitly includes ensemble behavioral data of people in the social-cyber-physical space, the rules or structures of human behaviors can be extracted from them, which may reflect human brain functions. Behavior of complex dynamic systems has so extensively been studied in mathematics, biology, and complex system sciences, that combination of these studies to big data has provided some important insights of ensemble behavior of people. For neuroscience and cognitive science, thus, utilization of the big data as stimulus sets has now provided new ways to better understanding of human brain functions and mechanisms. There are several studies carried out, in which stimulus sets from big data were used and a kind of reverse engineering of the human brain was performed [9, 10].

For example, neuroeconomical studies on decision-making in a social context have revealed the network of brain regions responsible to social decision making. Many of these studies have been carried out with using behavioral economics games [11]. Using these games, our research group also aims to construct the computational model of human decision making which enables us to predict future behaviors [12]. We are particularly interested in decision making in social settings, individual differences in decision making and learning mechanism of decision making. Results obtained with these studies will provide new aspects for analysis on big data and especially on social media such as SNS or twitters.

fMRI measurements provide a large amount of nodes and connections. The relationship between the nodes is analyzed by network analysis for building the model in which the degree of freedom is autonomously reduced [13]. Brain is the ensemble of transfer functions. We would like to know the transfer functions, the way of representation of information in brain, and transition between unconscious and conscious. For these studies, images and auditory stimuli, such as languages with tags will be useful as stimulus sets. The various stimuli are applied to a subject and measure the brain activity by fMRI. Another observation is that human thought is always the product of multiple collaborating brain centers linked by white matter tracts. Thinking is a network function and white matter is the unsung hero of human thought [14, 15].

To analyze the relationship between the input and patterns of neural activities, we can estimate the transfer function with using machine learning techniques. This is an example of the usage of big data for neuroscience. Nishimoto and colleagues collected various types of natural movies from the Internet and used them as stimulus sets [16]. These movies are presented to subjects. Then, evoked patterns in visual cortex are analyzed with machine learning and the way to reconstruct visual experiences from the brain activity has finally been found.

How should we collect neural activity during daily lives? To combine the huge non-invasive measurement systems and ordinary human activity, we need to fetch daily-life environment into these measurement systems and bring the brain activity measurements into social and daily lives. Although fMRI and MEG are versatile and precise imaging methods which non-invasively measure and image human brain activities, they require electromagnetic shield and vibration isolation system for their high accuracy at reasonable temporal resolutions. These requirements make the systems far from portability and being wearable and restrain persons as subjects in these machines. In addition, fMRI and MEG are too large to be moved and the subjects are under highly constraint conditions. This situation is very far from the daily life. Therefore, we have to develop a simple and mobile measuring system of neural activity, which is combined with measurements and records of other physical activities as shown in Fig. 15.2. These form big data of human activities. An example is to develop portable EEG which requires no paste or gel for electrodes and transmits the signals measured by wireless telecommunications.

The other option is to establish the daily lives in the fMRI with using big data. To combine the huge non-invasive measurement systems and ordinary human activity, we need to fetch daily-life environment into these measurement systems and bring the brain activity measurements into social and daily lives. Since the MRI is very noisy, you need ear plug. Two fMRIs are connected with a tube equipped by microphones for the natural dialogue inside MRI. For visual stimulation, 3D images and movies are represented to the subject inside fMRI. Haruno and Frith used dictator games to classify subjects as prosocial or selfish and then measured their brain activity with

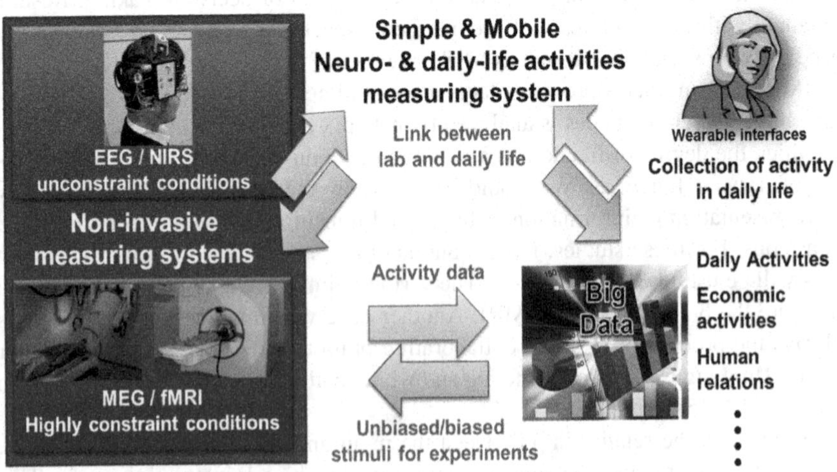

Fig. 15.2 How would brain big data be collected and used in the social-cyber-physical space

fMRI while the subjects rated the desirability of different reward pairs for self and other on a scale from one to four [12]. These developments have paved the way for the combination between precise measurements in laboratories and activities in ordinary lives.

15.4 Brain Big Data Based Wisdom Services

To demonstrate brain big data in the W2T applications, Fig. 15.3 gives an outline of a smart hospital service system for brain and mental disorders. Based on the previous prototype of the portable brain and mental health monitoring system that has been developed to support the monitoring of brain and mental disorders [3, 17], the development of such a smart hospital service system needs to consider various system-level and content-level demands. It is necessary to effectively integrate multi-level brain and mental health big data and provide multilevel and content-oriented services for different types of users by an open and extendable mode. Such a system is based on the WaaS architecture with a variety of data acquisition devices, the brain data center and LarKC semantic cloud platform [3, 18, 19]. Three types of data need to be collected from patients in a hospital:

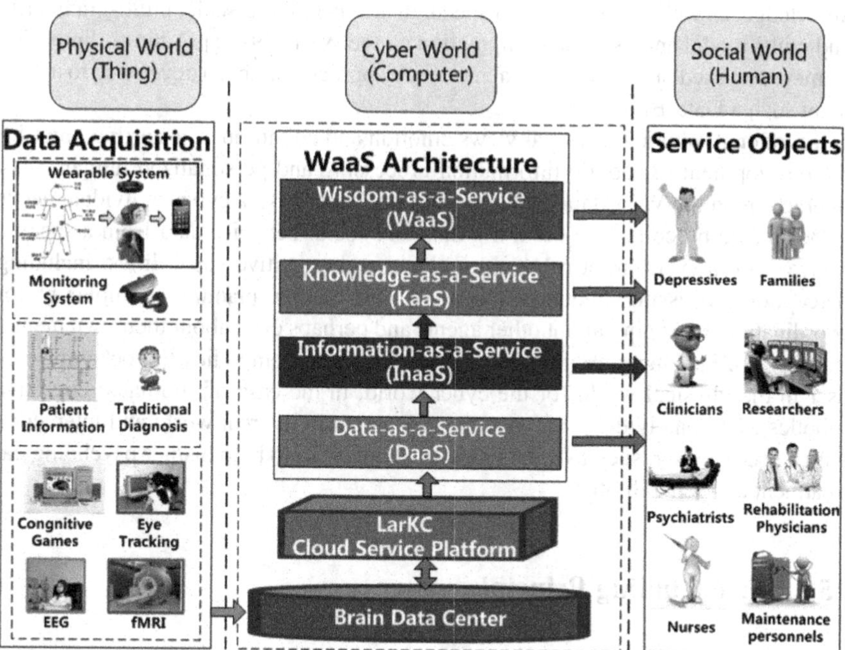

Fig. 15.3 The W2T based architecture of a smart hospital service system for brain and mental disorders

- Physiological data acquisition, based on wearable systems, as the method of long-term data acquisition to collect physiological data of patients;
- Behavior data acquisition, based on wearable and monitoring systems, as the method of long-term data acquisition to collect behavior data of patients;
- Data acquisition from traditional diagnosis and physiological measuring of patients, centered on scale rating, as the method of non-periodic data acquisition to collect psychological and physiological data of patients.

Various wearable health devices, such as the wearable EEG belt, wearable voice, wearable heart rate and tremor, wearable sleeping monitoring system, are used as new physical examination devices to obtain macro and meso levels of brain and mental data. These wearable health data are analyzed and integrated with clinical physical examination data, as well as various medical information and knowledge sources, including medical records, experimental reports, LOD (Linked Open Data) medical datasets, such as ICD-10, SNOMED CT, PubMed, and DrugBank. Furthermore, these integrated sources are combined with personalized models of patients for providing DaaS (Data as a Service), IaaS (Information as a Service), KaaS (Knowledge as a Service) and WaaS (Wisdom as a Service) to various types of users [3].

A powerful brain data center needs to be developed on the W2T as the global platform to support the whole systematic brain informatics research process and real-world applications [2, 19]. As the core of brain big data cycle system, the Data-Brain represents a radically new way of storing and sharing data, information and knowledge, as well as enables high speed, distributed, large-scale, multi-granularity and multi-modal analysis and computation on the W2T [19–21]. A multi-dimension framework based on the ontological modeling approach has been developed to implement such a Data-Brain [19].

Emotional robotic individual views emotion and cognition as a starting point for the development of robotic information processing and personalized human-robot interaction on the W2T data cycle system [1, 22]. At first, a cyber-individual needs to be created by collecting brain big data and social behavior data from a specific user, in addition to target robotic emotional and cognitive capabilities, including perception processing, attention allocation, anticipation, planning, complex motor coordination, reasoning about other agents and perhaps even about their own mental states [22, 23]. Then an emotional robotic individual embodies the behavior of a user in the physical world (or the cyber world, in the case of simulated cognitive robotics). Ultimately the robot must be able to act in the real world and interactive with a specific user, such as a patient with depression, to help his/her psychological treatment and rehabilitation.

15.5 Five Guiding Principles

To prepare well for the massive progresses in brain big data in the social-cyber-physical space, technological innovation is necessary but not sufficient, we do need to have a deeper understanding of how technically brain/behavioral data can(not) be collected and the nature of human perception/behavior. To this end, we propose five guiding principles.

First, "*dynamic link* across brain-body-world" is the key. Just as an example, the "gaze cascade" effect illustrates how gaze shift interacts with perceptual processing and facilitation to form a dynamic positive feedback loop towards a conscious decision of visual preference [24].

Second, the *implicit* cognitive process (of "tacit knowing") needs to be understood. The brain/mind processes that are consciously aware of is just a tip of iceberg—the vast majority of neural processing remains implicit, including the critical mechanisms underlying decision making. To prove this, we showed that the nucleus accumbens (a subcortical structure well known to be a part of the dopaminergic cirtuit) is activated to the more preferable face image than the less, not only in the explicit preference judgment task but also in an emotionally-neutral, control task on the same face images (i.e. to judge which face is rounder).

Third, perception and action are *interactive & ubiquitous* from the outset. Most directly demonstrating this point is the well-known snake illusion. In this and several related illusions, an entirely static image yields a strong impression of motion (rotations, in this case), typically contingent upon saccadic eye movements. While the critical factors and the underlying mechanisms are still under a debate [25], it is obvious that active approach from the observer to the object triggers a vigorous interaction to yield dynamic perception, and this is true everywhere even in the natural (non-technological) environment. As for yet another line of evidence, there are studies indicating that a locomotion or a body movement vigorously changes perception [26].

Fourth, predicting-past is easy, predicting-future is hard. This is so fundamentally because the brain and behavior/decision of the human is strongly *situation-dependent*. There are many lines of evidence, mostly in behavioral, EEG, and fMRI studies, indicating that the data obtained from the same brain with the same stimulus materials/tasks are necessary to perform reliable decoding, with saying larger than 90 % correct rate, including our own EEG study of decoding facial preference decision [27]. One may also expect a reasonable and feasible ethical border here, to deal with related ethical issues in the near future.

Fifth and finally, we would like to emphasize that creativity is "waiting" in the environment. Just to intuitively illustrate this point, imagine the following (gedanken) folktale. Two towns were facing against each other beyond a very deep valley. People travel miles of mountain road to trade with each other. Constructing a bridge was an obvious solution, but until one rich man came up with the idea and actually implemented it, nobody ever thought of it, so one may call it a creative insight. One may add that this was the first bridge ever created in the human history, to make it more persuasive. But at the same time, one may also argue that the environment (*i.e.* landscape) had been structured such that this creative idea was implicitly awaited.

To conclude, technical attempts and discussion around brain big data should be based on the keen realization of the vigorous interaction and interdependence of brain-body-environment.

Acknowledgments This work was supported by grants from the National Basic Research Program of China (2014CB744600), the International Science & Technology Cooperation Program of China (2013DFA32180), the National Natural Science Foundation of China (61420106005 and 61272345), the Beijing Natural Science Foundation (4132023), and the JSPS Grants-in-Aid for Scientific Research of Japan (26350994).

References

1. N. Zhong, J.H. Ma, R.H. Huang, J.M. Liu, Y.Y. Yao, Y.X. Zhang, J.H. Chen, Research challenges and perspectives on wisdom Web of things (W2T). The Journal of Supercomputing **64**(3), 862882 (2013)
2. N. Zhong, J.M. Bradshaw, J. Liu, J.G. Taylor, Brain informatics. IEEE Intelligent Systems **26**(5), 16–21 (2011)
3. J. Chen, J.H. Ma, N. Zhong, Y.Y. Yao, J. Liu, R.H. Huang, W. Li, Z. Huang, Y. Gao, J. Cao, WaaS—Wisdom as a service. IEEE Intelligent Systems **29**(6), 40–47 (2014)
4. D. Douglas, The limits of intelligence. Scientific American **37–43**, (July 2011)
5. F. Heylighen, The global superorganism: an evolutionary-cybernetic model of the emerging network society. Social Evolution & History **6**(1), 58119 (2007)
6. T. Murata, N. Matsui, S. Miyauchi, Y. Kakita, T. Yanagida, Discrete stochastic process underlying perceptual rivalry. NeuroReport **14**, 1347–1352 (2003)
7. O. Sporns, Making sense of brain network data. Nature Methods **10**(6), 491–493 (2013)
8. H.-J. Park, Karl Friston, Structural and functional brain networks: From connections to cognition. Science **342**, 1238411 (2013)
9. T. Horikawa, M. Tamaki, Y. Miyawaki, Y. Kamitani, Neural decoding of visual imagery during sleep. Science **340**, 639–642 (2013)
10. T. Cukur, S. Nishimoto, A.G. Huth, J.L. Gallant, Attention during natural vision warps semantic representation across the human brain. Nature Neuroscience **16**, 763–770 (2013)
11. V.K. Lee, L.T. Harris, How social cognition can inform social decision making. Front Neuroscience. (2013). doi:10.3389/fnins
12. M. Haruno, C. Frith, Activity in the amygdala elicited by unfair divisions predicts social value orientation. Nature Neuroscience **13**, 160–161 (2013)
13. N. Turk-Browne, Functional interactions as big data in the human brain. Science **342**, 580–584 (2013)
14. T.M. Mitchell, S.V. Shinkareva, A. Carlson, K.M. Chang, V.L. Malave, R.A. Mason, M.A. Just, Predicting human brain activity associated with the meanings of nouns. Science **320**, 1191–1195 (2008)
15. T.A. Keller, M.A. Just, Altering cortical connectivity: Remediation-induced changes in the white matter of poor readers. Neuron **64**, 624–631 (2009)
16. S. Nishimoto, A. T. Vu, T. Naselaris, Y. Benjamini, B. Yu, J. L. Gallant. Reconstructing visual experiences from brain activity evoked by natural movies. Current Biology **21**, 1641–1646 (2011)
17. B. Hu, D. Majoe, M. Ratcliffe, Y. Qi, Q. Zhao, H. Peng, D. Fan, F. Zheng, M. Jackson, P. Moore, EEG-based cognitive interfaces for ubiquitous applications: developments and challenges. IEEE Intelligent Systems **26**(5), 46–53 (2011)
18. D. Fensel, F. van Harmelen, B. Andersson, P. Brennan, H. Cunningham, E.D. Valle, F. Fischer, Z.S. Huang, A. Kiryakov, T.K.-I. Lee, L. Schooler, V. Tresp, S. Wesner, M. Witbrock, N. Zhong, Towards LarKC: a platform for Web-scale reasoning. Proc. ICSC **524–529**, 2008 (2008)
19. N. Zhong, J. Chen, Constructing a new-style conceptual model of brain data for systematic brain informatics. IEEE Transactions on Knowledge and Data Engineering **24**(12), 2127–2142 (2012)

20. G.Y. Wang, J. Xu, Granular computing with multiple granular layers for brain big data processing. Brain Informatics (2014). doi:10.1007/s40708-014-0001-z
21. G.E. Hinton, R.R. Salakhutdinov, Reducing the dimensionality of data with neural networks. Science **313**, 504–507 (2006)
22. Y. Anzai, Human-robot interaction by information sharing. Proc. HRI **65–66**, 2013 (2013)
23. J.H. Ma, J. Wen, R.H. Huang, B.X. Huang, Cyber-individual meets brain informatics. IEEE Intelligent Systems **26**(5), 30–37 (2011)
24. S. Shimojo, C. Simion, E. Shimojo, C. Scheier, Gaze bias both reflects and influences preference. Nature Neuroscience **6**, 1317 (2003)
25. I. Murakami, A. Kitaoka, H. Ashida, A positive correlation between fixation instability and the strength of illusory motion in a static display. Vision Research **46**, 24212431 (2006)
26. G. Ishimura and S. Shimojo. Voluntary action captures visual motion. Investigative Ophthalmology and Visual Science (Suppl.), **35**: 1275, 1994
27. J.P. Lindsen, R. Jones, S. Shimojo, J. Bhattachary, Neural components underlying subjective preferential decision making. NeuroImage **50**, 16261632 (2010)

Printed in the United States
By Bookmasters

Printed in the United States
By Bookmasters